Aromatherapy For Dummies®

W9-BRN-765

Cheat Sheet

What Essential Oils Do for You

Essential oils enhance both the health and beauty of skin, hair, and nails. Plus, they have healing benefits for your body and mind. As an added bonus, they smell wonderful when applied to the body. Here's a list of the most important properties found most often in essential oils.

- Kill bacterial, viral, and fungal infections
- Seal wounds
- Reduce inflammation
- Regulate hormones
- Tone and moisturize skin
- Stimulate the immune system
- Repel bugs
- Attract a mate
- Heat the skin in a liniment
- Aid blood circulation and digestion
- Decrease sinus and lung congestion

Eight Advantages of Using Medical Aromatherapy

Instead of using an over-the-counter drug to ease a cold, headache, indigestion, or bee sting — the simple complaints that you already take care of yourself without consulting your doctor — turn to aromatherapy as a natural alternative. After all, that's what aroma*therapy* is — a healing therapy. The *aroma* part of the word refers is to the aromatic plants that are used in this therapy.

- Inexpensive
- Compact to carry
- Work with, not against you
- Go directly to the affliction
- Work quickly once they're there
- Can use with drugs
- Leave your body quickly without residues
- Have few side effects

Having the Scents to Relax

Relaxing fragrances help you deal better with stress. They also tend to produce slower frequency brain waves. You may not need it, but these scents additionally have antidepressant properties when you smell them.

- Bergamot
- Chamomile
- Frankincense
- Geranium
- Lavender
- Neroli
- Petitgrain
- Rose
- Sandalwood
- Ylang ylang

...For Dummies®: Bestselling Book Series for Beginners

Aromatherapy For Dummies®

Cheat Sheet

Mental Scents to Thinking Better

The same essential oils that pep you up and reduce your drowsiness also decrease the likelihood of becoming irritable or of getting headaches. Here are the mind-stimulating scents.

- Angelica
- Basil
- Cardamom
- Cinnamon

- Clove
- Ginger
- Peppermint
- Sage

How to Buy Your Essential Oils

Your shopping days will be much easier if you follow these simple tips when choosing what essential oils to buy:

- Buy oils from companies who have an established reputation.
- Ask. Are they pure? Where do they originate? What are the botanical names?
- Be on the look out for synthetic essential oils such as carnation, lilac, strawberry, rain, or cucumber. If so, all the oils in that line may be synthetics.
- Check for purity. Put a drop of essential oil on a piece of paper. It should quickly evaporate, leaving no oily mark (an oily mark indicates it's cut with vegetable oil).

- Check for quality. Sniff out fuller and rounder scents. A little should go a long way.
- Purchase only a small amount of essential oil from a company you haven't tried before to test their quality.

IDG BOOKS WORLDWIDE

...For Dummies®: Bestselling Book Series for Beginners

Praise for Aromatherapy For Dummies

"Aromatherapy works! Physicians at American WholeHealth Centers regularly use aromatherapy techniques as part of the personally designed 'Healing Paths' for their patients. Now, under the expert tutelage of one of America's leading herbalists, you can bring the wonders of aromatherapy into your own life. If you're wondering which of the dozens of aromatherapy books to buy for yourself, this is the one."

— David Edelberg, M.D., Northwestern University

"With the current surge of availability information and aromatic products, so many individuals, from all walks of life, are embracing the enticing concept of scents being beneficial to well-being. In the United States, the development of aromatherapy has been mainly in small businesses. Larger corporations are now offering scent-oriented products, many of which are not true aromatherapy. Kathi Keville clarifies to the general public how true plant essences — not just sometimes synthetically scented products — can support body, mind, and spirit. The advice offered on how to select genuine aromatherapy products greatly increases the value of this much-needed source of essential knowledge. Always clever and charming, Kathi so clearly presents the safe and effective use of essential oils for true aromatherapy."

— Cheryl Hoard, President of the National
Association for Holistic Aromatherapy (NAHA),
Owner of Cheryl's Herbs

"Experienced researcher, educator, and botanical expert Kathi Keville has created the most useful guide ever written on aromatherapy. This flawlessly organized book has a wealth of practical information for everyone, from novice to accomplished practitioner. She provides clear, concise, and scientifically rational information, unraveling what some might see as a confusing and complicated subject into an engaging and easy-to-read book full of common sense advice on everything from therapeutics and cosmetics to the recreational uses of essential oils."

— Mindy Green, Aromatherapist,
Director of Education, Herb Research Foundation

Other Books Authored by Kathi Keville

Women's Herbs, Women's Health, coauthor Christopher Hobbs, Interweave Press (1998)

Aromatherapy: For Healing the Body and Mind, Publications International (1998)

Complete Book of Herbs: Herbs to Enrich Your Garden, Home, and Health, Publications International (1997)

Herbs to Help Chronic Fatigue, Keats Publications (1997)

Herbs for Health & Healing, Rodale Press (1996)

Pocket Guide to Aromatherapy, The Crossing Press (1996). Also translated as *Aromatherapie,* Deltas, The Netherlands (1999) and *Aromaterapica: Guía Práctica,* Ediciones Obelisco, Spain (1998)

Ginseng, Keats Publications (1996)

Aromatherapy: The Complete Guide to the Healing Art, coauthor Mindy Green, The Crossing Press (1995). Also translated as *Die Seele der Pflanzen* (German). Deukalion (1997) and *Aromatherapie* Herder (1999)

Herbs, An Illustrated Encyclopedia, Friedman/Fairfax (1994). Also published as *The Illustrated Herb Encyclopedia,* Simon & Schuster, Australia (1991) and *The Illustrated Herb Encyclopedia,* The Grange, England (1991)

Herbs: American Country Living, Crescent/Random House (1991). Also translated as *Le Monde Merveilleux des Herbes,* Minerva (1991) and in *American Country Living: Ultimate Lifestyle Compendium,* Random House (1992)

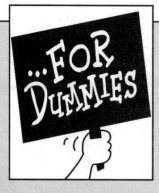 ™

References for the Rest of Us!™

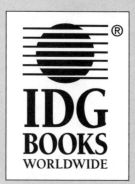

AROMATHERAPY FOR DUMMIES®

by Kathi Keville

IDG Books Worldwide, Inc.
An International Data Group Company

Foster City, CA ◆ Chicago, IL ◆ Indianapolis, IN ◆ New York, NY

Aromatherapy For Dummies®

Published by
IDG Books Worldwide, Inc.
An International Data Group Company
919 E. Hillsdale Blvd.
Suite 400
Foster City, CA 94404
www.idgbooks.com (IDG Books Worldwide Web site)
www.dummies.com (Dummies Press Web site)

Library of Congress Catalog Card No.: 99-65840

ISBN: 0-7645-5171-X

Printed in the United States of America

10 9 8 7 6 5 4 3 2 1

1B/SV/QY/ZZ/IN

Distributed in the United States by IDG Books Worldwide, Inc.

Distributed by CDG Books Canada Inc. for Canada; by Transworld Publishers Limited in the United Kingdom; by IDG Norge Books for Norway; by IDG Sweden Books for Sweden; by IDG Books Australia Publishing Corporation Pty. Ltd. for Australia and New Zealand; by TransQuest Publishers Pte Ltd. for Singapore, Malaysia, Thailand, Indonesia, and Hong Kong; by Gotop Information Inc. for Taiwan; by ICG Muse, Inc. for Japan; by Norma Comunicaciones S.A. for Colombia; by Intersoft for South Africa; by Eyrolles for France; by International Thomson Publishing for Germany, Austria and Switzerland; by Distribuidora Cuspide for Argentina; by LR International for Brazil; by Galileo Libros for Chile; by Ediciones ZETA S.C.R. Ltda. for Peru; by WS Computer Publishing Corporation, Inc., for the Philippines; by Contemporanea de Ediciones for Venezuela; by Express Computer Distributors for the Caribbean and West Indies; by Micronesia Media Distributor, Inc. for Micronesia; by Grupo Editorial Norma S.A. for Guatemala; by Chips Computadoras S.A. de C.V. for Mexico; by Editorial Norma de Panama S.A. for Panama; by American Bookshops for Finland. Authorized Sales Agent: Anthony Rudkin Associates for the Middle East and North Africa.

For general information on IDG Books Worldwide's books in the U.S., please call our Consumer Customer Service department at 800-762-2974. For reseller information, including discounts and premium sales, please call our Reseller Customer Service department at 800-434-3422.

For information on where to purchase IDG Books Worldwide's books outside the U.S., please contact our International Sales department at 317-596-5530 or fax 317-596-5692.

For consumer information on foreign language translations, please contact our Customer Service department at 1-800-434-3422, fax 317-596-5692, or e-mail rights@idgbooks.com.

For information on licensing foreign or domestic rights, please phone +1-650-655-3109.

For sales inquiries and special prices for bulk quantities, please contact our Sales department at 650-655-3200 or write to the address above.

For information on using IDG Books Worldwide's books in the classroom or for ordering examination copies, please contact our Educational Sales department at 800-434-2086 or fax 317-596-5499.

For press review copies, author interviews, or other publicity information, please contact our Public Relations department at 650-655-3000 or fax 650-655-3299.

For authorization to photocopy items for corporate, personal, or educational use, please contact Copyright Clearance Center, 222 Rosewood Drive, Danvers, MA 01923, or fax 978-750-4470.

About the Author

Kathi Keville is a nationally known herbalist, aromatherapist, and masseuse with over 30 years experience. She is director of the American Herb Association and editor of the AHA Quarterly Newsletter. Kathi is an honorary, founding member of both the American Herbalist's Guild and the National Association of Holistic Aromatherapy, the only national organization for aromatherapy in the U. S. She is also a member of United Plant Savers, an organization dedicated to preserving endangered medicinal herbs.

Kathi has the authored ten other popular herb and aromatherapy books and written over 150 articles for national magazines such as *Prevention, Vegetarian Times, Herbs for Health,* and *Let's Live,* consulted for *National Geographic, Newsweek,* and *Woman's Day,* and was associate editor with *Well-Being Magazine.*

For 14 years, Kathi co-operated a commercial herb farm that grew medicinal and aromatic plants. She now owns the mail-order herb and aromatherapy company Oak Valley Herb Farm, which carries many products made with herbs grown in her gardens and essential oils. She gives aromatherapy seminars at Herb Symposiums throughout North America and has taught seminars at 12 institutions in the U. S., including San Francisco State University; The University of San Francisco; University of California at Davis, Sierra College, American College of Ayurveda, and Omega Institute. Kathi currently conducts weekend aromatherapy courses at Oak Valley Herb Farm in Nevada City, California; Natural Healing Institute of Naturopathy in Encinitas, California; Blue Sky Educational Foundation in Grafton, Wisconsin; Gentle Strength University in Tempe, Arizona; and Phillip's School of Massage in Nevada City, California. (See the Appendix for these addresses.)

ABOUT IDG BOOKS WORLDWIDE

Welcome to the world of IDG Books Worldwide.

IDG Books Worldwide, Inc., is a subsidiary of International Data Group, the world's largest publisher of computer-related information and the leading global provider of information services on information technology. IDG was founded more than 30 years ago by Patrick J. McGovern and now employs more than 9,000 people worldwide. IDG publishes more than 290 computer publications in over 75 countries. More than 90 million people read one or more IDG publications each month.

Launched in 1990, IDG Books Worldwide is today the #1 publisher of best-selling computer books in the United States. We are proud to have received eight awards from the Computer Press Association in recognition of editorial excellence and three from Computer Currents' First Annual Readers' Choice Awards. Our best-selling ...For Dummies® series has more than 50 million copies in print with translations in 31 languages. IDG Books Worldwide, through a joint venture with IDG's Hi-Tech Beijing, became the first U.S. publisher to publish a computer book in the People's Republic of China. In record time, IDG Books Worldwide has become the first choice for millions of readers around the world who want to learn how to better manage their businesses.

Our mission is simple: Every one of our books is designed to bring extra value and skill-building instructions to the reader. Our books are written by experts who understand and care about our readers. The knowledge base of our editorial staff comes from years of experience in publishing, education, and journalism — experience we use to produce books to carry us into the new millennium. In short, we care about books, so we attract the best people. We devote special attention to details such as audience, interior design, use of icons, and illustrations. And because we use an efficient process of authoring, editing, and desktop publishing our books electronically, we can spend more time ensuring superior content and less time on the technicalities of making books.

You can count on our commitment to deliver high-quality books at competitive prices on topics you want to read about. At IDG Books Worldwide, we continue in the IDG tradition of delivering quality for more than 30 years. You'll find no better book on a subject than one from IDG Books Worldwide.

IDG
BOOKS
WORLDWIDE

John Kilcullen
Chairman and CEO
IDG Books Worldwide, Inc.

Steven Berkowitz
President and Publisher
IDG Books Worldwide, Inc.

WINNER

*Eighth Annual
Computer Press
Awards ≥1992*

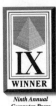

WINNER

*Ninth Annual
Computer Press
Awards ≥1993*

WINNER

*Tenth Annual
Computer Press
Awards ≥1994*

WINNER

*Eleventh Annual
Computer Press
Awards ≥1995*

IDG is the world's leading IT media, research and exposition company. Founded in 1964, IDG had 1997 revenues of $2.05 billion and has more than 9,000 employees worldwide. IDG offers the widest range of media options that reach IT buyers in 75 countries representing 95% of worldwide IT spending. IDG's diverse product and services portfolio spans six key areas including print publishing, online publishing, expositions and conferences, market research, education and training, and global marketing services. More than 90 million people read one or more of IDG's 290 magazines and newspapers, including IDG's leading global brands — Computerworld, PC World, Network World, Macworld and the Channel World family of publications. IDG Books Worldwide is one of the fastest-growing computer book publishers in the world, with more than 700 titles in 36 languages. The "...For Dummies®" series alone has more than 50 million copies in print. IDG offers online users the largest network of technology-specific Web sites around the world through IDG.net (http://www.idg.net), which comprises more than 225 targeted Web sites in 55 countries worldwide. International Data Corporation (IDC) is the world's largest provider of information technology data, analysis and consulting, with research centers in over 41 countries and more than 400 research analysts worldwide. IDG World Expo is a leading producer of more than 168 globally branded conferences and expositions in 35 countries including E3 (Electronic Entertainment Expo), Macworld Expo, ComNet, Windows World Expo, ICE (Internet Commerce Expo), Agenda, DEMO, and Spotlight. IDG's training subsidiary, ExecuTrain, is the world's largest computer training company, with more than 230 locations worldwide and 785 training courses. IDG Marketing Services helps industry-leading IT companies build international brand recognition by developing global integrated marketing programs via IDG's print, online and exposition products worldwide. Further information about the company can be found at www.idg.com. 1/24/99

Dedication

I dedicate this book to you, the reader, for being interested enough to pick it up. I hope you find it a fun and lively way to discover aromatherapy and the fascinating world of fragrance.

Acknowledgments

It's a big job writing a book. It means translating lots of ideas into words and then compiling them into the text you hold in your hand. None of us do it alone. Thanks to the many people at IDG who made it possible. It's been a sincere pleasure to work with Kelly Ewing, Brian Kramer, Karen Young, Tami Booth, as well as Pam Tanzey who illustrated this book so beautifully. Thanks, too, to everyone behind the scenes. I also greatly appreciate the dedicated work of my agent Carol Roth and the research and editorial assistance of Mary Greer. Mindy Green, a marvelous aromatherapist and herbalist, read every word and added her guidance and insights. Chemists Larry Jones and Jim Symes also looked over selected parts of the manuscript. My friends and colleagues Christopher Hobbs and Beth Baugh helped make this book happen in so many ways. Thanks also to Marion Wyckoff for massaging my desk-warped body and to my partner Ron Bertolucci for contributing far more than his share of making dinners and watering the garden and for his skillful blending of many of the aromatherapy formulas in this book.

Learning about aromatherapy hasn't been a lonely road. There are so many people who graciously shared their knowledge and friendships with me. I especially acknowledge aromatherapists Jeanne Rose, Shirley Price, Robert Tisserand, Kurt Schnaubelt, Marcel Lavabre, and John Steele for inspiring me and also for all they have contributed to modern aromatherapy. I also must applaud my fellow herbalists for their work with fragrant plants. Special thanks goes to my father, Jesse Keville, for teaching me so much about his passion and vocation — chemistry. (Read just a few pages of this book, and you'll find out why I'm so thankful for chemistry!)

Publisher's Acknowledgments

We're proud of this book; please register your comments through our IDG Books Worldwide Online Registration Form located at http://my2cents.dummies.com.

Some of the people who helped bring this book to market include the following:

Acquisitions, Editorial, and Media Development

Project Editor: Kelly Ewing

Executive Editor: Tammerly Booth

General Reviewer: Mindy Green

Editorial Coordinator: Maureen Kelly

Editorial Director: Kristin Cocks

Acquisitions Coordinator: Karen S. Young

Illustrator: Pam Tanzey

Production

Project Coordinator: Regina Snyder

Layout and Graphics: Amy Adrian, Angela F. Hunckler, Barry Offringa, Brent Savage, Janet Seib, Michael A. Sullivan, Brian Torwelle. Mary Jo Weis

Proofreaders: Nancy Price, Nancy L. Reinhardt, Maianne Santy, Rebecca Senninger, Ethel M. Winslow

Indexer: Sherry Massey

General and Administrative

IDG Books Worldwide, Inc.: John Kilcullen, CEO; Steven Berkowitz, President and Publisher

IDG Books Technology Publishing Group: Richard Swadley, Senior Vice President and Publisher; Walter Bruce III, Vice President and Associate Publisher; Steven Sayre, Associate Publisher; Joseph Wikert, Associate Publisher; Mary Bednarek, Branded Product Development Director; Mary Corder, Editorial Director

IDG Books Consumer Publishing Group: Roland Elgey, Senior Vice President and Publisher; Kathleen A. Welton, Vice President and Publisher; Kevin Thornton, Acquisitions Manager; Kristin A. Cocks, Editorial Director

IDG Books Internet Publishing Group: Brenda McLaughlin, Senior Vice President and Publisher; Diane Graves Steele, Vice President and Associate Publisher; Sofia Marchant, Online Marketing Manager

IDG Books Production for Dummies Press: Michael R. Britton, Vice President of Production; Debbie Stailey, Associate Director of Production; Cindy L. Phipps, Manager of Project Coordination, Production Proofreading, and Indexing; Tony Augsburger, Manager of Prepress, Reprints, and Systems; Laura Carpenter, Production Control Manager; Shelley Lea, Supervisor of Graphics and Design; Debbie J. Gates, Production Systems Specialist; Robert Springer, Supervisor of Proofreading; Kathie Schutte, Production Supervisor

Dummies Packaging and Book Design: Patty Page, Manager, Promotions Marketing

◆

The publisher would like to give special thanks to Patrick J. McGovern, without whom this book would not have been possible.

◆

Contents at a Glance

Cartoons at a Glance

By Rich Tennant

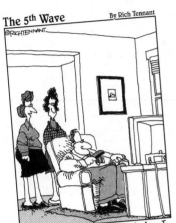

"When I know he's had a rough day, I always put a few drops of lavender on the TV remote before he gets home."

page 249

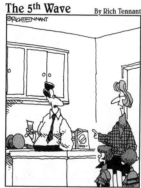

"Hand me that mallet and a box of chocolate chip cookies. The kids want to make up aroma sachets for their bedrooms."

page 235

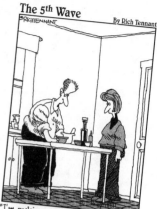

"I'm making my own scents with celery seed, almond oil, and rosemary. What we don't use in the bathtub I'll toss with lettuce and serve it for dinner."

page 101

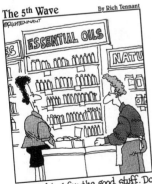

"I'm looking for the good stuff. Do you have any of this stuff that's extra virgin?"

page 9

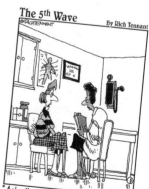

"Actually, I didn't become dizzy and nauseous until I started inhaling the scent strips in the waiting room magazines."

page 321

Fax: 978-546-7747 • E-mail: the5wave@tiac.net

Table of Contents

Introduction

*W*ho says that medicine has to be bitter to be effective? Aromatherapy offers a way that you can literally smell your way to good health. You can't beat a prescription that reads, "Bathe with scented oils twice a week." *Aromatherapy For Dummies* is your guide into a new way to stay healthy and fit and to also take care of yourself when you do get sick.

If you're like most people, you take the smell of a flower or the scent of freshly baked bread for granted. That's because fragrance is all around — everyday and everywhere. Scent may be common place, but you'll have to agree that it greatly enhances life. And, it does even more. As it's name implies, aromatherapy is indeed a *therapy* that uses *aroma* for healing. It works on many levels. It can treat emotional as well as physical problems and even help you think better or improve your athletic performance. There is even a "scentsual" form of aromatherapy that can improve your love — and your sex — life.

No wonder such a large selection of scented products are now available — everything from candles to facial cream to room freshener is promising to bring aromatherapy into your life. Obviously, aromatherapy covers a lot of territory, so I've written this book to guide you through all of the clouds of wafting aromas and show you how to make real sense out of it. I've been enjoying the benefits of aromatherapy for more than 30 years — and sharing them with others almost this long. Simply put, I'm impressed. I think you will be, too.

About This Book

In this book, you discover the world of fragrance and dozens of ways that aromatherapy enhances your health and general well being. *Aromatherapy For Dummies* helps you understand essential oils so that you can savor and enjoy the pleasures and benefits of aromatherapy. It's also a guide to using aromatherapy effectively and safely.

I show you how to bring aromatherapy into your home, how to take it to work with you, and even how to carry it with you. One of the best things about aromatherapy is that it's so easy to do. They are so simple, I include over a hundred aromatherapy recipes that I developed so that you can whip up everything for oily skin to indigestion. Most of these recipes take less than five minutes to make.

Conventions Used in This Book

Throughout this book, I use the common names of plants. These are the names with which you're most likely familiar, such as jasmine or rose. Common names are easy to recognize and pronounce, but they can be confusing because sometimes several plants share the same name. The way to know for certain which plant is being discussed is to use its Latin name (also called a *binomial*), along with the common name. The Latin name consists of two names. The genus represents a larger grouping, so it comes first (and is capitalized) The species, the second name, identifies a specific plant. I use Latin names in the Aroma Guide and occasionally in other parts of the book when discussing a plant that isn't identified in the Guide. (For more on Latin names and their usefulness, see Chapter 1.)

What You're Not to Read

I already know that you're busy. That's why I've written this book, because I want to introduce you to aromatherapy even though you've got a million other things to do. Thinking about you, I make it easy to find out what you need, and also what you don't need.

First of all, if you're going for basic information without the frills, then forget about the sidebars. They're highly visible, so you can always go back and read them when you've got the time and the interest. Or, at least just read the ones that catch your eye.

You also don't need to read this book cover to cover. You may not want to find out everything there is to know about aromatherapy, and anyway, there's no exam at the end. Instead, use this book as a reference to look up what you need, but only when you need it. For example, you might only want to know about aromatherapy skin care and couldn't care less about how to improve your work or sports performance. Whatever your interest in aromatherapy, you can find it here and can go right to it.

Do I Know You? Foolish Assumptions

Probably I do know you. You're already intrigued by aroma, so you can't help wondering what's all the fuss about aromatherapy. Maybe you're missing out on something that could really be a plus in your life and help a few physical, and maybe even some emotional, things that you're working on. Anyway, the idea to spice up your life with fragrance sounds like fun, and it surely can't hurt — or can it? And, that's not the only question on your list. You want to know if this is really a therapy, then how does it work? What will my doctor say? Hey, forget about doc, what will my friends say? Will they suspect that I've gone off the deep end and now will spray strange vapors into the air or walk around smelling as if I fell into a vat of perfume?

Well, have I got answers for you! I even provide some answers to questions that I bet you haven't thought of yet. In fact, if you're already on the fragrant path and using aromatherapy, you can find plenty of recipes and ideas about how to use them as a part of your healing program. If you've been using aromatherapy, you're likely already impressed with the results, and now you're wondering why it works so well. However, you're too busy to delve into studying botany and physiology and whatever other complicated subjects are involved with aromatherapy. If so, then I'm here to help you out. You can slide right through what's in this book and before you know it, you'll know everything that you need to use aromatherapy throughout your life.

Be Sure to Read This!

This book deals with the many aspects of aromatherapy, including its use to treat medical conditions. It's designed as a self-help guide to using simple, natural remedies to treat simple problems, such as a mild headache or sore throat — the conditions that you would take care of yourself anyway. However, this book is not a substitute for expert medical advice or treatment. You can use some suggestions in conjunction with other treatments for serious health problems, but do this under your doctor's supervision. You are unique from anyone else, so when you get really sick, the best treatment for someone else who has the same thing may not be ideal for you. There's nothing like individual care when you really need it. My general rule is when in doubt, don't. If you're not sure what you have or you don't know how to treat it, seek professional guidance. This will probably be your physician. In addition, many alternative practitioners, such as an acupuncturist, chiropractor, herbalist, or clinical aromatherapist, can help with certain problems. Always remember, don't take any chances with your health!

How This Book Is Organized

My philosophy is that if you really want to have a handle on a subject, you need to get to know all of its whys and hows. If you understand the building blocks, then you can figure out just about anything. Because this book addresses healing — and specifically a holistic form of healing — it's especially important for you to understand the basic principles so that you can make good choices about your health.

When I think about what makes aromatherapy tick, several topics come to mind. Aromatherapy involves some chemistry, dabbling in physiology, and a touch of psychology. These areas help you understand why aromatherapy works. Then there's also the nitty-gritty of aromatherapy. That's how to use it and the results that you can expect. These are the contents of this book, all broken down in clear, simple language.

Part I: Aromatherapy Essentials

Aroma follows a fascinating journey as it travels from the flower to your nose and then into the realms of your brain. Part I of this book explains what your sense of smell is, how different aromas can tap into your mind, and how your emotions can also affect your physical body. This is the science of aromatherapy, but I present it in simple terms, without any scientific jargon to slow down your reading. In this part, you find the tools that you need to distinguish the difference between good and poor aromatherapy products. I also give you hints so that you know the best items to choose on your next shopping spree. You'll want to read all of Part I if you're interested in making your own aromatherapy products. Then I give you many, many ways in which you can bring aromatherapy into your life.

Part II: "Inscentives" for Living: Aromatherapy in Your Life

In Part II, you'll find aromatherapy at use in your kitchen, in your bedroom, and in your study. I tell you ways that aromatherapy can help your all-around performance, whether you're at home, working out at the gym, busy at the office, or planning a romantic evening. I give you enough suggestions here to completely fill your life with healing aromas. This way, you can pick and choose the ones that most appeal to you. I also devote an entire chapter to discussing how aromatherapy can tone and heal your complexion. Again, I give you plenty of recommendations on selecting the best type of product for your particular skin. Chapter 11 even explains exactly how aromatherapy works to treat physical disorders. The focus is on the ways that aromatherapy heals and the seven most common methods of treatment.

Part III: The Part of Tens

For a quick reference to aromatherapy-related topics, turn to this fun section. In The Part of Tens, I take aromatherapy into the garden, into the kid's playroom, and then out and about the world. In this part, you find the top ten aromas that kid's like, plus projects to share aromatherapy with them. I explain how you can grow ten fragrant plants in your garden or on your balcony. If this book gets you excited about aromatherapy, you'll be especially interested in these ten aromatherapy experiences.

Part IV: The Guides

With this book, you get two bonus guides for quick reference. Because you may want to refer to these guides often, I've made them easy to find. They're the yellow pages that are near the back of this book.

Flip to the Symptom Guide to look up any symptom of condition that ails you. Here, you discover simple and easy remedies to treat all sorts of minor problems. This guide lists a hundred different conditions or disorders and how to tend to them yourself and a formula or two for you to try. These include sniffles, coughs, cramps, digestive woes, and various aches and pains, to name a few. I even tell you how aromatherapy can help you be less cranky and moody. You find how to use aromatherapy for healing.

Then, check out the Aroma Guide for detailed descriptions (including illustrations) of essential oils. This is an A-to-Z guide of fragrant plants that are used in aromatherapy. As you discover while reading this book, essential oils are the components that make plants fragrant, and they're the basis of aromatherapy. So you can also use this A-to-Z to look up the facts on essential oils. These essential oils are the ones most commonly used in aromatherapy and the ones that I discuss throughout this book. Whenever I mention an essential oil or plant and you're curious to find out more, then flip to the Aroma Guide.

Part V: The Appendix

You can find one appendix in this book.

The Appendix is a resource guide where you'll find places that sell all of the various aromatherapy supplies through the mail. This appendix is especially handy if you don't live near a store that supplies these items or if you don't have the time or transportation to get there.

Icons used in this book

This icon indicates sections in this book where you should pay close attention. They feature important facts or a place where I'm trying to get a point across. This icon usually marks the most technical part of the text, and it's what you need to know to talk aromatherapy.

I use this bull's eye to tip you off whenever I present a hint or expand upon the text. A lot of these are the tips that I've discovered by trial and error, so I save you the expense of learning the hard way.

There are some things that it just pays to remember. When you spot this icon, I'm telling you something that you'll probably want to know about aromatherapy in the future. This way, you can pay special attention when you read it and, just in case you do forget, you're able to quickly locate it again.

Experience is certainly one of the best teachers. It's one thing to imagine what a rose smells like and quite another to actually sniff one. Whenever possible, I think of ways that you can personally experience aromatherapy either by smelling something or by trying your own home experiment.

This icon marks information you should read carefully.

A Word about Holistic Healing

Aromatherapy is closely akin to herbalism. As an aromatherapist and herbalist, I find the two weave together very nicely in my practice. The two disciplines use many of the same medicinal herbs. Aromatherapy focuses on plants that are scented. Both herbalists and aromatherapists follow the principles of holistic medicine. The "holistic" part comes from "whole" and represents the biggest difference between it and standard (allopathic) medicine. Holistic medicine looks at the whole person and takes into consideration not just your symptoms, but your entire being, including your emotional self and how you conduct your life. How you think, what you eat, how much you exercise, what brings you joy, and what stresses you out are just a few of the things that are part of the whole picture of who you are. A holistic approach to health also works on healing all aspects of you and keeping you healthy so that hopefully you don't get sick again. I'm sure that you'll also discover in using this book that holistic aromatherapy offers you a tremendous opportunity for good health.

Where to Go from Here

Chances are that you've already experienced aromatherapy. If you've ever sipped a cup of chamomile tea, rubbed on rose or lavender scented hand lotion, or sniffed a cinnamon roll, you've already experienced aromatherapy. Where you go from here is into an adventure that combines enticing fragrances with good health. You hold in your hands a guide that can gently lead you to explore the many facets of this therapy.

Is some ailment bugging you? Then head straight to Chapter 11 to understand how aromatherapy works and then look up your specific problem in the Symptom Guide. Maybe you're feeling great physically, but you're too tired or need to have a little more focus? Then turn to Chapter 9 to help you stay alert. Want some hints on how to use aromatherapy? Then browse through Chapter 4.

Part I
Aromatherapy Essentials

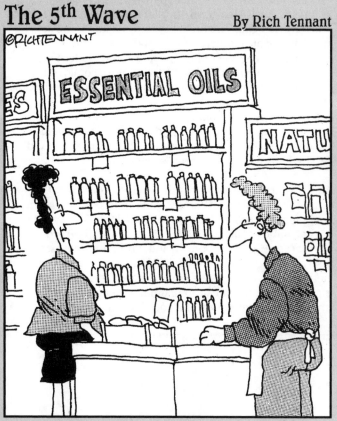

The 5th Wave   By Rich Tennant

"I'm looking for the good stuff. Do you have any of this stuff that's extra virgin?"

In this part

1 If aromatherapy conjures up for you the idea of a mystic art with a good sprinkling of hocus pocus, Part I will surprise you. The first chapter is all about the scientific basis of aromatherapy. It's good stuff to know, considering that most of the people in the modern world — and perhaps you, as well — feel a lot more comfortable treating their physical and emotional conditions with something that they feel confident works. Knowing that aromatherapy is a concrete science also makes it easier for you to explain what in the world you're doing running around the office or your home spritzing fragrance. And, aromatherapy makes perfect "scents."

Once you read about aromatherapy, you certainly will want to use it. Aromatherapy is big right now, so you'll find plenty of products that boldly claim it. The problem is that some of these are truly therapeutic-style aromatherapy: Good for your health, good for your skin, good to treat emotional imbalances. Then there are all the products labeled as aromatherapy that are just along for the ride. This is your one-stop manual to become a savvy shopper. So, jump in and fill your life with fragrance.

Chapter 1

Making Sense Out of Scents

. . . .

. . . .

*N*atural scents are everywhere; sniff a few aromatic plants, and you'll dis-cover how much fragrance is in the world. There's no doubt that fragrance enhances life, whether you're conscious of it or not. The scent of lilacs or violets that wafts in a spring day or the scent of freshly baked bread are the kind of smells that conjure up smiles in most anyone who encounters them. There are so many different smells in life that you probably don't give them a second thought. Or at least you may not yet. After you read this chap-ter, the world of aroma may take on an entirely different perspective.

I've always been fascinated by knowing how something works, and that extends to my interest in aromatherapy. Rather than just memorizing a list of scents that are useful for some disorder, I want to know why these particular ones are important. In that way, I can decide which scents are really the best choice for each situation. It also gives me a better perspective of which aroma I can substitute for another when necessary. In fact, it lets me make more edu-cated decisions about everything I do with aromatherapy. Another way that this understanding helps me is to convince folks who believe that aromather-apy is yet another "airy-fairy" practice (yes, these people are out there, and you will meet them) that it rests on a substantial, scientific foundation.

If you, too, are curious about aromatherapy, then there's no better place to start than discovering what creates scent in the first place. That's what this chapter is about. It's an often neglected topic in discussions of aromatherapy, but it's the nuts and bolts that can make more sense out of scents and help you see why they're so useful in therapy. In this chapter, I tell you all you need to know about these natural scents.

Defining Essential Oils

A plant's scent is produced by special oils — called *essential oils* — that it holds in special glands. Identifying plants that have these oils is an easy one-step process: Simply smell the plant. If the plant has a scent, it contains essential oils. Roses, violets, rosemary bushes, and even Christmas trees all owe their distinctive aromas to essential oils.

Essential oils are separated from a plant through several methods. (See the section "Producing Essential Oils," later in this chapter.) Once extracted, a pure essential oil is slightly oily to the touch. Although technically an oil, it is much thinner than vegetable oils used in cooking, such as canola or olive, or the motor oil that lubricates car engines. Essential oils are composed of such tiny compounds that the oil feels thin and seems to disappear when rubbed between the fingers. They also don't leave an oily stain on cloth and evaporate easily into the air. Because they dissipate so quickly, another name for essential oils is *volatile oils.* That name is a good description of them because volatile means "vaporous" or to be "like gas."

Special scent glands in a plant produce essential oils. These glands can occur anywhere, but are most likely in the flowers and leaves and least likely in the stems. Not all plants need essential oils to survive, but those that do put them to good use. For a long time, botanists couldn't figure out why plants contained these oils. Now they know that essential oils play several important roles:

✔ They attract bees and other pollinators.

✔ They repel harmful insects.

✔ They repel other plants so that they don't crowd the space.

✔ They kill bacterial, viral, and fungal infections.

Essential facts

Many centuries ago, the aromatic compounds in plants were named *essential* by poetic alchemists who believed that a plant's fragrance represented its "inner" nature. Fragrance is invisible, so people considered it magical and difficult to capture or define. These traits made it seem akin to a person's soul. Thus, fragrance was considered the *essential* part of a plant. It was thought that inhaling fragrance could bring you closer to heaven and inspire prayer. Indeed, one of the earliest uses of fragrant plants was as incense for religious ceremonies — an application still popular today throughout the world in Catholic churches, Hindu and Buddhist temples, in Japanese Taoist and Shinto practices, and in many Native American and African healing ceremonies.

- They seal the plant's wounds.
- They make the plant waterproof.
- They increase immunity to disease.
- They possibly influence reproduction as plant hormones.

Getting Physical: Simple Smell Science

Essential oils are valuable to people as well as plants, and for more than just enjoyment of their scent. Essential oils treat all sorts of physical and emotional conditions. In a perfect blend of aromatherapy's actions on body and mind, the billion-dollar beauty company also embraces aromatherapy because essential oils enhance both the health and beauty of skin, hair, and nails. As an added bonus, they smell wonderful when applied to the body. Such uses are what aromatherapy is all about. Here's a list of the most important medicinal properties found most often in essential oils.

- Kill bacterial, viral and fungal infections
- Heal wounds
- Reduce inflammation
- Regulate hormones
- Tone and moisturize skin
- Stimulate the immune system
- Repel bugs
- Possibly influence reproduction as plant hormones
- Attract mate
- Warm the skin in a hot massage oil (a *liniment*)
- Aid blood circulation and digestion
- Decrease sinus and lung congestion

I find it interesting that essential oils perform many of the same functions in people that they do in plants. In fact, if you refer to the preceding section, the roles of essential oils in plants is almost identical to this list. A few of the descriptions change — for example, "attracting pollinators" on the plant list appears as "attract mate" for the medicinal uses, although the two are not so different!

Essential oils have a lot in common when it comes to medicine. Due to their general makeup, most essential oils are highly antiseptic and able to kill an assortment of harmful microorganisms such as bacterial and viral infections. Many essential oils also reduce inflammation. This in turn often helps eliminate pain, which usually results when an inflamed or infected area pinches or presses on your nerves. Quite a few essential oils also encourage wounds to heal faster because they stimulate the repair of cells. All these actions combine into an excellent treatment for minor injuries, such as cuts, bruises, sprains, tight or cramped muscles, arthritis, headaches, inflammation, and infection. (For more on the therapeutic effects of essential oils, see Chapter 11 and the Symptom Guide.)

Getting Under Your Skin

The small size of essential oil molecules comes in handy to treat physical ailments. Tiny molecules such as these weigh in at less than 500. (That's molecular weight, not pounds! Although it may sound pretty hefty, this is really amazingly small.) That means they tend to pass through your skin without much trouble. Not every drop of oil is absorbed. A small amount of essential oil evaporates just from the heat of your skin, and some remains on the surface of your skin.

This absorption doesn't happen all at once. Essential oils are made up of many different compounds, and some pass faster through your skin than others. The most absorbable components in lavender, clove, and other essential oils appear in the blood 20 minutes after being rubbed on the skin. You can sniff bergamot, anise, and lemon on the breath 40 to 60 minutes after rubbing them on the skin. Geranium, citronella, peppermint, pine, and the heaviest compounds in lavender take just a little longer. Chemists say three things determine how fast a compound goes through skin: Its size, its shape, and how it functions (an example is how easily the oil mixes with water).

Test this one out at home. Cut a clove of garlic in half and rub the cut side liberally on the bottom of your foot. Put socks on and wait for the results of the experiment. It takes your blood system about 20 minutes to carry the essential oil of garlic throughout your body. You'll know because you'll be able to taste it! Not only can you taste garlic, but its powerful antiseptic action is going to work throughout your body! (*Caution:* Doing this experiment isn't recommended before attending a social event.)

The advantages in having essential oils go through your skin include the following:

> ✔ **The essential oils are right on target.** Essential oils go directly to the spot where you need them the most to work their healing magic. Say that you have a sore muscle and want to use an essential oil like chamomile to soothe muscle cramps. Rub on a massage oil that contains chamomile essential oil over a sore area, and you'll send the medicine into the underlying area — your tight muscle. Over and over, I've seen essential oils quickly knock out an infection, relieve a bruise, or ease a cramping muscle.

✔ **You'll have a happy liver.** Not only does the problem area get most of the medicinal dose when you put aromatherapy products on your skin, but less essential oil ends up in your blood stream. Not as much essential oil in your blood means less oil must be processed by your liver. That translates into less work for your liver and less chance of the oil producing a toxic reaction in your body.

Any aromatherapy product that contains vegetable oil — and that includes skin lotion, facial cream, salve, and massage oil — slows absorption of essential oil into your skin. In the long run, a little less essential oil is absorbed. What's happening is that large molecules in vegetable oils such as almond and olive oil are simply too big to slide through your skin, so they sit on top of your skin and hold on to some of the essential oil while they're at it. This is

Using the "Lizard Brain"

Once the nose gathers information about aroma, it sends a report to your brain. It bypasses the central nervous system and the areas of the brain that control reasoning. Instead, the nose sends its fragrance facts to a very old part of your brain called the *limbic system* for processing.

Considered ancient and primitive, the limbic system is sometimes called the "lizard brain" because it works in a similar fashion to the simple brain of a reptile. Similar to the brain of a reptile, your limbic system controls your basic survival. If you want to understand the limbic system better, think about what a lizard needs: To find food and a mate, be alerted to danger, remember a few survival skills, recognize its territory, and maintain its body's healthy equilibrium. All these requirements are more or less associated with the sense of smell.

One of the many jobs performed by the limbic system is to alert your body's warning system of potential danger. It signals the "fight or flight" response that causes your adrenals to provide a rush of adrenaline with its resulting burst of energy so that you can protect yourself or run from danger during an emergency. Another place that receives information about fragrances is the higher parts of your brain that control long-term memory.

The limbic system also directly communicates with glands called the *hypothalamus* and *pituitary*. Both of these are considered "master glands" because they regulate so many body functions. Through these glands, your sense of smell reaches all your various hormones and your immune system. Main areas where information is relayed are to those body functions that work automatically. These are ones not controlled by your will or reason: Appetite, digestion, sexual arousal, memory, body temperature, and heartbeat.

Anthropologists and psychologists are exploring why your sense of smell is closely linked to these particular areas. They assume that at one time smell played a very important role in survival. Perhaps five times more powerful in your ancestors than it is today, this super sense enabled them to smell spoiled food, the potency of their plant medicines, their kin, and friend or foe and to be attracted to a mate. This keen sense of smell also helped treat illnesses. It is likely that the use of aroma as therapy goes back to the earliest uses of plants as medicine. The first recorded uses of aromatherapy are from Egypt, Mesopotamia, and China just after 3000 B.C.

good for skin care because it gives the essential oils a chance to do their work directly on your skin. It also makes sense that more essential oils gets absorbed if your skin is cut or broken. Absorption may also be influenced by your skin type — for example, if you have dry or freshly washed skin, it's suspected that essential oils penetrate more easily.

During your exploration of aromatherapy, you're likely to encounter some differences of opinion. So, I should mention that another school of thought — although it's a different one than I attend — thinks that all the great results of aromatherapy come from breathing in the aromatic scents rather than what penetrates the skin. It's true that researcher haven't invented an experiment with aromatherapy in which the subjects don't smell the product as it's applied. Aromatherapy is much too fragrant for that! So, in the few studies that have been done, it's hard to say whether inhaling or rubbing the essential oil on the skin had more effect.

From Rose to Nose: Getting Emotional

One aspect of aromatherapy is how it affects the mind. Certain scents make you think better and faster, while others work on your emotions. Some mood-lifting aromas are antidepressants, while some are relaxants and still others act as stimulants. (If you're curious about which scents affect your mind, read the section "Reaping the Benefits of Aromatherapy," later in this chapter, and go to Chapter 9 and then to Chapter 4 to find more ways to bring these scents into your life. You can also find specific recipes under the individual emotions that I list in the Symptom Guide.)

I know that this all may seem a little mysterious — especially because the molecules responsible for producing aromas are too small to see with your eye. Actually, the route that fragrance uses to reach your emotions is really very scientific. If you could see the aromatic molecules that make up essential oils, you would discover that the air is filled with these microscopic particles of scent. Simply brushing against a fragrant plant or opening a vial of essential oil releases thousands of aromatic molecules into the air where they freely float to your nose (which is happening in Figure 1-1).

Every time you sniff something aromatic — say your favorite fragrant flower or perfume — thousands of tiny scent molecules tumble into your nose. High up in your nose, smell receptors await these compounds. They send information about what you smell to your *olfactory bulb*. (Olfactory is scientific lingo for smell.) These receptors are able to tell the difference between all of the various odor molecules. One way that they may differentiate the compounds is according to their shape. Much like your fingerprints, each aromatic molecule is unique.

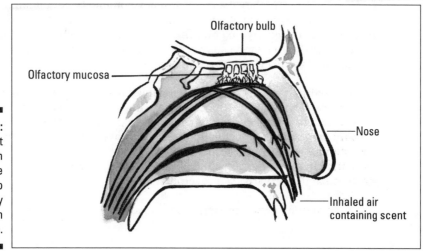

Olfactory bulb

Figure 1-1:
Scent
captured in
the nose
and sent to
the olfactory
bulb in
the brain.

Olfactory mucosa

Nose

Inhaled air
containing scent

Reaping the Benefits of Aromatherapy

The effect of fragrances on your mind and emotions may be subtle, but smell alone makes you feel better about yourself. It can improve your mood, reduce stress, cause you to become more energetic, or help you relax or fall asleep more easily. The bottom line is that you are happier. In this way, it achieves the goals set by most self-help books and seminars. After all, feeling good about yourself makes you less combative, jealous, and angry. You also feel more in control of your life, and that makes you less frustrated and more satisfied with life in general. Not bad results for a little sniff now and then of a pleasant fragrance!

Stimulants such as peppermint and eucalyptus intensify brain waves to sharpen the mind and quicken your reactions. This action is very similar to what happens if you drink coffee, but without caffeine's detrimental impact on your adrenal glands. A calming scent like chamomile has the opposite effect. It slows brain wave patterns to produce a relaxation that is similar to taking a sedative drug, but without side effects.

Pleasant smells put people into better moods and make them more willing to cooperate and compromise. Psychologists have had a field day testing this out! Dr. Susan Schiffman, professor of Medical Psychology at North Carolina's Duke University, really put the way that scent affects people's minds to the test. She got on the New York City subway and sprayed food scents in the cars. Under the influence of scent, passengers pushed and shoved each other

40 percent less, and they made fewer nasty comments per minute. At Memorial Sloan-Kettering Cancer Center, also in New York City, vanilla relaxed patients undergoing MRI (magnetic resonance imaging) scanning. Aromas piped into hospitals lower the anxiety of patients, staff, and the friends and families visiting patients.

Other conditions are currently being studied to find successful treatments that are just a sniff away. Researchers are hoping to uncover aromas that counter fatigue, headaches, food cravings, depression, anxiety, schizophrenia, and irregular heartbeat. If not cures, they at least want aromatherapy to improve the quality of life for people who suffer from these disorders. One thing that aromatherapy may offer is the ability to take less pharmaceutical drugs when the two are used together.

Don't try to reduce your prescription drugs without your doctor's approval.

Journeying into Aromatherapy: The Magic behind the Plants

You don't have to study chemistry to enjoy aromatherapy, but understand a thing or two about the makeup of fragrant plants, and you'll find your journey into aromatherapy suddenly gets much easier. Simple chemistry helps you select the best aromatic plants for the job. It guides you in creating blends that are effective *and* smell great — an important consideration since aromatherapy is so much about fragrance!

The magic molecules of aroma

Essential oils are not just one thing, but can be broken down into smaller parts. Each oil is composed of many very tiny aromatic molecules. Nature mixes and matches these compounds in various combinations. It is similar to a giant jigsaw puzzle in which all the pieces are interchangeable. Every time Nature rearranges the pieces, she comes up with a new design. In this case, it is a new smell as each different grouping makes yet another unique fragrance.

Variety is called the "spice of life," and that is certainly true of fragrance. I never cease being amazed at how many different natural scents exist. Take a whiff as you walk through a flower or herb garden, and you'll see that Nature has been busy. Rose, lilac, honeysuckle, gardenia, lemon, lavender, sage, rosemary . . . the number of aromas seems endless.

A rose by any other name would smell so sweet. . . .

Researchers are busy exploring aromatherapy to discover how fragrance can heal your body and mind. If you're talking to a cosmetic chemist or a psychologist (most of the studies on how aromatherapy affects the mind and emotions are found in psychology journals) or looking up research, you'll often find aromatherapy called *aromacology.* You have to admit that this scientifically correct name does have more of an official ring to it. Sometimes, instead of being used interchangeably, the two terms are used to differentiate the science and the theory (aromacology) from its application by clinicians and aromatherapists (aromatherapy).

Imagine that you are blindfolded, and someone leads you through a garden filled with fragrant plants such as roses, lilacs, lavender, and jasmine. One by one, a highly aromatic leaf or flower is held under your nose. Even if you can't distinguish them by name, you'll recognize that each one smells distinctively different.

An amazing number of different aromatic compounds exist. So far, more than 30,000 have been identified. In some cases, one essential oil contains hundreds of different ones — each contributing its own scent and therapeutic properties! Do the math if you want, but take it from me — a mind-boggling number of possible combinations exist. Plants with similar aromas are likely to also share some of the same aromatic compounds.

You can sniff out a lot about which individual molecules are in a plant just by smelling it. Compare the smell of a lemon peel to lemon verbena, melissa (also called lemon balm), lemongrass, lemon thyme, or lemon eucalyptus — either the essential oil or from the plant itself. You've probably guessed from their names, before even inhaling their scent, that all these plants smell like lemon. They do. That's because the essential oil in each one contains at least one type of lemon-scented component. But that's only the beginning. These six plants still smell distinctly different because their essential oils contain other aromatic components in addition to the lemon-scented ones. For example, the essential oil of lemon thyme contains both a component that makes it smell lemon-scented and thymol, which makes it smell like thyme. The leaves of the lemon eucalyptus tree contain the component *eucalyptol* and a lemony compound, giving it the combined smell of lemon and eucalyptus together. Different chemistry mixes such as these provide each plant with its own unique slant on the lemon theme.

Medicinal compounds in essential oils

Ask a chemist what makes chamomile relaxing or why thyme is such a strong antiseptic, and he or she will point to the individual compounds in an essential oil. Chemists know the properties of many aromatic compounds because researchers have determined their molecular structure and have done studies to discover how they work on the body. They found that some aromatic compounds improve digestion or are antiseptic, while others produce sedative effects.

The same aromatic compounds that give essential oils such a diversity of fragrances are responsible for their medicinal properties. An essential oil's therapeutic uses depend on which compounds it contains. The particular compounds and combinations determine which essential oils are more potent than others.

Here are the major categories of the chemical families found in essential oils. You don't have to memorize this list to be a good aromatherapist, but reading it helps you realize why essential oils are medicinal. Keep in mind when looking at this list that essential oils have complex chemistry so that they can contain more than one type of component and fall into more than one category.

Acids kill bacterial and viral infections and reduce inflammation. They are moisturizing to the skin. Examples of essential oils that contain acids are

- Birch
- Niaouli

Alcohols destroy bacterial and viral infections and are skin toners. Their scent is considered a tonic to the nervous system. Most alcohols are very safe to use. Examples of essential oils that contain alcohols are

- Carrot seed
- Clary sage
- Coriander
- Geranium
- Ginger
- Marjoram
- Neroli (orange blossom)
- Palmarosa
- Patchouli
- Peppermint
- Petitgrain

- ✓ Rose
- ✓ Sandalwood
- ✓ Vetivert

Aldehydes reduce inflammation and destroy bacterial infections. They produce a light sedative effect when inhaled. Many citruses fall under this category. Some aldehydes need to be used cautiously because they can cause allergies or irritate the skin. Examples of essential oils that contain aldehydes are

- ✓ Cinnamon
- ✓ Citronella
- ✓ Cumin
- ✓ Lemon eucalyptus
- ✓ Lemongrass
- ✓ Lemon verbena
- ✓ Melissa (lemon balm)

Coumarins thin the blood and are also calming and uplifting emotionally when inhaled. Many coumarins can make your skin sensitive to the sun, so use them carefully. Examples of essential oils that contain coumarins are

- ✓ Angelica
- ✓ Bergamot
- ✓ Citruses

Esters soothe muscle spasms and irritated skin and kill fungal infections. Most of them are strongly aromatic and are very relaxing when inhaled. Examples of essential oils that contain esters are

- ✓ Bergamot
- ✓ Clary sage
- ✓ Geranium
- ✓ Lavender
- ✓ Marjoram
- ✓ Neroli
- ✓ Roman chamomile
- ✓ Ylang ylang

Ester oxides release lung congestion. Many oxides are stimulating mentally when inhaled. They tend to have a camphorlike scent. Some potentially toxic oils in this group are not suggested for use, such as calamus and wormseed essential oils. Examples of essential oils that contain ester oxides are

- Bay
- Eucalyptus
- Hyssop variety decumbens
- Rosemary
- Tea tree

Hydrocarbons (such as terpenes) reduce bacterial infections, inflammation, and intestinal gas. They tend to be mentally stimulating. These are one of the two most common chemical types found in essential oils. Examples of essential oils that contain terpenes and sesquiterpenes are

- Carrot seed
- Cypress
- Fir
- German chamomile
- Ginger
- Grapefruit
- Lemon
- Nutmeg
- Orange
- Patchouli
- Pine
- Sandalwood

Ketones promote wound healing and thin out lung and bronchial congestion. A few of them are thought to stimulate fat metabolism. Some ketones are not easily metabolized in the body, so they pass unchanged, and unused, into the urine. Some of them, such as camphor, wormwood, tansy, and hyssop, are potentially toxic. Examples of essential oils that contain ketones are

- Caraway
- Fennel
- Hyssop
- Pennyroyal

- ✔ Rosemary
- ✔ Sage
- ✔ Thuja

Phenols are powerful antibacterials that also warm the skin and stimulate blood flow. They are mentally stimulating when inhaled. Many of the phenols are so heating that they irritant skin and need to be used in small amounts. Due to their heating action, they are used in liniments. Note that this phenol is not the same as the toxic phenol derived from petroleum. Phenols are one of the two most common chemical types found in essential oils. Examples of essential oils that contain phenols are

- ✔ Basil
- ✔ Clove
- ✔ Oregano
- ✔ Thyme (various varieties)

Organizing Plants: Variations on a Theme

In aromatherapy, you'll sometimes come across two or more essential oils that have the same name, yet they are designated as different. This can be understandably frustrating. Just when you think you know what you're looking for in an essential oil or aromatherapy product, you're confronted with still more choices. One confusing example is chamomile. A catalog or store that sells essential oil may give you the option of buying blue, gold, German, or Roman chamomile. A question that I often hear asked in my aromatherapy seminars is, "What's the difference, anyway?"

To explain exactly what's going on, I need to first talk a little more about science. This time it's botany. Plants come in many different sizes, shapes, and colors. To organize them, botanists divide them into categories according to the plant's physical characteristics. A large, major grouping is the family, with smaller categories under that.

When botanists sort plants into families, it's not unlike your own family tree. Here's how it looks:

A Plant's Family Tree

Family

Genus

Species

Variety Chemotype

Quick facts about plant names

Here's a few quick facts about plant names. This information comes in handy when you purchase essential oils to help you know exactly what you're getting.

- Botanical names are in Latin. They're often based on Latin and Greek words that describe one of the plant's distinctive characteristics, where it grows, or the name of someone associated with that plant. The names are written in italics to distinguish them as scientific names.

- Botanists write a plant name as var. variety *Genus species*. If this were Mary Smith's name, in botany, it is written *Smith mary*.

This differentiates her from her sister, *Smith sue.* If Mary is a twin and the two have the same name (just pretend this might happen, okay?) but different colored hair, then Mary would be *Smith mary* variety red hair.

- In botanical Latin, hyssop is written as *Hyssopus officinalis.*

- A variety of hyssop is written as *Hyssopus officinalis* var. *decumbens.*

- Common thyme is written as *Thymus vulgaris.*

- The chemotype "thymol" is written as *Thymus vulgaris* thymol.

I like to think of a plant's family as similar to your extended family — everyone who has the same last name. That makes the genus comparable to your closer kin. The species are your brothers and sisters. A variety or chemotype are the twins (very similar, but with at least one differentiating characteristic.)

One of the last classifications, chemotype, isn't used by botanists, but by chemists. (The name refers to a "chem-ical type.") A botanist classifies "variety" according to the plant's physical characteristics, but a chemist classifies a chemotype according to its chemical compounds. These two terms aren't interchangeable because it's an entirely different way of looking at things.

Most plants stop at species, and they aren't divided down to the point of being labeled a variety or a chemotype. However, these distinctions do come up in aromatherapy. In a few cases, it can make the difference between a potentially toxic essential oil and a therapeutic one. Because both terms come up when you're buying essential oils, I want you to be prepared. That way, if these terms are new to you, they don't send your head spinning when you see them in an aromatherapy catalog.

Although you may not be able to tell chemotypes apart by looking at them, you can smell a slight difference due to tiny alterations in their essential oils. A chemotype doesn't occur very often, but when it does, the essential oil it produces is definitely a little different. This quirk of nature is sometimes due to different growing situations such as the soil quality, climate, altitude, or amount of rainfall, but some chemotypes can be transplanted to a totally different area and still retain their altered chemistry.

Using different species

The species in the same genus not only look like they're related, they often have a comparable chemistry. This gives the plants a similar smell, as well as a similar use. However, the slight chemical alterations can make a difference in how you use the essential oils, as you see as you read the following descriptions of different species.

Chamomile essential oil is produced from several species, although their action and uses are similar. German chamomile reduces inflammation slightly better than Roman chamomile, which is one of the best muscle relaxants.

Cinnamon essential oil usually comes from a less expensive species called cassia rather than from true cinnamon. Cassia flavors colalike soft drinks, soaps, and pharmaceutical medicines and scents incense. Both the closely related camphor and Ceylon cinnamon are other species that are rarely used because they can easily irritate skin.

Eucalyptus has several species that are made into essential oil. Lemon eucalyptus contains so much of the compound called citrpnellal that it is a great bug repellent with a delightful lemony scent. *Eucalyptus radiata* is specific to treat sinus and herpes infections, while *Eucalyptus australiana* takes care of lung congestion and sore throat. *Eucalyptus smithii* is extra gentle, so it's used for children and sensitive individuals.

Fir essential oil comes from a few different species: Balsam fir, Canadian fir, and Siberian fir. They are used interchangeably, although they have a slightly different scent.

Lavender essential oil is most commonly "lavandin" from an easy-to-grow hybrid of English lavender crossed with spike lavender. It is less refined, but also less expensive, than English lavender essential oil, so at least 20 times more lavandin is sold. The essential oil from spike lavender smells more camphorous, but it is especially good for treating sinus and lung congestion and acne. *Lavendula stoechas* is a strong wound-healer that reduces inflammation and is also safe to use.

Sage essential oil is derived not only from common sage, but also Spanish sage, which has a distinctive lavender fragrance and is less irritating to skin. Both are strong antiseptics. Clary sage is less antiseptic, but its scent produces more of a heavy, relaxing effect.

Tea tree is derived from a few very similar species that are sometimes pooled together and sold as one oil. The type of tea tree called niaouli *(Melaleuca quinquenervia)* is considered the most antiviral species and has a sweeter, more pleasant scent. Cajeput, on the other hand, is very harsh.

Using different varieties

Not all species are further divided into varieties, but this designation is sometimes needed to distinguish two very similar plants. The two plants are closer than just being siblings. Think of them as twins. They're very much alike, yet still have distinct differences. The difference that's important to an aromatherapist is their different actions. I only have only one example of an essential oil that is commonly sold, but the difference between it and its "twin" is like night and day.

Hyssop essential oil is so strong, most aromatherapists use it sparingly if at all. Yet a variety of hyssop called "decumbens" is very gentle because it contains none of regular hyssop's potentially toxic ketones (see "Medical compounds in essential oils" in this chapter) that can increase blood pressure, stimulate the nervous system, and trigger asthma or epilepsy attacks. That's quite a difference and enough of one to make sure that you know which one you're using.

Using different chemotypes

Sometimes plants are so close, they look like identical twins that only a mother — or in the case of essential oils, a chemist — can tell apart. Their chemistry is the deciding factor. It's amazing the difference that changing a few molecules here or there can make! The following plants in each category look very much alike, but their individual smells give them away so that you can tell with one sniff that they are indeed different. In fact, chemotypes are so close, this category is a relatively new one that is made possible by advanced science. It's a designation used by chemists more than by botanists to distinguish the fine line between these plants.

Basil develops easily into chemotypes. The "Réunion" type contains mostly methyl chavicol, which has a harsh smell and can irritate skin, but very little of the linalol found in standard basil. East Indian basil comes with either a large amount of thymol (also found in thyme) or eugenol (also found in clove buds) and two distinctly different scents. Both compounds are strongly antiseptic, but they can irritate the skin.

Thyme has more than eight chemotypes. When thyme is grown at sea level in alkaline soil, it contains much more thymol, which is a very strong antiseptic, but is also very harsh and irritates skin. Although not as antiseptic, thyme that contains a large amount of geraniol or linalol is gentle to skin. A chemotype that is gentle and potent is the "thuyanol" type.

Eucalyptus has several species that produce chemotypes. Blue malle produces a "cryptone" type that specifically treats urinary and vaginal infections, while the "cineol" type is used for sinus and bronchial congestion. *Eucalyptus dives* is slightly toxic when it is the "piperitone" type, but a specific acne treatment when it is the "cineol" type. The two trees look identical, but they smell different.

Rosemary has the sweeter and gentler "verbenone" and "cineol" chemotypes and the harsher camphor type.

Essential oils made from different species, varieties, and chemotypes and aromatherapy products made with them are rarely sold in stores, except in those that cater just to aromatherapy. Most essential oil and aromatherapy manufacturers feel that aromatherapy is already confusing enough without trying to explain the different species and chemotypes on their labels. Where you will encounter them is in mail-order catalogs (see the Appendix). Most mail-order essential oils companies offer a wider selection of oils and products. These oils are also used by aromatherapists in their own practices and products.

Producing Essential Oils

Essential oils are extracted several ways. To obtain them in their pure form requires elaborate laboratory equipment that separates the oil from the fresh plant. The method used depends upon the plant, but steam distillation is most common. Most essential oils are not produced for aromatherapy. They mainly go to either the perfume industry or minute amounts flavor prepackaged foods. Many essential oils also scent all sorts of products that you buy, either to make them more appealing to consumers or to cover up an objectionable smell, say of plastic, a preservative, or a glue that is used in the product. Only about five percent of the essential oils produced today are used in aromatherapy, but this leaves plenty to choose from.

- ✔ **Water/Steam distillation** uses steam to pull essential oils from the plant. The plant is suspended over boiling water in a closed container so that the steam rises through it. The essential oils are quick to hitchhike a ride with the steam, which carries them up a long tube that is surrounded by a cold water bath. The cold forces the steam to rapidly cool and condense back into water. Water and most essential oils do not mix, so the two go their separate ways; the essential oil into a small collection vial and the water into a large vat. (A variation of this technique is *steam distillation,* which uses no water but instead pumps steam directly into a chamber holding the plant material. This technique, especially when done under pressure, is faster and more efficient.) See the diagram of a steam distiller in Figure 1-2.

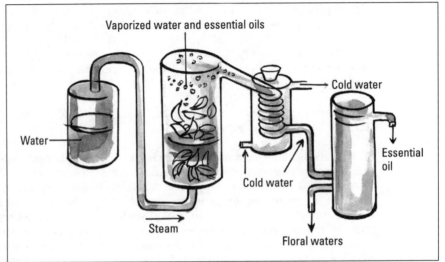

Vaporized water and essential oils

Cold water

Water

Essential oil

Cold water

Steam

Floral waters

Different processing techniques produce distinctly different versions of the same essential oils. Peppermint oil, for example, is commonly *redistilled* — run twice through a steam distiller to extract the oil. When distilled the first time, peppermint oil smells like peppermint, but the scent is harsh, and so is the taste. Distill this peppermint oil a second time, and the harshness disappears in favor of the lighter, fresher smell (and taste) that most people associate with peppermint chewing gum and candy. The lighter version is considered superior and worth the extra work to distill the oil twice. Almost all peppermint oil that is offered for sale is redistilled.

✓ **Expression** presses essential oils from the peels and seeds of citruses, such as orange, lemon, lime, and grapefruit. These are usually left over from manufacturing citrus juice. The technique is similar to pressing olive oil.

✓ **Enfleurage** is an ancient method of extracting oils that is rarely used today except in a few places in France. It's no wonder because it is a long, complicated, and expensive process. Fragrant blossoms are placed on solid sheets of warm fat, which absorb the essential oil. (The sheets were originally made from animal fat or lard, but now are solid vegetable fat.) Jasmine and tuberose flowers are the primary candidates for enfleurage because they continue to exude fragrance after they are picked. (However, the jasmine and tuberose that you'll find for sale are almost always solvent extracted.) When all the fragrance is transferred from the flowers to the fat, the "exhausted" flowers are removed and replaced with fresh ones. The process is repeated several times until the fat is saturated with scent. Then it is separated from the oil with solvents, leaving just the essential oil.

✔ **Carbon dioxide** is a new method of extraction using carbon dioxide gas (and sometimes also solvent) to extract the essential oil. The gas is kept under high pressure at a constant temperature. The equipment for this process is very expensive, and so are the resulting essential oils. Therefore, only the most expensive essential oils are extracted with carbon dioxide. However, it does produce a scent that is very close to the plant's scent because high heat is not used during the process. There is a similar and equally expensive process that uses even lower temperatures, but it uses fluorocarbons, which are potentially harmful to the environment, to extract the essential oils.

✔ **Solvent extraction** uses very little heat, so it's able to produce essential oils whose fragrance would otherwise be destroyed or altered during steam distillation. The plant is dissolved in a liquid solvent solution of hepane, hexane, or methylene chloride. These chemicals pull the essential oil from the plant. The plant is removed, and the solvent is boiled off under a vacuum or in a centrifugal force machine to help separate it from the essential oil. Because the solvent has a lower boiling point than the essential oil, it evaporates before the oil. The solvent is cooled back into liquid and reclaimed to be reused. Along with the essential oil, the fats, waxes, and heavier oils may also be extracted. This produces a semi-solid substance appropriately called a *concrete*. You can sometimes find these sold as is. Usually, the process is continued by dissolving oils into warm alcohol. Then the alcohol is removed under a vacuum. What's left is pure essential oil (although a little of the oil is lost during the process). This process is expensive, so it is reserved for costly oils, many of which cannot be distilled, such as jasmine and vanilla. Rose that is extracted with solvents is slightly less expensive than the steam distilled oil. A solvent-extracted essential oil is called an *absolute*.

Producing your own essential oils

If you want to produce your own essential oils, you need to buy a steam distiller. You can purchase ready-made stills through chemistry equipment supply houses listed in a big city phone directory. Some distillers are designed for home oil distillation. (See the Appendix for addresses.) You can rig up a makeshift distiller in your kitchen, but it isn't very efficient at producing much essential oil.

You also need a healthy supply of fresh plant material to distill. Even the plants that contain abundant amounts of essential oils, such as eucalyptus and rosemary, require several bucketfuls of plant matter to produce just 1 ounce essential oil.

Hydrosols

A *hydrosol* is a byproduct of distillation. It is called a hydrosol, meaning a "water solution." A lot of water runs through the still when essential oils are produced during steam distillation. Usually, the water and the essential oil separate, but a few essential oils contain water soluble compounds that refuse to separate during this process. Instead, these aromatic compounds stay in the water and make it very fragrant and therapeutic.

Hydrosols have many uses. And, they have the advantage of being ready to use. Unlike essential oil, you can put hydrosols directly on your skin undiluted and even use them in cooking. They are usually dispensed in a spray bottle so that you can spritz them on your skin or around the room. I carry hydrosols on my many seminar trips to freshen me and the places that I stay. Their uses vary according to which one you choose. Common uses of hydrosols include

- Aftershave
- Animal flea spray
- Breath freshener
- Cosmetic ingredient
- Face moisturizer
- Freshener for sheets and towels
- Fruit rinse
- House plant spray
- Ironing spray
- Room freshener
- Sore throat spray
- Spray disinfectant
- Therapeutic mist for massage

The most common hydrosol is rose water. Along with orange water, it is sold in East Indian groceries (found in large cities all across the country) and liquor stores to flavor mixed alcoholic drinks. The quality is usually only fair, but they work fine for cooking. Rose water also flavors the Indian yogurt drink lassi and the candy Turkish delight, and it is added to cosmetics as a skin moisturizer.

Quality hydrosols were only recently introduced commercially, and you still need to look around to find them. (See the Appendix for suppliers.) They are most often sold in spray bottles. The following hydrosols are available.

- ✔ Chamomile
- ✔ Geranium
- ✔ Lavender
- ✔ Lime
- ✔ Orange blossom
- ✔ Rose
- ✔ Rosemary
- ✔ Sandalwood
- ✔ Lemon verbena
- ✔ Yarrow

Aromatic waters

An *aromatic water* is made by adding essential oils to water to produce a fragrant water. The oil and water don't readily mix but after a few days and lots of shaking, some of the water will be scented while the remainder of the oil floats on top. Commercial aromatic waters usually contain an emulsifier that helps to keep the two blended together.

Aromatic waters are often confused with hydrosols because both are water based and they are used for the same purposes. (See the preceding section for a list of hydrosol uses.) They are manufactured by adding an essential oil to distilled water. Unlike hydrosols, they do tend to separate, so you have to shake the bottle well before each use. Aromatic waters are also considered less moisturizing to the skin because the essential oil molecules float around in the water instead of being fully broken down and incorporated with it.

On the plus side, aromatic waters are less expensive than hydrosols to buy and a real good deal if you make your own. You can also make a much larger selection. I call them aromatic waters to differentiate this product from hydrosols, but they go by several different names. You also may see hydrosols called aromatic waters, and both are called just plain rose water or orange water. The best way to tell the difference is to see whether the container states that it is a distilled water or *produced* during distillation. If not, you probably have the copycat.

More on solvent-extracted essential oils

Although solvent-extracted essential oils — either an absolute or a concrete — come from plants, many aromatherapists shy away from them. They worry that slight traces of the solvent may remain in the final product, even though it is supposedly completely removed. The following are solvent-extracted essential oils. (The asterisk next to some oils indicates that these oils are also steam-distilled and what you most often find for sale are the distilled version. These distilled oils are much less expensive.)

- Calendula
- Carnation
- Champaca (from India)
- Clary sage* (rarely solvent extracted)
- Clove bud* (rarely solvent extracted)
- Fenugreek
- Gardenia
- Helichrysum*
- Immortale
- Jasmine
- Labdanum
- Lavender* (rarely solvent extracted)
- Maile fern (from Hawaii)
- Mimosa
- Narcissus
- Oak moss
- Orange blossom*
- Rose*
- Rosemary* (rarely solvent extracted)
- Tuberose
- Vanilla
- Ylang ylang*

Chapter 2

Sniffing the Diff: What to Look for in a Scent

• •

• •

*I*f you're sold on the idea of aromatherapy, you may be ready to head to the nearest store and stock up on some products. But you may want to read this chapter first. To find quality scents, you need to make your way through a marketing jungle. To find what you're looking for, you need to distinguish between true and phony oils and understand that even the purest and most natural essential oils can come in several different qualities.

Don't fret — by using the guidelines in this chapter, the task of choosing oils and products wisely is not as monumental as it may seem. In this chapter, I tell you how to differentiate between top-of-the-line essential oils and the run-of-the-mill variety, as well as the downright stinky.

Your Nose Knows: The Good, the Bad, and the Stinky

An *aromatherapy product* is one that contains essential oils. Therefore, you need to focus your attention on the quality of these oils. At first glance, all essential oils may appear equal. The truth is that many variables affect the quality of essential oils, such as how the plant is grown, how its essential oil is processed, and how well the oil is then stored.

Unfortunately, you can't always tell what you're buying just by reading the label. An oil identified as essential oil or a product that lists essential oil as an ingredient gives you no assurance that you're purchasing the real thing. Oils can be cut with something or completely replaced with another oil that smells similar. Some essential oils are even made from completely different materials in a laboratory. (See the section "Avoiding imitations: Sinful synthetics," later in this chapter.)

Sniffing 101

Because you rely on your nose to lead you through the aromatherapy marketing maze, you need to teach it the tricks of the trade. First, you need to discover how to smell. When smelling a finished aromatherapy product, such as shampoo or body oil, you can just sniff away because only a small amount of the essential oil is already mixed into the finished product.

However, undiluted essential oil is another story. Undiluted oil is too strong to sniff directly from bottle. The olfactory overdose from inhaling straight essential oil while holding the bottle directly under your nose will probably do no worse than make you lightheaded or give you a headache, but why suffer these consequences? Anyway, oil this potent is also too strong to give you an idea of what it will really smell like in a finished product.

To safely sniff essential oils:

✔ Smell the scent of the oil from the lid rather than the bottle.

✔ When sniffing an undiluted essential oil, hold the lid about 6 to 10 inches from your nose.

✔ Move the bottle or lid back and forth through the air to dilute the aromatic molecules.

✔ After smelling several essential oils, clear your nose palate so that you can keep on sniffing. For tips on how to clear your nose, check out the following section.

Clearing your nose

Your capacity to smell begins to decline after about six or seven good sniffs in succession. Along with it goes your ability to distinguish an oil's subtle characteristics — an obvious problem when you're trying to determine an oil's quality. Keep sniffing, and eventually your nose gives out altogether so that you can't smell a thing.

Quality control and chemisty

In the world of aromatherapy, quality control means getting down to the nuts and bolts of fragrance. That translates to chemistry (see Chapter 1). You don't need a graduate course in science, but knowing a thing or two about aromatic molecules is good way to be a savvy consumer. It also helps your skill in designing your own aromatherapy blends. (For more on creating your own blends, see Chapters 1 and 5.)

Essential oils contain many different compounds (see Chapter 1). Considering the multitude of possible combinations, each type of essential oil has its own unique fragrance. A change in chemistry means a change in the scent. A poor mix of compounds can smell weak, as if something is missing, decidedly inferior, or just plain lousy. And, it isn't just the smell that is altered — different proportions of these molecules also modify the essential oil's healing properties.

Scientists determine essential oil quality in their laboratories by measuring the amount and proportions of compounds that an oil contains. Granted, you probably don't have access to a fancy scientific lab. However, you're already carrying a highly sophisticated and fairly reliable meter with you: your nose. An experienced nose need only a sniff to distinguish the good, the bad, and the stinky.

To regain your sense of smell, you can simply take a break and stop smelling the oils for 10 minutes, or until your sense of smell returns. If you don't want to wait that long, you can recover your sense of smell in less than a minute by:

- **Walking outside and deeply breathing fresh air.** Here's a good way to clear your nose of all those scent molecules bouncing around in there. Think of this as an air "wash."

- **Sniffing coffee beans or hovering over a cup of coffee.** Yes, you read this correctly; I did say coffee. And you thought it was just for a pick-me-up? Exactly why coffee works on your ability to perceive scent is a bit of a mystery, but it definitely does the trick.

- **Taking several breaths through a wool scarf or cap.** There's something about the smell of wool that changes your smell perception. This trick also works well to filter out the scents that linger in a room when you work with essential oils. Not any cap or scarf will do; make sure that it's a wool one.

- **Putting a few grains of salt on the tip of your tongue.** This is not only a good way to regain your sense of smell, it also illustrates the close connection between sense of smell and your taste buds. The salt cuts short the smell information reaching your brain and sets an empty stage that is ready for a new scent experience.

Talking Scents: Language of Fragrance

This section is all about describing a scent. Although it may seem complex, it is a useful skill. Try to define different scents using this "language" to compare one fragrance to another. This helps you distinguish what you like in a scent, as well as what you don't like. That's important if you're trying to develop a discriminating nose and pick out quality products and essential oils.

Try borrowing three ideas from the experts of smell, the perfumers: Become more familiar with various scents, determine quality, and eventually create your own blends.

Perfumers — often called *noses* as a compliment to their trade — place essential oils into many categories. For your aromatherapy work, you can place scents into three categories, which I describe in the following sections:

✔ Scent type

✔ Scent quality

✔ Scent notes

Using the three categories I describe, you can develop fragrance "talk." For example, an essential oil may smell to you like a sharp wood. Another may seem like a strong, sour citrus. After you begin using phrases like these, they come to you automatically when you come across any fragrance. Of course, unless you encounter someone else who works with aromatherapy, you may not be talking to anyone else but yourself. It doesn't matter. Mumble away. The point is that by putting a name on it, you better identify what you're smelling.

Scent type

I start with type of scent because it's the easiest and most familiar way to categorize scents. In fact, you probably already know the type of scent categories well enough to imagine them. Table 2-1 introduces and explains the basic types of scent produced by nature.

Table 2-1	Types of Scent	
Scent	*Description*	*Oil Example*
Floral	Think of the fragrance exuded by a bouquet of flowers	Rose, lavender
Wood	Think of the smell of freshly cut wood	Cedar, cypress, firs, sandalwood

Scent	Description	Oil Example
Citrus	Imagine the fresh scent of an orange, lemon, or lime.	Grapefruit, lemon, orange, petitgrain, tangerine
Herbal	Think of something yummy to eat that contains herbs, like the smell of a pizza, freshly toasted herb bread, or stuffing cooking at Thanksgiving.	Marjoram, rosemary, sage
Spicy	Go to the kitchen for a spicy scent: You can find it in cinnamon-flavored oatmeal or hot cinnamon rolls.	Cinnamon, cloves
Minty	Mint is another obvious smell, one of chewing gum and mint breath sweeteners.	Peppermint, spearmint
Camphor	Imagine the pungent, sharp smell of camphor. Think of the smell of mothballs, although the aromatic wood of the camphor tree itself smells sweeter and much more pleasant. A camphorous smell seems to go directly to the top of your head when you sniff it.	Camphor, pine

Any of these six types of scents can be overbearing if they dominate the scent that you smell. This is especially true of camphor — a little goes a long way. A strong camphorous scent in geranium, pine, and rosemary can be unpleasant. Give someone a camphorous pine oil to sniff, and her first reaction is to wrinkle her nose and pull her head back. When you see a reaction like that, you know you've dealing with an essential oil that leans too heavily in the direction of a scent that is unpleasant when it's in full force — in this situation the scent of camphor.

If you sniff an essential oil and it seems to literally float back and forth between more than one scent type, don't worry. Your nose is doing a great job detecting the complex makeup of an essential oil that falls into more than one type. For example, I list pine as camphorous, but it also is definitely woodsy. Although lavender is floral as listed, it also smells very herbal. As a result, both pine and lavender fall under two categories, with one more predominant than the other.

Geranium is even more complicated. It smells like several familiar scents rolled into one, which is exactly what it is. In fact, one sniff and anyone unfamiliar with geranium will think it is a blend of several oils mixed together. Geranium has five distinct scent types. The two most distinct aromas in geranium are citrus and rose. There is also an herby aroma. You can also sense a subtle, underlying woodsy scent. Finally, a pinelike scent makes the oil smell slightly camphorous. As far as quality goes, geranium essential oil that carries a stronger rose scent is considered better than one that is predominately citrus. A strong camphorous scent in geranium is even more undesirable, especially if it is overbearing.

Scent quality

Describing a scent's quality is a little more difficult, but not too hard after you get the hang of it. Good essential oils are described as *full bodied.* Full body means that the scent carries more intensity and a richer, more rounded "bouquet" of fragrance because it contain more aromatic compounds. On the other hand, you can describe the same but lower quality oil as smelling "flat," "one-sided," or just plain weak. You can even call it boring.

Trying to define a term like *rounded* or *flat* in regards to scent isn't exactly easy, but one way is to compare it to taste. Think of this comparison. You bite into a cheese sandwich that is made with a slice of cheese between two pieces of plain bread without butter, mayonnaise, or anything. Your taste buds probably don't get very excited about that lunch! Now envision eating the tastiest sandwich that you can that has all your favorites; perhaps it includes pickles, mustard, and tomatoes. Now, that's the difference between a flat taste and a full taste.

Try another experiment. This time compare your sense of smell to hearing. Imagine that you're listening to music. Someone is hitting the same piano key over and over. You have no interest in continuing to listen. In fact, you wish they would stop. It's very *one-sided.* Compare this to hearing a full piano concerto played. Many notes are involved, and it moves all around the scale. There is a much richer sound, definitely a full bouquet of notes that sound musical to your ear.

Also, you may notice that poorer quality oils tend to smell sharper, harsher, or even bitter. For example, citrus oils smell a little sour, but the best ones also smell sweet. If this scent-describing sounds like wine-tasting, that's because it is — the only difference is that you're smelling rather than tasting.

The following are a list of qualities to detect in essential oils. Think about each of the following descriptive pairs when smelling an oil. In other words, try to categorize an oil as more mellow or more sharp and then move on to detecting whether it's smooth or harsh. You won't necessarily find all these qualities in each oil, but see how many are obvious.

- ✔ Soft or strong
- ✔ Mellow or sharp
- ✔ Smooth or harsh
- ✔ Sweet or bitter or sour
- ✔ Full or flat

Scent notes

A third category classifies fragrance as a high, middle, or low *note*. Scent is so analogous to music, that perfumers borrowed the idea of fragrance notes from musicians. They place different scents on a scale, similar to a musical score, and designate them as top, middle, or base notes. A fragrance can just have one note, but more notes in the scent create a richer experience. When you're looking at a good smelling essential oil or aromatherapy product, recognizing the note isn't as important as the scent type or the quality, but I include it to round out your nose education. (You can try to determine the top, middle and base notes for extra credit.)

- A **top (high) note** smells light and is described as airy. A high note is the flirty aspects of smell. It's the first one to greet your nose, but then dissipates quickly. Examples are lemon, grapefruit, lime, and peppermint.

- A **middle note** is trickier to detect because it falls somewhere in between the high and low notes. A middle note can confuse your nose by seeming to bounce between the high and low note or take on different notes depending upon what other essential oils are mixed with it. Examples are chamomile, fennel, and marjoram.

- A **base (low) note** is just the opposite of a high note. It smells "heavy" and has staying power. Examples are cedarwood, jasmine, and sandalwood.

Choosing Wisely

When sniffing your way around essential oils, you often find that two bottles of the same type of oil smell differently. This does not necessarily mean that one is better than the other. Like someone judging fine wine, music, or movies, even the experts don't always agree on their favorites.

However, sometimes two bottles of the "same" oils don't smell the same at all. You need to watch out for a variety of things while choosing essential oils. The most common are manmade oils, adulterated oils, and diluted oils (see my explanations in the following sections).

Avoiding imitations: Sinful synthetics

Whipped up in a laboratory, *synthetic* essential oils are a brew of derived chemicals that are mostly manmade and often produced from petroleum. Creating a new compound is similar to making a puzzle. Pretend that the chemical is cardboard and that you cut it into dozens of intricate shapes. Then you take out just a few pieces and instead of putting them back, you force them to fit into an entirely new puzzle, or in the case of a chemical, a new compound. Because the pieces aren't designed to fit together, it takes some work to get them to do so. You might have to knock off a corner before you can push it together. This is not unlike what a chemist does in her laboratory. She often takes a natural compound to form the building blocks and then adds on a petroleum-derived substance. Petroleum is one of the "natural" compounds that can be manipulated into hundreds of different directions.

Smellwise, some synthetics are better than others as one sniff will tell you, but you have to pay for the quality duplicates. Healthwise, they're all probably pretty lousy. No one knows why for sure, but nothing does it better than nature. Aromatherapists agree that natural oils get far better results with their clients (having a better and quicker response) than with synthetic. This certainly has been my experience. As an added benefit, natural oils cause far fewer allergic reactions and sensitivities. All aromatherapists I know use natural essential oils.

Pricewise, you tend to save a little by buying synthetics with most oils, except for expensive essential oils such as rose and vanilla. As far as selection goes, it's much greater with synthetics because a chemistry lab can manufacture anything; it may not smell very good, but they can make it.

However, scientists who research aromatherapy are not as fussy as aromatherapists. They experiment with synthetics such as strawberry and apple, as well as natural oils. The same is true for perfume manufacturers who love the vast array of new, cheaper, and otherwise unobtainable fragrances offered by synthetics. Many, many companies — making everything from candles to cream rinse — claim that they sell aromatherapy products even though they use cheaper synthetic essential oils. Even quite a few lotions, hair conditioners, creams, and other body-care products sold in natural-food stores are not all that natural when it comes to the essential oils used to scent them.

So, what's the problem with synthetics, you may ask. The answer, like so many other things, isn't black and white. Aromatherapists insist on using only natural essential oils because synthetics are very different from those found in nature. For example:

- ✔ Synthetics don't smell or work the same as natural essential oils, because they consist of a different set of molecules than a natural oil. They even have a different smell.

- ✔ Any aromatherapist or herbalist can tell you that synthetics cause far more allergic reactions — such as skin rashes, sneezing, headaches, and puffy eyes — than natural oils. There haven't been any studies or surveys that I know of on the negative effects of synthetic fragrance, but we aromatherapists see problems from them all the time. No one knows exactly why, but it may have something to do with the chemical mix of the synthetics and that our bodies seem to adapt better to natural medicines than manmade ones.

✔ I also worry because synthetic molecules are tiny enough to be absorbed by the skin and enter the blood stream. While oils derived from medicinal plants contain therapeutic properties when absorbed into your body, petroleum-based molecules are a very different story. Of course, I can't say for sure, but most holistic healers suspect that the overload of petroleum-derived products in the environment in the last few decades may contribute to a corresponding increase in cancer rates. Researchers are busy investigating this connection, but until they come up with an answer, aromatherapists choose to not put the synthetic oils on skin or to inhale them.

If you haven't smelled rose essential oil, then you're in for a treat, although inhaling this divine aroma is sure to spoil you for life! When someone tells me that rose oil smells a little "soapy" or simply "nice," I suspect that he or she has never encountered the real thing. This doesn't surprise me, considering that synthetics are everywhere. Most skin lotions, creams, and other body-care items — even those sold in natural-food and herb stores — use synthetic scents. Rose is the most popular body-care fragrance — and it is also one of the most expensive. It's so common that I usually have at least a few students in my seminars tell me that they're either allergic to rose or they hate the smell. However, when they sniff the real thing, none of them have ever reacted adversely, and even the rose-haters love it. (Wondering where to find some real rose oil to sniff? The Appendix lists suppliers of natural essential oils.)

Some synthetics need nature's help to come even close to a natural fragrance. To do so, chemists mix synthetic and naturally derived molecules together. Rose is especially difficult to duplicate with synthetics alone because it contains so many different aromatic molecules. Instead of making a pure synthetic, chemists find it easier to make compounds that smell like rose out of geranium oil and mix them with synthetics. The final product mimics, although never duplicates, true rose, and is still considered a synthetic and aromatherapists don't use them.

Here's the confusing part for shoppers: Synthetic and natural essential oils can both be called essential oils. This means you can't trust labels to inform you about what you're buying. Making it even harder to tell the difference, synthetics look and feel very similar to the natural essential oils produced from plants. Plus, there aren't any labeling restrictions on essential oils. This leaves it all up to the data you collect on essential oils and your nose.

What gives synthetics away is their scent. No matter how hard chemists try, they never completely duplicate nature. The poorest quality synthetic oils are the easiest to detect, but even the best synthetics you can buy still don't smell quite right.

If differentiating between good and poor natural essential oil seems a formidable enough task for you, spotting a synthetic may seem impossible. It's not. I'm not talking about detecting the difference between diamonds and fake stones or anything requiring lots of expertise. The fact is, science hasn't perfected the manufacture of synthetic essential oils, and most of them don't even come close to smelling like the real thing.

One way to sort the real from the fake is to visit a store that sells essential oils and check out its display rack. You can find out a lot with a quick glance at the merchandise. The following are a list of things to watch out for. Find just one of these, and the other oils in the rack are likely to also be synthetic or adulterated.

✔ If you see a very expensive oil, such as rose or jasmine, sold at a ridiculously low price — say less than $50 for a quarter ounce — figure that it can't be a pure, natural essential oil.

✔ Look at the other essential oils on the same rack. Popular scents such as peach, lilac, strawberry, and coconut (the essential oil, not coconut vegetable oil) can't be produced naturally, only as synthetics.

✔ Extracting a real essential oil from carnation or violet flower is so expensive that you'll never see it for sale. Vanilla is available as a natural essential oil, but it sells for around $40 for a little quarter ounce bottle. As a result, most vanilla scent relies on the synthetic version.

✔ Look at the names given to oils in the rack. Certainly, an essential oil labeled "Rain" or "Oriental Gardens" or "New Mown Hay" are not real essential oils. When you find a brand that carries these obvious pretenders, assume that their entire essential oil line is fake.

Natural versus synthetic: What's the fuss?

Sixty years ago, most chemists were pretty darned excited about the new development of manmade (or synthetic) chemicals. It was the wave of the future, and it was theirs. It expanded their field greatly, and the new chemistry also offered the hope of creating all sorts of new compounds, including drugs. Back then, a chemist could fairly well duplicate many of the compounds that are found in nature — or at least they thought so. The modern, state-of-the-art equipment that is now available to analyze essential oils shows us a different story. What once looked fairly similar now displays different traits from a supposedly identical natural compound. And, different traits can mean different activity.

I talked this over with Larry Jones, a chemist who spends his working hours analyzing the purity of essential oils for his business, Spectrix. Larry can tell the difference between natural compounds and the manmade ones that show up in synthetic essential oils and also ones that are adulterated (see more on this in the section on "Substitution and adulteration," later in this chapter). What he sees is a visual difference in the molecules when they're displayed on the screens of his lab equipment.

When you do find synthetic oils, take the opportunity to smell a few. You'll notice that the fragrance of synthetic oils is often "too much." They're too sweet, too overpowering, and too blatantly fake. If you get a chance, smell a synthetic essential oil, say a jasmine or rose, and then compare it to a natural essential oil. This little experiment can help you further distinguish the difference between synthetics and naturals.

Also, try this test to find quality aromatherapy products: Check the label to see whether it lists essential oils that are available only as synthetics. If you spot even one synthetic oil lurking in a formula, then aromatherapists don't consider this a true aromatherapy product. The most popular synthetic essential oils include

- ✔ Apple
- ✔ Carnation
- ✔ Coconut
- ✔ Gardenia
- ✔ Lilac
- ✔ Magnolia
- ✔ New mown hay
- ✔ Oriental garden
- ✔ Peach
- ✔ Rain
- ✔ Raspberry
- ✔ Strawberry
- ✔ Violet flower (a natural violet leaf is sold)

Dilution

Sometimes, other materials are added to an essential oil to make it more affordable. There is nothing wrong with *diluting* an essential oil with either vegetable oil or alcohol. In fact, you need to dilute essential oils before you can use them. Essential oils are often intentionally diluted to save you the trouble of doing it yourself or to make them more affordable. (Jojoba oil is a popular choice for diluting essential oils because it doesn't spoil.) The label is supposed to list all the ingredients — including essential oils and vegetable oils such as almond or grapeseed — with the largest amounts listed first. That way, you can tell whether the product that you're considering buying has more essential oils or something like a vegetable oil.

The problem with diluting comes when oils are mislabeled as pure essential oil — and it's even worse if they have the price tag to go with it. Some essential oils are quite expensive, so it's no surprise that unscrupulous dealers dilute them to extend the oil and get more for their money. Inexpensive oils are seldom altered, but the practice is all too common with more expensive oils, especially those that are in high demand. Any alteration can drastically affect the oil's scent and its healing properties.

Dilution is usually done with alcohol, vegetable oil, or a chemical solution. You can't easily tell they contain a potential health hazard because the chemicals are absorbed into your body when rubbed on your skin or inhaled through your lungs. That's not good because most of these chemicals are suspected of causing health problems.

You can use a few tricks to help you detect a diluted essential oil. One clue is that diluted oils smell much weaker than pure essential oil. You can also use some other tips to identify specific types of dilution:

- **Vegetable oil:** Adding vegetable oil to an essential oil is the easiest type of dilution to detect. Try this test. Take a small piece of paper. Place a couple drops of the essential oil on the cloth. Wait a few minutes for the oil to evaporate. If it leaves an oily stain, it is probably diluted with vegetable oil. On the other hand, a pure essential oil evaporates, leaving no stain behind. (A few highly pigmented oils such as the deep blue German chamomile and the dark brown patchouli do slightly discolor the paper, but aren't oily.)

- **Alcohol:** It is more difficult to detect an essential oil that is diluted with alcohol than with vegetable oil. However, it does have a slight alcohol odor that smells like vodka. After you become familiar with what an essential oil should smell like, the alcohol is easier to detect.

- **Chemicals:** Essential oils diluted with solvents are the most difficult to recognize because the solvents are clear, non-oily, do not have a significant odor, and usually feel very similar to essential oil. Just about all that you can do is to recognize that the oil smells too weak to be a pure essential oil.

Substitution and adulteration

Some companies stretch their dollars, and their ethics, by replacing some or all of an expensive essential oil with a less expensive essential oil.

- Inexpensive lemongrass, citronella, or lemon eucalyptus sometimes masquerade as the very expensive melissa (lemon balm) oil. This is an example of *substitution*. Although the end products from substitution contain only pure, natural essential oils, it is not the essential oil it is supposed to be. And, it may not have the therapeutic properties you need.

✔ An expensive oil like rose essential oil may be cut with the much cheaper rose geranium oil to extend and make it go farther. This is *adulteration*. A second way to do adulteration is to "spike" an essential by adding a small amount of a compound that the oil already contains. This is a snap to do for a chemist with either a compound that has been extracted from a plant or made in the lab. This type of adulteration can buff up a poor quality essential oil that contains too little of some important ingredient so that it smells better. It's as if you make some lemonade from scratch, but the lemons taste weak and company is on its way over, so you add lemon flavoring to make it taste more like it should. The flavoring you use may be extracted from real lemons or a manmade compound that resembles the taste of lemon. If you do this kitchen version of adulteration carefully and add just the right amount, only the lemonade connoisseur will detect your secret.

Substitution and adulteration are problems in the essential oil business because they're harder to pick up with your nose than the more obvious synthetic, until you've been around lots of different essential oils. The company that bottles the essential oil you buy may not know much about its origins. Even if they know that an oil is adulterated, it's not something that a company is inclined to talk about unless you ask. The best thing that you can do is to find an essential oil dealer that you can trust.

To try to purchase pure, natural essential oil:

✔ Buy essential oils from a reputable company that you can trust. (You can find companies that sell true essential oils or products made with them in the Appendix.)

✔ Ask for an essential oil by its Latin name. This still doesn't always guarantee that you get what you want, but the few companies that bother to put these scientific names tend to be more reliable.

The following oils are often adulterated, substituted, or diluted because they're very popular and also very expensive. Be on guard when you purchase them.

✔ Bergamot

✔ Frankincense

✔ Jasmine

✔ Melissa (lemon balm)

✔ Myrrh

✔ Neroli (orange blossom)

✔ Rose

✔ Sandalwood

- ✔ Vanilla
- ✔ Ylang ylang

The following oils are seldom adulterated, substituted, or diluted.

- ✔ Cedarwood
- ✔ Citronella
- ✔ Eucalyptus
- ✔ Fennel
- ✔ Lemongrass
- ✔ Orange
- ✔ Tea tree

Making the Grade

Winning the oil quality game involves more than just differentiating between natural and synthetic oils. A variety of factors that occur between the time that they're produced in the plant and the time that you purchase them can influence natural essential oils. Of course, you can't do much about an essential oil that was poorly grown or produced, except to not buy it. If you do end up with a poor essential or a product that contains inferior oils, then you just don't get the results you should.

Buying quality certainly has its advantages. Not only does the oil has better fragrance, but you can use less. In addition, the oil is often more medicinal (although the difference can be slight).You'd think logically that the grade of an essential oil would be reflected in its price. This is often the case, but not always. A lot of people are out to make a buck, so you'll find inferior essential oils sold for more than they're worth. Some unscrupulous companies are hoping that you haven't read this book.

In case you're wondering what can happen to an essential oil to make it so undesirable, here are some problems that decrease the quality of an essential oil before you ever see it.

- ✔ As much as folks love her, Mother Nature is not always consistent. All nature's quirks, like weather and the types of soil, can alter an aromatic plant's chemistry. So can changes in temperature and rainfall in the area where an aromatic plant is grown. Growing conditions not only vary from year to year, but from one location to another. The oil's scent is altered along with these changes, sometimes for the better, but sometimes for the worse.

✔ For an optimum oil, most fragrant plants are harvested just before they flower. However, some oil harvesters are fussier than others about picking plants at their peak.

Sniff things out for yourself. Pick out any plant with aromatic leaves in your own yard or in a nearby park. Rub a leaf between your fingers and then take a good sniff. Visit this plant several times during the growing season and give it additional sniffs. You'll notice that the fragrance of most aromatic leaves increases and improves just when their flower buds start to form. After flowering, the fragrance declines.

✔ The type of equipment and the temperature used to extract the oil is another consideration. I've encountered essential oils that smelled burnt or all too light simply due to a poor production techniques.

✔ After an essential oil is produced, it still needs to be carefully stored — away from heat and light — to retain quality.

Some aromatherapists and aromatherapy companies who claim to have the best aromatherapy products or essential oil line say that only the highest grade are medicinal. This is not necessarily so. Aromatherapist Jane Buckle, R.N., did an interesting experiment using two different grades of lavender essential oil with patients who had just had heart operations. The idea was to help them relax during their stressful recovery period and to see whether the quality of essential oil made any difference. The results surprised Buckle because the lesser, inexpensive grade of lavender oil, called lavandin, proved the most effective.

So, don't go dumping out all of the essential oils you've already purchased in fear that you didn't choose the supreme example. Don't feel that you need to spend a fortune to practice aromatherapy. Base your decision on how you intend to use the oil. You might be a lot fussier about what you put on your skin, say in a hand lotion or a massage or bath oil, compared to what oil you use to scent your candles or soap when you're thinking about how much you should spend. This is a big consideration, especially when you see how much oil it takes to scent soap, potpourri, and candles! Just make sure the oils are natural and not synthetic.

To decide the grade of aromatherapy products and essential oils to use, ask yourself these questions:

✔ How am I using the essential oil or the finished product?

✔ How important is to achieve maximum results?

✔ How substantial is the price difference among the various qualities?

✔ Does the more expensive brand really smell that much better?

✔ Do I need to use more of the poor quality essential oil to get the desired scent and benefits?

Having an organic experience: Organically grown oils

Only a small selection of organically grown essential oils are available. These come from plants that aren't grown with chemical pesticides (or chemical fertilizers). Because these oils are quite a bit more expensive, here's the scoop on organically grown essential oils so that you can decide for yourself if they're worth it.

- **Certification varies.** Certifying organically grown oils varies from state to state in the United States. Essential oils are produced all over the world, but many countries don't have such a designation, or they have it but can't regulate it. The result is that the term *organically grown* has many different meanings depending upon where the plant is grown.

- **Designation isn't regulated.** Calling an essential oil certified organically grown isn't very well regulated. No committee reviews the catalogs to check that the oils they claim are certified are indeed produced from organically grown plants.

- **Some plants are wild anyway.** Quite a few plants that produce essential oils are collected from the wild, so they don't require any pesticides. Pesticides certainly aren't sprayed on the eucalyptus trees that yield eucalyptus essential oil or on the cedar trees that produce cedarwood oil. (Actually, the majority of essential oils are pesticides themselves and work better than chemical ones — in particular, see Chapters 1 and 6.)

- **Pesticides don't easily distill.** Essential oil chemists agree that pesticides contain mostly big molecules that are simply too heavy to be distilled, which is the method used to produce most aromatherapy essential oils. (See Chapter 1 for a description of this process.) Instead, any pesticides stay behind in the plant material (unless the oil is distilled with poor equipment that produces too much steam, which allows larger compounds into the oil). Citrus essential oils, such as orange and lemon, are more of a concern. The oil is pressed from the rinds of these fruit in a different type of extraction (again, refer to Chapter 1) that can pass large pesticide molecules into the essential oil. Except for pressed oil, most of the chemists I talk to think that buying organically grown essential oils is not a big concern. They're far more worried about essential oils being adulterated after they are produced.

- **Quality of organically grown plants varies.** Finally, an organically grown oil isn't necessarily a better smelling essential oil. It depends on the same things that determines the quality of any essential oil: The climate, how well it's harvested and stored, how the essential oil is extracted, and how well the final oil is stored. (See Chapter 3 for more on this.) I've heard some interesting theories expressed that a plant grown without pesticides produces more essential oils because it has to defend itself against predators.

- **Support organic growers.** So far, this list sounds like it leans more toward the cons than the pros of using organically grown essential oils, but I admit that I'm an avid organic grower myself. I think that it's great to support organically grown essential oils if you can afford it just on the principle alone. Also, many organically grown plants are tended by people who are on a mission to see that their plants are of exceptionally high quality, as well as the essential oil they produce.

Chapter 3

On the Scented Trail:
Shopping and Storing

*T*here is no doubt about it; fragrance sells. Enticing scents waft from the bakery, thanks to a strategically placed fan that sprays the scent of freshly baked bread toward you as you enter the store. Used car dealers use a "new car" spray to convince you that the dashboard isn't really faded because the car *smells* new. You can't stop thinking about that apartment or house you're thinking of buying because something (maybe the vanilla and cinnamon scents that the realtor dabbed on the light bulbs?) made it seem so homey.

Savvy companies are smelling the sweet scent of success as they pick up the aromatherapy lead with all kinds of merchandise jumping on the scented bandwagon. Multimillion dollar cosmetic companies promise to change your mood if you simply wash your hair with their aromatherapy shampoos or dab on an aromatic shower gel. The "squeaky clean" scent of lemon or pine is a must in your laundry detergent and dish soap. Camping supply catalogs even offer candles so that aromatherapy can accompany you out into the wild and deter insects at the same time.

Marketing surveys do show that you, if you're like most consumers, prefer buying a pleasantly scented product over an unscented one. Dr. Alan R. Hirsch, Director of the Smell and Taste Treatment and Research Foundation in Chicago, tested this idea out on consumers. He found them willing to spend more when advertising is presented to them in a scented room — at least that's what happened in his study on Nike running shoes. When Hirsch circulated a pleasant scent through the air-conditioning system of a Las Vegas casino, a similar reaction occurred. Slot machines sales soared an impressive 40 percent. Well-known U.S. department stores, impressed by these studies, now use fragrance to its fullest as they pump scents through their heating and air-conditioning systems in an attempt to encourage their customers to buy more.

 Aromatherapy is big right now. With its popularity, the availability of essential oils and aromatherapy products has greatly expanded. The word catches my eye almost everywhere I go. Aromatherapy is sold in natural-food stores, herb stores, specialty mail-order and Internet catalogs, and, of course, aromatherapy and skin care outlets. Every mainstream department, houseware, drug, and large discount store features it. (See the Appendix for suggestions for sources.)

Aromatherapy's new popularity and availability is fantastic. The only problem is, with so many products, how do you decide which one to choose? You may *need* to use an aromatherapy antistress formula just to get through all the decisions you encounter when you go shopping. In this chapter, however, I tell you all you need to know to make it through the aromatherapy shopping maze.

Figuring Out Who to Believe

The first thing to do when you start your shopping quest is to seek out an aromatherapy company you can rely on. Like anything, the quality of aromatherapy products and essential oils varies greatly from one product line to the next. Companies are inclined to use the same grade of essential oils for their entire line. For some businesses, this means using only top-of-the-line essential oils, while another company is satisfied with pretty-good quality. Then you always have those companies who stick to the cheapest, let's-make-a-buck ingredients. Still other companies throw all discrimination aside and use synthetic essential oils, but still brand them as aromatherapy.

 One place *not* to turn for advice on quality are the aromatherapy companies themselves. Expect to find, as with other types of products, a lot of marketing hype as one company declares its products better than its competitor. Sure, some companies care about honesty and the medicinal and cosmetic uses of their products, but to play it safe, regard any advertising and merchandising bravado cautiously. Read the advertising material with a discriminating eye and don't let those fancy ads and elaborate packages sway you. Watch out for declarations that "this" product line is superior to all others. I know through connections in the industry that some companies claim superiority even though they get many of their essential oils from the same place as their competitor.

Also, be wary of claims that an entire line of essential oils or that all the essential oils that are used in a line of aromatherapy products originates exclusively from the company's own farm. A tremendous amount of plant material is needed to produce essential oils; it takes literally acres to grow enough plants for just one type of oil. The only way a company can carry a broad selection of home-grown essential oils is to maintain dozens of farms worldwide, along with a few forests. Sandalwood trees are grown commercially only in tropical Indonesia and on government-regulated land in India. Clove trees and ylang ylang vines are grown in Madagascar, and cinnamon comes from trees grown in Ceylon or Java. Tea tree grows in Florida, but it is only harvested commercially in Australia.

It never hurts to discuss quality with store clerks, but weigh everything they tell you against what you already know. On your next aromatherapy shopping spree, educate yourself first and then come to the store armed with information and ask questions. That way, you'll be able to tell from the clerk's responses whether he or she knows much about aromatherapy. Many people learn everything they know from product advertising or a company's education seminars.

The very best way to determine quality in aroamatherapy products and essential oils is to learn to spot differences in oils yourself. So educate your nose. It's not too hard to tell the difference between grades of essential oils if you use the guidelines I provide in Chapter 2.

Sniffing Out the Best Deals

Price can be a helpful guideline when you're on the lookout for quality, although don't totally rely on cost alone. Some good deals are available on quality oils that are sold without fancy packaging and advertising. The high expense of an aromatherapy product or of an essential oil may reflect the best quality, or it may be a just-so-so oil sold by a company that is out to make a big profit and hoping you won't be a consumer who "nose" the difference.

Mail-order catalogs tend to offer good prices because they have less overhead than a store. However, ordering through the mail can be a little more tricky because you don't get a chance to smell the product until the first time that you buy it. If it isn't right, then you have the hassle of returning it, if this is even accepted. You'll also need to know what you need ahead of time. With mail-order companies, it makes even more sense to trust your source.

Essential oils are priced according to how much work it takes from plant to the vial of oil you hold in your hand. How difficult they are to cultivate, harvest, and extract, and their availability are all reflected in the final price. A single ounce of oil requires about 600 pounds of rose petals, making pure rose oil a pricey commodity at about $300 an ounce! Contrast this with the easily obtainable essential oils, such as eucalyptus at a meager $4 an ounce. The difference is that rose is labor intensive to cultivate and harvest. After all that, it only yields a precariously small amount of essential oil. Eucalyptus, on the other hand, is a big tree that yields a lot of oil. Sandalwood is also a tree, but a small one that demands elaborate processing to obtain its essential oil. Because sandalwood is only grown for its oil in a few places in the world, its already high price went up even higher after a fire occurred in India's main sandalwood land tracts?.

After making such a big deal about the importance of using quality essential oils, I should mention that there are times when you probably don't need to use the top-of-the-line essential oil or aromatherapy products. If an oil is pure and natural, sometimes that is good enough — it depends on the purpose. Room fresheners and candles don't necessarily require the same high quality oil as you use in your facial cream. If you make your own candles, you'll find that they require so much essential oil, the price can get out of hand if you stick to only the best oils.

Of course, it is possible that using cheaper essential oils can actually end up costing you more. One of my friends manufactures a delightful facial cream that smells just like fresh lemons. Once she had to resort to using a completely natural but low-grade lemon oil. She couldn't get enough scent with her regular recipe, so she started adding more lemon oil. It took four times what her recipe called for, and more than twice the usual cost, to achieve the right scent.

Buying Essential Oils

Your shopping days will be so much easier if you follow these simple tips:

- ✔ **Buy essential oils from companies who have an established reputation for quality.** (See the Appendix for a list.)

- ✔ **Ask the company about essential oils.** Are they pure? Where do they originate? Can the company supply you with the botanical names and assure that their essential oils came from those plants? Remember that you can't always trust what a company tells you, but it never hurts to ask. Be especially suspicious if they can't give you straight answers.

- ✔ **Check for authenticity.** Make sure that the line of essential oils doesn't include any blatantly synthetic essential oils such as carnation, lilac, strawberry, rain, or cucumber. If so, all their oils may be synthetics. (For more on synthetics, see Chapter 2.)

✔ **Check for purity.** Put 1 drop of the essential oil on a piece of paper. It should quickly evaporate, leaving no oily mark, which is indicative of being cut with vegetable oil. Sniff for any alcohol overtones that indicate the oil is diluted with alcohol.

✔ **Check for quality**. Sniff out scents that are fuller, rounder, and more complex. A little should go a long way. (For more on what to look for in a scent, see Chapter 2.)

✔ **Don't buy too much the first time you deal with a company.** Initially purchase a small amount (a quarter ounce, dram, or even less) of essential oil that you are familiar with from a new company as an example of their quality.

To a Long Life!: Storing Aromatherapy

Once you've selected your high quality aromatherapy products and essential oils, you'll want to keep them that way. Because the basis of any aromatherapy product is the essential oils it contains, I focus on the oils. Also consider the quality of the product's other ingredients. You can do this in part by reading the ingredients on the label (see Chapter 7).

Do oils spoil?

Essential oils don't exactly spoil. For example, you don't have to worry about them going rancid like vegetable cooking oil. They are themselves natural preservatives, so they keep for a long time in their pure, undiluted state. They also help the other ingredients in aromatherapy products to last longer. The problem is that an essential oil's scent eventually fades. This is true for both pure essential oils and the aromatherapy products that contain them. How long that takes depends on how well you store them. Done properly, most essential oils last several years.

What you want to avoid in your essential oils and the products that contain them is *oxidation*. This change occurs when oxygen combines with the aromatic compounds in an essential oil, changing them chemically. The result is that the compounds break down and the scent that they carry diminishes. Along with this destruction, the essential oil's therapeutic properties also decrease.

Preserving fragile fragrances

Considering that the air is filled with oxygen, the most obvious route to preserving essential oils and aromatherapy products is to expose them to as little air as possible. That means keeping them in containers with tightly sealed lids. Sunlight and heat are the culprits that encourage oxidation. The trick is to store your essential oils in glass bottles in a dark, cool place. Store them in either dark glass or keep clear bottles in the cupboard. Most essential oils are sold in amber or blue glass. With products that contain essential oils, the type of container isn't quite so critical because the essential oils are diluted, but glass is still much preferred over plastic to retain the scent and also the quality of all the ingredients.

If you're looking at long-term storage, you can be fanatic by making sure that there is as little air in the container as possible. Rebottle your oils and products into smaller containers instead of keeping a little bit in the bottom of a jar or bottle. While you're at it, also make sure that whatever container you use to rebottle is sparkling clean — run it through the dishwasher or boil it — to make sure that you don't introduce any bacteria. And be sure the container is thoroughly dry inside.

Storing pure essential oils in plastic can result in a real disaster. The problem with it is that essential oils are so powerful that they eventually dissolve plastic. This means double trouble. For one thing, molecules from the dissolving plastic contaminate the essential oil, so you end up with a lot more than you bargained for in your oil. And then, it is possible that a plastic container of essential oil will completely dissolve. I've heard some funny and then some not-so-funny stories about this happening.

Essential oils also break down the rubberlike droppers used in medicine bottles and some types of rubber inserts that fit in the lids of bottles with glass rods or other types of applicators. As tempting as it is to keep your essential oils in a dropper bottle for handy dispensing, it takes a type that is specially designed for use with essential oils to resist essential oil meltdown. Anything that isn't glass can slowly dissolve into a gooey mess. (Don't ask how I discovered this important fact!)

Keeping aromatherapy products in plastic is not so much of a problem. Of course, because they contain essential oils, they are best kept in glass containers. However, essential oils aren't so much of a problem when they're diluted in a lotion, hair rinse, or some other body-care product. You'll probably find it much more convenient to travel with your aromatherapy lotion in a plastic bottle, to keep your aromatherapy hair rinse in an unbreakable container, or to use a plastic squeeze bottle while giving a massage. If so, by all means go ahead and use plastic containers. Besides, a lot of products come only in plastic, and you won't want to run home and change the container of every aromatherapy product that you buy.

The most vulnerable essential oils are the citruses. After about a year, the strength of their scent begins to decline and becomes more noticeable after two years. One way to store citrus scents longer is to keep them refrigerated, or at least store them in a cool place. These are examples of the citrus oils:

- ✔ Grapefruit
- ✔ Lemon
- ✔ Mandarin
- ✔ Orange
- ✔ Tangerine

The party's over: Dumping old scents

It is always a tough decision when the time comes to toss out old essential oils. There is no cut-off date when an oil's effectiveness expires. Any essential oil that you've had for several years or that hasn't been stored properly has probably lost at least some of its smell and its therapeutic properties. Fortunately, you can tell by the smell, so use the sniff-and-tell rule as a guideline. If the smell has declined, so have the essential oil's properties. This might be a good time to use them to clean your floors and countertops. (See Chapter 6 for recipes to make household cleaners.)

Aging gracefully: Fixatives

After all the fuss about oxidation, some essential oils do something everyone dreams of: They improve with age. Even better, the older some essential oils are, the more valuable they become. Their scent is actually enhanced when they oxidize due to air exposure.

If you've made potpourri, you're already familiar with the following oils because when added to potpourri, they keep, or *fix,* the scent longer. Potpourri makers refer to this special class of long-lasting essential oils as *fixatives*. The fixative essential oils also enhance potpourri's fragrance. All of them also become darker, richer, and even change their consistency, becoming more syrupy as they age. My bottle of 30-year-old patchouli barely resembles the pale scent and color of freshly extracted patchouli oil. This oil is purposely aged before it is ready for sale.

- ✔ Benzoin
- ✔ Clary sage
- ✔ Myrrh

> ✔ Patchouli
> ✔ Sandalwood
> ✔ Vetivert

Playing It Safe: Going Nontoxic

Essential oils are very concentrated. This makes them potent medicine, but also means that they need to be used responsibly. The potential hazards of essential oils are determined by the compounds found in an oil, the dosage and frequency used, and the method of application. I can't emphasize safety enough times. Remain aware of how potent essential oils are so that you can use them in an educated and responsible manner. Here are some guidelines to ensure the safe and effective use of essential oils.

✔ Use only pure quality essential oils made from plants, never synthetics, and check the botanical name to be sure that you have what you want.

✔ Always use essential oils diluted (in oil, a bath, diffused through the air, and so on). Don't use them undiluted on your skin.

✔ Keep essential oils away from your eyes and ears.

✔ Don't take essential oils internally unless you really know what you're doing, except for small amounts used to flavor foods, such as peppermint oil in candy.

✔ Use essential oils cautiously, or not at all, if elderly, convalescing, or if you have a serious health problem such as epilepsy or liver or kidney damage.

✔ Don't use photosensitizing essential oils, such as the citrus oils, especially bergamot, before spending time in the sun or in a tanning booth.

✔ Use only the very safest and gentlest oils for pregnant women and children.

✔ Do a patch test (see the next section) the next section if you suspect that you are sensitive to an essential oil.

✔ Keep essential oils out of the reach of children.

Essential oils and the aromatherapy products that contain them offer wonderful therapeutic results. If you are ill, have a worn-out immune system, are pregnant, or are very elderly, stick to aromatherapy products that contain the safest and most gentle essential oils. This is also true of children, especially young kids and babies.

"Scentsitivities"

Most people who are sensitive to synthetic fragrances face no problems using high quality essential oils made from natural sources.

If you have a tendency to be overly sensitive to anything or if you have allergies, try a patch test first. To do so, rub a little in the crook of your arm or on the back of your neck at the hairline. (If you're testing an aromatherapy product, then use a little dab of it straight. If you're testing a straight essential oil, then dilute 1 drop of a suspect essential oil in ¼ teaspoon vegetable oil and apply this.) If your skin slightly reddens, you're having a mild reaction, and you may be able to use the oil or product if it's diluted more or in small amounts. (Because a product contains many ingredients, there's no way to know if you're reacting to the essential oils or another ingredient.) If the spot where you dabbed on the oil burns, itches, or turns your skin seriously red, this essential oil or product is not for you. (Wash off the oil immediately with warm, soapy water if you have a reaction.) Seek an alternative oil and then do another patch test before using it.

Sun-Shy Oils

A few essential oils cause a skin reaction in sensitive people when they go out in the sun after using the oil. This reaction is most often an uneven pigmentation that may look like a rash. Called *photosensitization,* it occurs on the same place where the oil or a product containing it was applied. Use anything that contains the photosensitizing essential oils with caution and never use them in a suntan lotion. Bergamot is the most notorious of the photosensitizing oils due to a compound called bergaptene. However, it is available as a bergaptenefree oil. Products that use this special type indicate it on the label. Here is a list of the photosensitizing oils roughly in order of their strength, beginning with the strongest one.

- ✔ Angelica root
- ✔ Bergamot
- ✔ Cumin
- ✔ Grapefruit
- ✔ Lemon (unless distilled instead of pressed)
- ✔ Lime (unless distilled instead of pressed)
- ✔ Bitter orange (not sweet orange)
- ✔ Lemon verbena

Essential oils for mother and child

Aromatherapy can greatly enhance pregnancy, just go easy. Be very cautious about using essential oils during pregnancy, especially during the first trimester when so much early development is happening. Even the most gentle essential oils may be too stimulating for some women who are prone to miscarriage. Instead, drink the safe and gentle herb teas and use aromatherapy just for sniffing to keep your emotions balanced.

Choose already-made products that are especially designed for pregnancy or babies. If you're making your own aromatherapy products for pregnant women and young children, then use about half the usual amount of essential oils. For babies, use one-quarter the adult dose; they do best with aromatherapy products that contain the gentlest essential oils, such as lavender and chamomile.

The essential oils that most children say are their favorites are the citruses, such as lemon, tangerine, mandarin, grapefruit, and orange. These oils are fine for kids, but be sure that they are properly diluted because the citrus essential oils that are too concentrated can burn delicate skin. It's usually a good idea to not use citruses on babies. These are essential oils that are okay to use on young children.

- ✔ Chamomile
- ✔ Citruses
- ✔ Frankincense
- ✔ Geranium
- ✔ Jasmine
- ✔ Lavender (but not *stoechas* lavander)
- ✔ Neroli
- ✔ Rose
- ✔ Sandalwood
- ✔ Spearmint
- ✔ Ylang ylang

Don't mess with me: Avoiding toxic oils

Natural doesn't always mean safe. Some essential oils are simply too toxic to use. Other oils should be used with care: in small amounts and always diluted properly. Don't confuse the limited use of these essential oils with the herbs that they come from. Certainly cinnamon buns and oregano on your pizza present no problem. The problem with using essential oils is that they're so concentrated. A few drops easily equals several cups of the herb tea. I divide the essential oils that you need to use with care into three sections. If I don't include the essential oils in the Aroma Guide or elsewhere in this book, I list their botanical names in these sections to help you with proper identification.

Okay, but go easy: Be wary of these oils

These essential oils are fine to use, but they can all cause skin irritations, and even burn your skin if used improperly, so use them carefully.

- Allspice *(Pimenta dioica)*
- Camphor, white *(Cinnamomum camphora)*
- Cinnamon
- Clove (especially clove leaf)
- Oregano *(Oregano vulgare)*
- Savory
- Thuja *(Thuja occidentalis)*
- Thyme (except the gentle linalol type)
- Turmeric *(Curcuma longa)*
- Wintergreen/birch

A note on wintergreen and birch. Birch essential oil from the North American tree is typically sold as "wintergreen" because the two oils are so similar chemically. Both are potentially toxic, so they need to be used in very small amounts. On the other hand, North European birch has nearly the same properties with less toxicity (because it contains less of the toxic chemicals).

Forget it: Downright scary oils

Here's a list of essential oils that are so strong, your best bet is not to use them at all.

- Arnica *(Arnica montana)*
- Bitter almond *(Prunus amygdalus var. amara)*
- Calamus *(Acorus calamus)*
- French tarragon *(Artemisia dracunculus)*
- Hyssop *(Hyssopus officinalis),* except the gentle variety decumbens
- Mugwort *(Artemesia vulgaris)*
- Mustard *(Brassica nigra)*
- Pennyroyal *(Mentha pulegium)*
- Sassafras *(Sassafras albidum)*

Don't even think about it: Way too strong oils

The following potentially toxic oils are *really* strong. Avoid using them at all and certainly stay away from any aromatherapy products that contain them. So many useful essential oils are available that you have plenty of alternatives. Some oils in this list have limited use externally, and some are used for treating emotional problems or for perfumery.

- ✔ Horseradish *(Armoracia rusticana)*
- ✔ Jaborandi *(Pilocarpus jaborand)*
- ✔ Narcissus *(Narcissus poeticus)*
- ✔ Parsley *(Petroselinum sativum)*
- ✔ Rue *(Ruta graveolens)*
- ✔ Santolina *(Santolina chamaecyparissus)*
- ✔ Tansy *(Tanacetum vulgare)*
- ✔ Tonka *(Dipteryx odorata)*
- ✔ Wormwood *(Artemisia absinthium)*

It Goes More Than Skin Deep: Preventing Toxicity

The big concern about using potentially toxic essential oils such as the ones I list in the preceding section is that their use can be injurious to you. Any essential oil that is used improperly can cause problems. The idea in aromatherapy is to heal, not harm. Here are some things to watch out for.

- ✔ **Your kidneys:** It's obvious when you burn your skin using essential oils that you're experiencing a toxic reaction. What's not so obvious is what essential oils do once they're in your body. Both your liver and kidneys must deal with essential oils once they hit your bloodstream, and they can be overly taxed if you use too much essential oil. Essential oils are rather quickly cleared out of your body, generally in a few hours, and that job can only fall to your kidneys, which are susceptible to being damaged from excessive use of essential oils.

- ✔ **Your liver:** It's up to your liver to break down the essential oils that enter your body either when you inhale them or when you rub them on your skin, or you ingest them in foods and tea. Large amounts of essential oils can slow down the liver's ability to do its many important jobs. It's hard to imagine that you could absorb enough essential oil to damage your liver using any of the suggestions in this book, but it's still good to know the dangers that can occur when using too much oil.

Take pennyroyal and probably French tarragon as examples. During the liver's transformation of the oil, compounds in these oils bind to its cells to destroy them. (Pennyroyal's ancient reputation to induce miscarriage is overrated considering that even large amounts of the essential oil tend to poison a woman, but not even then cause miscarriage.) That's why these two oils are in the section "Forget it: Downright scary oils," earlier in this chapter.

✔ **Your head:** Lots of people develop a slight headache or feel a little dizzy when working with essential oils. Sometimes it even happens to some students during one of my all-day aromatherapy seminars. I consider this sensory overload your body's little warning that enough is enough. My recommendation is to go somewhere to breathe fresh air and stop sniffing the oils until your headache or dizziness is long gone. If your dizziness or headache persists long after excessive essential oil exposure, then the problem may involve your kidneys.

✔ **Your skin:** I know that it's common sense, but I'll go ahead and say that applying such a high concentration of essential oil on your skin so that it causes it to burn it is a big no-no. The answer is to follow the recommended dilutions in this book and, if you've got very sensitive skin, use half the recommended amount.

Potential drug interactions with essential oils

Very few studies are available on the interactions of essential oils with drugs. The ones that do exist use much larger amounts than the therapeutic doses you use for essential oils, so it's less likely that you'll experience the same interactions. So far, I've not heard of any problems with aromatherapy/drug reactions — although interactions do occasionally occur with herbs. (When they do, European physicians use it to their patient's advantage by reducing the medication, but that's nothing you should try to do on your own, considering the serious consequences if you misjudge the dosage.) Your best bet is to play is safe by following these general rules.

- If you take sleeping pills, watch out for relaxing aromatherapy products increasing their tranquilizing effect.

- Notice whether aromatherapy increases the action of a stimulating drug or cuts back those of a sedative drug.

I compiled information from the studies that do exist on the effect of combining essential oils and drugs. What happens in these studies is not necessarily what goes on in the real world, so how much of a problem exists with using these combination isn't known. However, it's always best to be on the safe side, so avoid using the following combinations unless you're being supervised by a health care professional.

- **Pentobarbital:** Melissa (lemon balm) and valerian oils can increase the effects, including your sleeping time, of sedative barbituate drugs. Inhaling cedarwood oil's aroma is stimulating and possibly counteracts the sedative effects of these drugs.

- **Acetaminophen:** Clove bud and leaf, bay rum, and cinnamon bark may counter some effects of these sedative drugs.

- **Quinidine:** Peppermint oil may interfere with this drug's actions to stabilize heart beat.

- **Warfarin, aspirin, heparin, and possibly other anticoagulant drugs:** Birch, wintergreen, clove, and garlic can thin the blood too much when used along with these drugs.

Essential oils to avoid if you have the following conditions:

- **Epilepsy, seizures:** Rosemary, lavandin, sage, "spike" lavender, thuja, and hyssop

- **Estrogen-related disorders** (breast and cervical cancer, endometriosis, and enlarged prostate): Anise, basil, clary sage, fennel, and myrtle as a precaution since their hormonal action on the body isn't known.

- **Glaucoma:** Melissa (lemon balm) and lemongrass (may increase pressure in eyes as it does in monkeys)

- **Heart fibrillation:** Peppermint

- **Kidney disease:** Anticoagulants such as birch and wintergreen, clove, garlic, and limited use of all essential oils

- **Liver disease, alcoholism:** Anise, basil, cinnamon, clove bud and leaf, and fennel (may be too strong for a weak liver to process)

- **Skin irritation or delicate skin:** Anise, citronella, clove bud and leaf, lemon eucalyptus, bay, lemongrass, lemon balm (melissa), oregano, and thyme (all potential skin irritants)

Chapter 4

Surrounding Yourself with Scents

. . . .

In This Chapter

▶ Exploring fragrances for work and play

▶ Blending scents

▶ Scenting a room

▶ Creating fragrant potpourri

▶ Making aromatherapy candles

▶ Scenting your light bulbs

▶ Using an aroma diffuser

▶ Spraying the air

▶ Burning incense

Recipes in This Chapter

▶ Aromatic Spray
▶ Disinfectant Room Spray

. . . .

Fragrance makes any environment more enjoyable and inviting, and it creates a comfortable place to work and play. So why not bring aromatherapy into every room of your house and into your workplace? You have probably heard of mood lighting that dims lights for relaxation or mimics sunlight to keep you alert and happy. How about trying mood scents that enhance the "feeling" of your personal space?

Creating mood fragrances is easy. In this chapter, I show you how to select the best scent. Then I explain quick ways — all simple and practical — to fill a room with the fragrance you choose. To help with your decision, refer to the list of possible fragrances in the Aroma Guide and Table 4-2 on the pros and cons of aromatherapy techniques that appears later in this chapter.

Choosing Your Environment's Scents

To fill your environment with fragrance, you first need to choose your scent. Choosing your scent is easier than it sounds. There are very few rules. Although you can find many suitable fragrances to scent your abode, you can follow your nose and go with what you like best. What particular scent you choose may not matter, as long as the room smells good to you. When aroma researchers in the United States and Japan put people in scented rooms and observed their behavior, a variety of different fragrances were tried. All the scents that the room's occupants found pleasing put them in a feel-good mood. Simply put, smells that you enjoy make you feel great.

Good scents also tend to make people feel more sociable and inclined to get along better. It's all in your head, say the researchers. That's because aromatherapy influences the way you think. Fragrance makes you more positive about yourself and your environment. A room containing a light, pleasing scent even makes people more friendly and improves their dispositions. Aromas can inspire confidence and self-motivation and improve thinking. And imagine, all of this is just a sniff away! (If this all seems too good to be true, refer to Chapter 2 to find out what science says about the way aromas affect the mind.) So, your first assignment is to sniff a selection of aromas and discover your favorites.

Specifically, what you're sniffing are essential oils — the components in plants that make them fragrant. Most of the aromatherapy techniques in this chapter use the essential oils already extracted from the plant because they provide ready-to-go fragrance. (You can find an explanation of how essential oils are extracted in Chapter 1.)

Essential oils are very concentrated, so they come in small vials. The best quality are sold in natural-food stores, herb and aromatherapy shops, and by mail-order. (To find out where to purchase essential oils, look in the Appendix.) Even if you end up buying your essential oils through the mail, you may want to sniff your way through a store's display to discover which ones you like the best.

You may be thinking that making your living space smell good sounds very pleasant, but what you really want is to create a special mood: You want to put the "therapy" of aromatherapy to work.

Go natural

You may already be scenting home and work with fragrance, but why not be sure that the scents you choose have healing properties? With any aromatherapy product, you get better therapeutic results — say to cheer you up or make you feel more energized — if you use true essential oils. With pure essential oils your home smells great, *and* everyone who enters it benefits.

Many of the overly sweet floral, fruity, and berry fragrances used in commercial products like scented candles and potpourri are synthetic essential oils produced by a chemist in a laboratory rather than coming from plants. They may have natural-sounding names, but that is where any resemblance to nature ends. Having trouble telling the difference between natural and synthetic oils? Turn to Chapter 2.

Some scents make you feel alert, while others are relaxing. Other aromas can ease depression or create a romantic atmosphere. An aromatic room helps you overcome low energy or poor self-esteem. To see how well these aromas work, use the information in Table 4-1 to choose scents known to have an effect on the emotions. These 14 popular room fragrances will get you started. Simply choose what you want to do with your environment. Say that someone in your household has been feeling down in the dumps. Then use one or more of the scents suggested for depression and give everyone an emotional lift. If you're having a party or you need to get an important project done that day, how about choosing something to pick up everyone's energy? When you get a bout of insomnia, then fill your bedroom with at least one of the aromas suggested for that problem. Maybe you have romance in mind instead. In that case, choose your fragrance! If you just can't decide, it's okay to mix and match different scents into an aromatic blend for your environment that will do everything you need.

If this is your first plunge into aromatherapy, approach the therapy part as simply as possible. Decide what emotional quality you want and the scent in that category that you like the best (or that you happen to already have on hand).

Table 4-1	Emotional Condition that You Want to Treat				
Scent	*Stress/ Depression*	*Imbalance*	*Energy*	*Romance*	*Insomnia*
Bergamot	X	X			
Chamomile	X				X
Cinnamon			X	X	
Eucalyptus			X		
Fir		X	X		
Jasmine			X	X	
Lavender	X	X			X
Lemon	X				X
Orange	X				X
Peppermint			X		

(continued)

Table 4-1 (continued)

Scent	Stress/ Depression	Imbalance	Energy	Romance	Insomnia
Rose	X	X		X	X
Rose Geranium	X	X			X
Spearmint			X		
Ylang Ylang				X	X

You may be asking yourself, "What are the best essential oils to buy so I can get started trying some of the recipes in this book?" The 14 great scents listed in Table 4-1 make a good starter kit. These essential oils are used over and over in this book. You can find out even more about each of the selected oils by turning to the Aroma Guide. When you're ready to move beyond these starter scents, then you can look through the other 33 scents that the Aroma Guide covers to select something new and different.

Scenting Your Home Sweet Home

After you have an idea of the aromas you can use to fill your rooms with good smells, the next step is to decide the best way to get it there. In this section, I give you the eight easiest and most popular methods.

- ✔ Dried potpourri in a container
- ✔ Potpourri cooker
- ✔ Scented candle
- ✔ Incense
- ✔ Light bulb ring
- ✔ Aromatherapy diffuser
- ✔ Steam
- ✔ Fan
- ✔ Spray

Potpourri

Potpourri is a an attractive mix of different dried herbs, flowers, and foliage that is heavily scented. Placed in a glass container, a basket, or in a bowl and set in a room, potpourri offers twofold charm as both an eye-catching and pleasingly fragrant center of attention. In an open container, potpourri scents the air around it. In a closed container, it invites the visitor to open it and experience a sudden burst of fragrance.

Place potpourri where people can notice it: By an entrance, close to the couch, or next to a bathroom sink. Wherever you decide to put it, potpourri adds a special charm to your home.

Potpourri is very popular these days. You can easily buy it in almost any store. Drugstores, household stores, gift shops, and even camping and hardware stores now usually carry something filled with potpourri.

Making your own potpourri

Potpourri is so easy to buy, you may not want to bother making your own. However, if you feel like being creative, you can make your own potpourri. And, it's as easy to make as one, two, three. Plus, you can

- ✔ Bring the colors and fragrances of the garden indoors — if you have your own garden or have access to colorful fresh or dried plant materials.
- ✔ Produce the best potpourri possible made from quality plants and essential oils.
- ✔ Choose whatever scents, colors, and textures you want to use.
- ✔ Match the scent to the mood you want.
- ✔ Coordinate the colors with your room.
- ✔ Create an inexpensive, handmade gift. (Potpourri makes a thoughtful gift for a bedridden individual when scented with a pick-me-up essential oil.)
- ✔ Keep enjoying cut flowers from a special occasion, such as a wedding, birthday, or an anniversary.
- ✔ Be creative and have fun.

Flowers and greenery dry best at room temperature or warmer. Be sure to keep them out of direct sunlight while they dry because the sun will blacken the various colors and destroy the scent. When the plant material feels very dry — brittle enough so that the pieces snap in your hands — toss them into an attractive container as potpourri or add them to a potpourri you already have.

All in a name

Potpourri is a French word pronounced "pô pour re." It means a collection of anything thrown together. This can be a vegetable stew, a musical medley, or a collection of disconnected literary pieces. The most common modern meaning is this usage: A mixture of dried flowers and spices.

To preserve cut flowers from your garden or a special occasion, cut them just before the fresh flowers and greens begin to wilt or lose their colors. Spread the plants thinly on a piece of newspaper, cookie sheet, or cutting board to dry them. Or, tie them at their base with either string or a rubber band around the stems and hang them upside down decoratively in your kitchen or pantry. Either method provides enough air circulation to allow the plants to dry. You will be amazed at the beauty that cut flowers give to a potpourri. I have many jars filled with memories, as well as potpourri.

When you're ready to make potpourri, go to the bulk herb section of your local natural-food store, choose several different dried herbs, and follow these steps:

1. **Mix several types of dried plant material together in a bowl.**

   You simply want the ingredients to look good together. Don't worry about the smell yet; that comes later. Look for interesting colors and textures. One way to do this is to mix dark colors with light colors to create visual contrasts. For example, yellow and white chamomile flowers contrast with dark green rosemary leaves or brown cinnamon sticks. You can even select colors that match your home's decor.

2. **Drop by drop, add ⅛ teaspoon essential oil for every cup of the herb blend.**

   Select one or more essential oils. (The amount called for in this step is for all the essential oils combined, not for each oil you add.) For help in your selection, refer to Table 4-1 earlier in this chapter, or for more lengthy descriptions of scents, check out the Aroma Guide.

3. **Place your newly made potpourri in a sealed plastic bag or in a jar with a tight lid for at least five days.**

   This gives the essential oils a chance to penetrate all the herbs and the various fragrances time to blend together, so that the scent "matures."

4. **After five days, put your potpourri in an attractive container — say a basket, fancy glass jar, or handmade bowl — and display.**

   You'll want to try all sorts of gorgeous containers to show off your potpourri.

Keep in mind the following tips about potpourri:

- ✔ **Once made, the scent of potpourri lasts for months in a closed container and for several weeks in an open container.** When the scent eventually does grow faint, revive it by placing a few drops of essential oil directly on the dried plants.

- ✔ **To make your potpourri's scent last longer, add ½ teaspoon of dried, finely chopped orris root to every cup of dried plants.** This fragrant root comes from the root (technically a *rhizome*) of a white-flowered iris. Called a *fixative,* the orris root's special chemistry makes it hold the scent of the essential oils longer. The root is readily available in herb and craft stores for use in potpourri. A few people are allergic to orris root, so craft stores also sell a manufactured alternative fixative made from cellulose, which absorbs and retains the smell of essential oils.

- ✔ **If you decided to send your potpourri off to a distant place as a gift and don't have time to let it sit for five days for the aromas to mature, go ahead and send it.** By the time it arrives at its destination, your potpourri will be done.

- ✔ **Potpourri is a great project to do with kids.** Give each one a plastic, sealable baggy and have them partially fill it with a selection of dried plant material, perhaps some things that they collected themselves. They love selecting the ingredients, and then you can add the essential oil of their choice. Make potpourri as a school or special club project, or with your children at home. (For more ideas on projects to do with kids, see Chapter 13.)

Using a potpourri cooker

Simmering potpourri cookers have been popular gift items for several years. The cooker typically stands less than a foot high and has a small bowl or basin over a candle or electric heat source. Water and potpourri are placed in the bowl. When the candle is lit or the electricity turned on, it heats the water and releases the fragrant essential oils in the potpourri. The scent goes out into the room for about an hour. After that, it should linger for at least another couple hours.

Most potpourri cookers are ceramic, but there are also metal and even glass versions. They come in variety of styles, usually selling for less than $10 in the U.S. unless they're handcrafted by a potter or metalsmith.

In a potpourri cooker, potpourri acts mostly as a carrier for the essential oils that scent it. In fact, it is often the essential oils that produce all the scent. If you want, you can skip the potpourri all together. Instead, put a small amount of water in the cooker's basin and add 8 drops of pure essential oil. The oil is your choice — use either a single oil or a blend.

If you use a blend of several oils in a cooker, use 8 drops *total,* not 8 drops of each one. You don't want to overdo the amount of essential oil in a potpourri cooker, or you risk creating such a strong fragrance that you may end up chasing visitors away instead of drawing them in!

Scenting candles

The popularity of scented candles is rapidly increasing. In fact, scented candles have become so popular, you find them not only in gift shops, but sold in mail-order catalogs and housewares stores. Even backpacking supply outlets sell compact aromatherapy candles to take camping!

Actually, there are scented candles, and then there are aromatherapy candles. The quality of the essential oils used in each type varies greatly, with some containing good quality aromatherapy oils and others using synthetics. If you're unsure how to sniff the difference, then turn to Chapter 2. Once you smell a quality aromatherapy candle, you'll have a difficult time going back to the overly sweet, fruity scents of a lesser quality or a synthetic. (See Appendix A for suggestions on where to buy aromatherapy candles.)

How to use a scented candle is no mystery. Simply light the wick and enjoy the fragrance. Certainly one advantage of using a scented candle is the pleasing atmosphere it creates as it burns.

To transform any candle into a fragrant one, try the following method. It is a great way to give that tired box of unscented candles a makeover. If you have a favorite style of candle, but alas, it comes without a scent, no problem. Scent it yourself.

One drawback to scenting candles yourself is that, unlike candles that are already scented, you need to re-scent them every time you use them. A candle with a scented wick releases its scent for about half an hour, and the scent lingers in the room for another hour or so. On the other hand, an aromatherapy candle that has essential oil already incorporated into the wax puts out continuous aroma.

The other problem with scenting your own candles is that the essential oil initially produces black smoke as it burns for the first minute.

To transform your tapers:

1. **Trim the wick of an unburned candle to ½ inch.**

2. **Place 10 drops of an essential oil (or a blend) around the base of the remaining wick.**

   That way, the liquid wax that puddles around the wick mixes with the oil and delivers it to the wick gradually.

You can choose the oil or oils from Table 4-1. A candle's wick is very absorbent and "pulls" the scent down into the center of the candle.

3. **Wait at least 15 minutes before lighting the candle and enjoy.**

If you want to scent a candle that has already been burned, you need to trim off the burnt wick because this part is no longer able to absorb the essential oil. Then dig down into the wax to expose ½ inch of the unburned, white wick. Scent this wick the same way you do an unburned wick.

When not using any scented candles, keep them sealed in a plastic bag or other airtight container so that they retain their fragrance.

Incense

Incense is made from a blend of essential oils mixed with charcoal and a little *saltpeter* — a combustible compound — so that it ignites and continues to burn. Most incense also contains some adhesive plant material to help it stick together. All this is mixed together and wrapped around a slender stick or formed into a roll, coil, or cone and baked, usually in the sun, to a hard consistency. When lit, the incense releases the scent of the essential oils as it burns.

Incense was one of the earliest forms of aromatherapy. Anthropologists guess that its use goes back long before recorded civilization, when fragrant barks, leaves, and saps of plants were tossed into the fire for purification and to appease the gods and goddesses.

The smoke from burning incense is strongly fragrant and lingers in a room for hours, making it a good method of using aromatherapy. Incense is easy because all you do is light the tip and find somewhere that you do not mind a little ash falling off as the stick burns. However, the down side is that the smoke itself bothers many people.

If you decide to go for incense, you can find a wide range of accents available. Incense is usually sold in stores that sell aromatherapy, herbs, natural foods, or gifts.

If you associate incense with hippies, do not feel that you have to dress in beads and wear long hair to burn it. In fact, the hippies got the idea of burning incense from the Buddhists and Hindus who use it, as do the Catholic and Greek Orthodox churches, to inspire prayer and meditation in their religious ceremonies. Incense is a highly refined art in Japan and part of the celebrated Japanese tea ceremony. Guessing games are traditionally played as part of the ceremony to determine the scent.

Making your own incense

To make your own incense, I suggest that you cheat and buy premade unscented incense sticks. Sometimes you can find incense blanks at natural-food or herb stores or craft stores, but you may have to order them through the mail (see the Appendix). They're called *blanks* because they have no scent and are produced so that you can make your own incense. This technique is much easier than making your incense sticks from scratch. (I have done it, and it means working with messy, powdered charcoal, and you and your work space are not pretty sights afterward!)

Making your own incense is really a fairly simple process:

1. **Place the incense "blank" on a pie pan or cookie sheet.**

2. **Take a glass dropper (like the ones sold at a drugstore) and fill it partly with the essential oil of your choice.**

3. **Apply 3 drops for every inch of the stick.**

   I did the math for you: On an average 8-inch stick of incense, use 32 drops. Apply the oil slowly, giving it time to absorb into the stick.

4. **Let the stick dry for one hour and then put it in a tall glass jar.**

   Don't put homemade incense in a plastic bag because it is too oily and will gum up the plastic.

   Your incense is ready to use the next day.

When you're feeling creative, you can make your own incense — see the sidebar "Making your own it." An advantage to this plan is that you aren't limited to the choices of incense already available. Instead, you can make a wide range of different scented varieties. You can also recycle old incense sticks that have lost most of their original fragrance by re-scenting them.

 Whether you make or buy your incense, be sure that the scent lasts a long time. To assure that it does, keep it in an airtight container. Although incense is usually sold in a plastic or cellophane bag, glass is best.

North American Indians still use an early form of incense once used by many cultures throughout the world and most likely a forerunner to incense: They burn the leaves of fragrant plants. Called a *smudge stick,* small branches of highly aromatic plants such as juniper and sage are tightly wrapped while still fresh into a broad stick around 8 inches long. When dry, the end of these sticks are lit so that they burn to release a profuse amount of fragrance and smoke. (If you use a smudge stick indoors, be sure to have the windows open!) The stick is traditionally used outside or in a hut or sweat lodge devoted to healing to "clear" the air and to dispel negative feelings in those who smell it. The essential oils that are released are also very antiseptic. The entire stick isn't burned, but is generally extinguished in water often after only a few minutes of burning. Smudge sticks are especially popular in the southwestern United States — they're sold in the Phoenix, Arizona, airport! — but are sold across the United States in many gift shops and natural-food stores. A similar item from the Plains Indians is a sweetgrass braid made from a vanilla-scented grass. It's used just like a smudge stick.

Light bulb rings

I borrowed this aromatherapy trick from realtors who know how to make a home more attractive to a potential buyer or have a work space appeal to renter. Place 4 drops essential oil directly on a low-watt light bulb. When you turn the light on — presto! — a subtle fragrance floats through the air and lingers. Make the kitchen smell sparkling clean with lemon and pine, the study studious with cedarwood, the bedroom exotic with jasmine, and the living room friendly and comfortable with rose geranium.

You can achieve an even longer lasting effect with a light bulb ring (see Figure 4-1). Place an inexpensive ceramic or metal ring on the top of a light bulb. Put it conveniently on the top of the rounded bulb. For a light bulb that is screwed into the ceiling, take the bulb out, place the ring over the neck, and then screw the bulb back in. You can purchase a light bulb ring almost anywhere that sells essential oils, such as natural-food, craft, gift, and in some department stores.

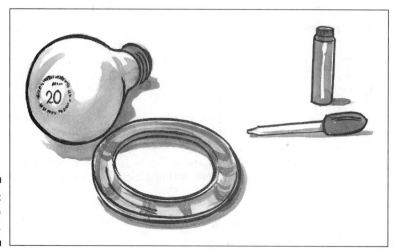

Figure 4-1:
A light bulb
ring.

Place 5 drops of essential oil on the light bulb ring with a dropper or *pipette* (a plastic dropper that is specially designed for liquids like essential oils), and the fragrance slowly releases as the light bulb heats the ring. (Most rings have a deep depression in them, but *do not fill* the ring up with essential oil unless you want your home to smell like a perfume shop. You'll end up using about 50 times the amount of oil than you need. Restrain yourself and use only a few drops.) You can leave the ring on the light bulb even if you decide to change scents because the last fragrance will totally disappear.

You can leave the ring on the light bulb even if you decide to change scents because the heat of the light bulb makes the oil disappear totally.

Both ceramic and metal light bulb rings work, but the ceramic ones have an advantage because they heat more slowly. As a result, they release the scent for a longer period of time — about an hour compared to less than 30 minutes for a metal ring. For the same reason, use very low wattage bulbs, preferably 20 watts or less, because the cooler the light bulb, the more gradually it releases the scent. Higher wattage bulbs tend to overheat the oil, making the essential oils smell almost burnt.

How long the aroma lingers in the room afterward depends on the amount of air flow through the room, but you can expect at least a light scent to stay for an hour or so.

A light bulb ring, especially the metal kind, gets very hot, so don't touch it until the light is off and the ring has cooled! It is also best to wait until the ring cools enough to touch it before adding more essential oil. Otherwise, the oil dissipates into the air almost as quickly as you pour it on.

Diffuser

One way to fill a room with scent is with a specially constructed *diffuser*. The three types of diffusers all run on electricity, so you need to have an outlet nearby.

Diffusers are designed to sit on a table or shelf, or you can place them on an out-of-the-way the corner of the room. A diffuser provides a continuous scent for several hours, making it a good choice for times when you need a longer lasting scent, say when entertaining guests. It is also ideal for a professional office or other situations when burning a candle or using a light bulb ring is not practical.

The unit is called a *diffuser* because the scent that it emits is *diffused* into the air.

A good way to decide which diffuser is best for you is to find a store that carries several different models and compare them. A store with a section devoted to aromatherapy is your best bet. Such stores are springing up everywhere. Search your local phonebook and call around to find stores that carry diffusers. Some natural-food stores also have aromatherapy departments, or they can special order a diffuser. Also, see the Appendix for mail-order and Internet suppliers.

The use of diffusers varies with the make and model, so follow the directions that come with the one you purchase. The procedure is pretty simple in all cases: Place a few drops of essential oil in or on the diffuser and then switch it on. After it warms for a few minutes, you can begin to smell the scent of the essential oil.

The following list describes the different types of diffusers in detail. Figure 4-2 shows you what they look like.

✔ **Glass diffuser:** These models resemble laboratory glass equipment. They use a small pump, which is usually a modified fish-tank pump, to continually puff light scent into a room. An advantage of this type of diffuser is that it does not use heat to dissipate the scent of essential oils into the air, and the unheated oil has a purer aroma.

If you buy a "fish pump" diffuser, be sure that you get a quiet one. Some pumps are so loud that they can ruin the relaxing mood you want to create.

✔ **Hard-plastic diffusers:** This type is a plastic unit that is usually a little larger than a coffee mug. An opening emits the scent when the unit is switched on. Some models rely on very low electric heat instead of a pump, which makes them quiet, but that means that they also heat the essential oil and slightly alter its scent. This type is probably the most popular diffuser because it's so easy to use. It also comes in quite a few different styles and sizes.

✔ **Electric outlet diffusers:** The least expensive, this model also uses heat to dissipate the aroma of essential oils in the immediate area. These diffusers come with absorbent pads on which you place a few drops of the essential oil. Then you insert the pad into the unit. When plugged in to an electric outlet, the pad heats and releases the scent. An innovative version of this type of diffuser plugs into your car's cigarette lighter to make your journeys more pleasant and relaxing.

The price of a diffuser varies with the style and the model. The glass/pump models run from $80 to well over $100, while the plastic versions range from $25 to $50 in the United States.

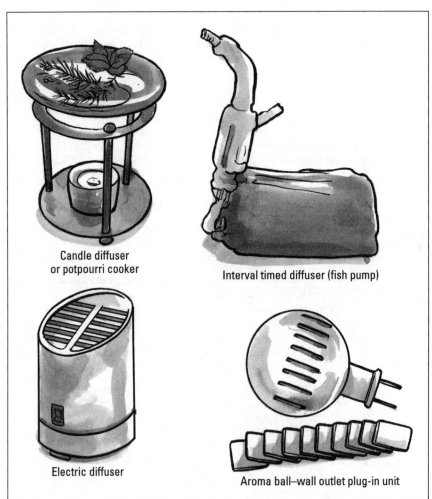

Candle diffuser
or potpourri cooker

Interval timed diffuser (fish pump)

Electric diffuser

Aroma ball–wall outlet plug-in unit

Figure 4-2:
Various
types of
aroma-
therapy
diffusers.

Table 4-2	Diffusers: What's the Diff?	
Type of Diffuser	*Advantages*	*Disadvantages*
Glass	Looks elegant Only model to not heat the oil Continuous release of scent	Most expensive type Can be noisy Must monitor so does not run out Needs special care Has breakable glass

Type of Diffuser	Advantages	Disadvantages
		Takes a while to begin working Usually must mail-order
Hard-plastic	Quiet Easy to use	Heats the oil, which can alter the scent
	Moderately expensive Fairly often sold in stores Continuous release of scent	
Plug-in-the-wall	Very easy to use Inexpensive	Uses the most heat, thus distorting the scent
	Very easy to find in stores Continuous release of scent	Oils must be replaced often

Make your own makeshift diffuser with a fan or heater

This quick method adds scent to your house. While you're cooling down with a fan on a hot summer day, take advantage of all that air flow to scent the room. Place about 6 drops of essential oil on a small strip of fabric or paper and tie or tape this on the grill in front of a fan. When you turn on the fan, air rushes past the scented cloth or paper to sweep the aroma into the room. This same technique works with an air-conditioner, a swamp cooler, or an air-flow heater. You can even use it with the air-flow control in your car. Absorbent pads, designed to scent with essential oil and placed in your house's heater vents, are even available. (With the new popularity of aromatherapy, just about everything that you can imagine has been invented.) On hot summer days, I always have a bottle of essential oil and my fan next to my desk.

With all of that air flow, the scent blows off fairly quickly, within half an hour, and then it lingers about another half hour. However, it's a simple matter to keep reapplying some essential oil — either the same or something different in case you're experiencing changeable moods.

Caring and feeding for your glass diffuser

Glass diffusers require some maintenance. For starters, they're quite fragile, so be careful when moving or refilling one. This type of diffuser also needs to be cleaned out by running rubbing alcohol through it each time you want to switch from one scent to another, unless you do not mind the old and new scents mixing together. (Sometimes oils smell okay together, sometimes not, depending on which ones they are.)

Even if you don't mind mixing scents together, you still need to clean out a glass diffuser after every few hours of use to keep it the delicate glassware tubing from becoming clogged. And, speaking of clogging, don't even try using thick essential oils such as patchouli, myrrh, benzoin, or vanilla unless you dilute them. These oils are sure to clog the works and make a mess inside that may be difficult to clean with.

Steam

One of the easiest methods to scent a room is with steam. The rising steam carries the fragrance into the air. The essential oils quickly go out of the steaming water into the surrounding air, but the lingering scent should fill the room for at least an hour or two.

To steam essential oils:

1. **Place 3 to 6 drops essential oil or essential oil blend in 2 or more cups of water in a pan.**

2. **Place the pan on the stove and bring to a light simmer.**

3. **Turn the heat off when the scent is released (about 3 minutes).**

If you don't have any essential oils yet, but are anxious to try an aromatherapy technique, you can try steaming aromatic herbs. Steaming can be done with fragrant herbs instead of the pure oils. (After all, all fragrant herbs contain essential oils because that is what makes them smell.)

To steam fragrant herbs:

1. **Place 1 to 2 heaping tablespoons of a fragrant herb, such as lavender flowers or cinnamon powder, into a quart or more of water in a pan.**

2. **Place the pan on the stove and bring to a light simmer.**

3. **Turn the heat off when the scent is released (about 20 minutes).**

A variation on the diffuser

One unique item is a porous clay made into a figurine, miniature pot, or design. It's labeled a diffuser, although it doesn't pump the fragrance into the air. Instead, the clay absorbs the oil, which then slowly dissipates into the air. The clay is so absorbent that it takes about 20 drops each time you scent it. The aroma lingers on the clay for several hours and scents the immediate area around it (but not a whole room), so it's good for small spaces or somewhere your nose will be close by. (I keep a clay flower wall disk fastened on the edge of my computer screen, scented with a fragrance to keep me alert, of course.) How much area is scented depends upon the size of your room and the amount of air flow in it. These diffuser make nice, relatively inexpensive gift items when you want to share aromatherapy with someone. If you want to go the simple route, a low-fired red clay flower pot works similarly. Place a clay diffuser where essential oils won't injure wood finishing or fine fabric and out of the reach of children who may suck on them.

Steaming is ideal if you use a wood stove to heat your home in the winter. You may already place water on your stove to humidify the dry air produced from burning wood. You can put the pan of water on the stove with essential oils or aromatic herbs and let it slowly release the aroma as it simmers. Want another good wintertime suggestion? A combination of equal amounts of cinnamon and orange peel will warm your spirit. Use either essential oils or the herbs.

Sprays

A room freshener spray instantly transforms your room with fragrance. The freshener is comprised of an essential oil to supply the scent mixed in a carrier such as water and placed in a spray bottle. When you spray the mist into a room, the essential oils float throughout the air and are lightly distributed on the furnishings. In this way, everything becomes lightly scented.

You can buy aromatic room freshener sprays, although the assortment of scents is limited with the emphasis heavy on citrus. Of course, some smell better than others. Again, let your nose help you out and choose what smells good to you.

Now that aromatherapy is so popular, quite a few companies offer sprays in either aerosol cans or pump-style spray bottles. (I suggest not buying fresheners in the type of aerosol cans that are detrimental to the environment. The can will tell you if it's a safe one.) Some room freshener sprays need shaking before they're used; others do not. It depends upon what other ingredients they contain besides water and essential oil. Follow the directions on the label. (And don't forget to watch out for those synthetic air fresheners. For more on the problems with synthetics, refer to Chapter 3.)

The most common type of room spray contains either water that contains essential oils and possibly a few other ingredients. Basically, it's scented water. You can also use a hydrosol to spritz around a room. This water and essential oil combination comes from producing essential oils by distillation. (See Chapter 1 for a more detailed explanation and Appendix A for places that sell them.)

Do not worry about staining furniture and curtains, unless water is injurious to the material. If that is the case, keep the mist a safe distance away. Be particularly careful to keep your distance from fabrics such as silk and satin because water can stain them. Some oil droplets can also make stains on varnish or lacquer finish on wood furniture.

Spraying a room freshener does not last long, often no more than a hour, but it is a quick way to freshen or disinfectant the air, get rid of unpleasant odors, set a particular mood, or simply make your house smell wonderful. Freshener sprays are versatile and come in handy for a variety of uses. I use them everywhere. Following are some ideas to get you started:

✔ A sparkling citrus on the towels in your bathroom.

✔ Lavender on your bed sheets to assure peaceful sleep.

✔ Eucalyptus on the kitchen counter to ward off pesky ants.

✔ Cedar on your dog's bed as a flea repellent — and on the dog herself!

✔ One mom says that she sprays her kids' bedrooms every evening with a relaxing mix of a chamomile and lavender — and it works to get them to sleep quickly!

✔ Peppermint in ashtrays at home and in the car.

✔ On trips, a room freshener spray is a must so that you can scent your home away from home. Try these:

  • A wake-up-and-keep-sightseeing spray like peppermint.

  • A calm-down-and-sleep-now scent like chamomile.

  • An enough-of-these-bugs (or mold) eucalyptus spray.

  • A something's-a-little-fishy spritz for your boat.

  • An all-purpose, home-on-wheels freshener for the kitchen and bathroom of your motor home.

If you're a teacher or nurse or have another type of job in which you work close to people, use aromatic room freshener sprays on the job — not just because room fresheners are quick and easy, but because they are already acceptable. That means not going through all of the official red tape to get their use approved by superiors.

You can take it with you: Aromatherapy in your auto

There's a good chance that whatever you do, you spend a lot of time in your car. You may commute a long way to work or travel in your job, or perhaps you chalk up a pile of miles just driving the kids back and forth to all their activities. Cars have become a home away from home and considering all the time people spend in them, cars deserve to be scented as much as houses.

Use scent to keep you calm when you're stuck in traffic or late for an appointment. It also comes in handy to cover up musty car smells, cigarette smoke, or the smoggy or fume-filled air outside. And, when you go to sell your car, who can resist the aroma, especially if you spray the "new car" scent available from auto parts stores near that torn seat and the cracking dashboard?

The aroma dissipates into the air fairly rapidly. How long it lasts depends on whether you have your car windows up or down and whether you have the outside air flow on. Of course, the tighter your car is sealed, the longer the scent hangs in the air, so it will stay put for a couple hours when you're using the air-conditioning or the heater. If your car is wide open and you're flying down the expressway, then your car needs an additional spray every 15 minutes or so. Techniques from this chapter that you can use in your car are

✔ **Aromatherapy spray:** I carry a selection of several mood-changing and refreshing sprays in my car and keep them in between the driver's and the front passenger seat.

✔ **Plug-in diffuser:** These small, plastic models are designed to fit in your cigarette lighter. Like their larger counterparts, these units hold a small, absorbent pad that has essential oil on it. As it heats up, so does the oil on the pad to fill your car. (Use your discretion about refilling while driving. Even a small distraction like that can make you look long enough to cause an accident.) You can get a lot of mileage out of this idea because it's easier to spray the air in the car than to change a tape in the tape player. As with the spray, how long the scent lingers depends on how open you have your car.

✔ **Incense:** This technique works to scent your car, but just be sure that the hot ashes don't fall on you or your upholstery. The safest incense to burn while driving are the cones that fit nicely in your ashtray.

✔ **Potpourri:** If a potpourri is aromatic enough, then it'll scent your car. I keep a small box of a solid perfume from India that's sold as "amber" in my ash tray because it keeps a light scent in the car. (I also have a handy supply of fragrance if I'm ever feeling the need for perfume.)

✔ **Car jewelry:** "What?" you may ask, but jewelry is the best description to describe the scented objects that hang from your car's rearview mirror. You can buy tacky cardboard ones that smell like overly sweet strawberry at the drugstore, but I prefer the aromatherapy versions. Most are tiny figurines, miniature vases, or designs made from porous clay that look decorative as well as scent the car. The low firing makes the clay absorbent enough to hold a few drops of essential oil.

Do-it-yourself sprays

You may want to make your own aromatic room freshener spray because store-bought sprays tend to be expensive, and so that you can have a custom-designed spray with the scents of your choice.

Making an aromatic spray is simple, as well as cheap. All you need is essential oil, distilled water, and a spray bottle for your final creation. Obviously, the idea of making aromatic sprays is catching on because you can get lightweight plastic or glass bottles, which often come in colored glass, to add a touch of elegance to your decor. (You can find spray bottles at large drugstores, many natural-food stores, and some craft stores. There are also mail-order suppliers of containers. See the Appendix for more info.)

What makes an aromatic room freshener spray inexpensive is the base; it's just water with essential oils in it. The spray method overcomes the problem that water and oil (and this includes essential oil) do not mix. Most essential oils float on the water's surface. The trick is to shake your bottle of aromatic room freshener very well before spraying. This distributes the essential oil in the water. Spray bottles have a tube that goes down close to the bottom of the bottle, so they release a good mix of water and oil. If you set your bottle down, most of the essential oils will again float to the surface in less than a minute, so shake it every time before you use it.

After a few days or several bouts of shaking have passed, the essential oils will mix into the water a little bit, but you still need to shake the bottle. The ease with which the oil blends with the water depends upon the essential oils you use. For example, rose blends with water fairly easily, while citrus oils such as orange and lemon do not. Go ahead and use them, just remember to shake the bottle well beforehand. On the other hand, heavy, resinous essential oils such as patchouli, benzoin, myrrh, and vanilla are especially stubborn mixing with water and may require more shaking than it's worth. These are the same ones that clog up a diffuser. When using resinous oils, first add 1 teaspoon of them to a tablespoon of vodka and then add the amount of water suggested in the following recipe.

Aromatic Spray

This recipe uses lavender, but feel free to replace it with another essential oil.

Preparation time: *5 minutes*

Yield: *4 ounces of spray*

40 drops lavender oil   *4 ounces distilled water*

1 Add the essential oils to the water in the spray bottle.

2 Keep the mixture in a spray bottle.

3 Shake before using.

Disinfectant Room Spray

A disinfectant spray is good to have around. Spray it in the bathroom or kitchen, or in the sickroom to help prevent the caregivers from getting sick. The following is a multi-purpose room disinfectant.

Preparation time: *5 minutes*

Yield: *4 ounces of spray*

12 drops lavender oil   *5 drops white thyme oil*

12 drops eucalyptus oil   *4 ounces distilled water*

12 drops orange oil

1 Add the essential oils to the water in the spray bottle.

2 Keep the mixture in a spray bottle.

3 Shake before using.

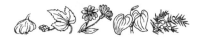

Aromatic fashion statements: Wearing your scents

One way to scent the immediate environment around you is to scent yourself. Of course, you can wear a drop of essential oil for perfume, but you can carry a scent in other innovative ways. Aromatherapy jewelry is specially designed to emit a slight fragrance. This saves putting essential oils directly on your skin and also makes an attractive and aromatic fashion statement. You can purchase anything from small goddess replicas that come with a vial of a blend to elegant stones suspended from gold chains with a small depression in which to put your favorite essential oils. You can find filigree hearts and globes that open so that you can insert a tiny piece of blotter paper that is drenched in a scent and tiny vial suspended on gemstones. I have several of these aromatherapy necklaces. My favorite is a silver engraved heart with a stopper on top. The scent of rose emanates from it only when I pop open the top. (See the Appendix for some companies that offer aroma jewelry.)

Aromatherapy is the wave of the future, so expect to see more and more personal items. If you think that there's a limit to aromatic creativity, check out this list. Some of these things hedge the line on aromatherapy due to the use of fake scents. Here are some items that are already patented or out on the market and may be coming to a store near you eventually:

- ✔ **Scented pantyhose** imbedded with time-release capsules.

- ✔ **Men's ties** in your choice of spice, leather, or — I kid you not — tobacco.

Chapter 5

Aromatherapy Alchemy: Making Your Own Scents

In This Chapter

▶ Converting your kitchen into a laboratory

▶ Diluting essential oils to make an aromatherapy product

▶ Blending scents so that they smell good

▶ Extracting fragrant herbs into vegetable oil

▶ Figuring out proportions

*Y*ou can turn your kitchen into a laboratory and play mad scientist. I warn you, though, that it's a fascinating hobby that can take over your life. That's what happened to me. And, it not only has taken over my life, but also my kitchen. I devote vast stretches of kitchen cupboards and even a section of my refrigerator to aromatherapy supplies and projects. In fact, I don't cook as much as I'd like to because I'm too busy concocting my newest brainstorm of an aromatherapy idea. Instead of creating a carrot cake or soufflé, my kitchen's more likely to feature a neroli-rose facial cream or a lemon-oatmeal skin scrub.

Thirty years ago when I began using aromatherapy products made with natural ingredients, none were available, period. I know that seems hard to believe considering the abundance of products that you can buy nowadays, but it's true. There was only one thing for me to do; I made them myself. One thing led to another and pretty soon I was sharing my creations with friends and then selling them to natural-food stores and by mail-order.

In this chapter, I tell you all you need to know to get started creating your own aromatherapy blends — and to make sure that they smell good. (That's certainly an important part of aromatherapy! The therapy's never going to work if you don't want to smell it!) I also tell you what to do with it once you have your fabulous blend. Okay, ready to roll up your sleeves and get to work?

Getting in Touch with Your Inner Mad Scientist

Consider yourself lucky. Nowadays, you can find a wonderful selection of aromatherapy products in stores and by mail. (I list plenty of sources for products that you can order from your home in the Appendix.) If you're busy (and who isn't!), you might want to purchase everything you need for aromatherapy body care and medicine and maintaining emotional balance.

I do enjoy sampling the array of aromatherapy that's available, but I still make my own. It's as easy as it is fun. Then, some aromatherapy projects are just so simple, the only way is to make them is yourself. They usually involve no more than adding a prescribed number of drops to vegetable oil or water. You can find many examples of these simple recipes in the Symptom Guide.

Making your aromatherapy creations is as simple as one, two, three.

1. **Turn your kitchen into a lab.**

2. **Blend your essential oils if you're using more than one.**

3. **Decide which base to use to dilute them.**

That's what I want to show you in this chapter. But, before you get started, read the basics on essential oils in Chapter 2 along with safety tips from Chapter 3. Then you'll have a good foundation to stand on.

Converting your kitchen into your lab

It only takes a second to turn your kitchen into an aromatherapy laboratory.

A glass measuring cup, stainless steel measuring spoons, and some small funnels, and you're ready to go into aromatherapy production. Also have on hand paper towels and some rubbing alcohol for clean up or spills.

Most of your supplies — vegetable oil, distilled water, rubbing alcohol, and vodka — are available from a grocery store. You can buy or order fancier vegetable oils such as almond, apricot, and grapeseed at most natural-food stores. Except for the essential oils, you probably have all the equipment and most of the supplies already in your kitchen.

You need a way to measure small amounts of the essential oils and transfer them from the vial to your project. Some essential oils are sold in bottles that have an insert called a *reducer* that has a small hole in the middle to let out only a drop of oil at a time. Allow yourself a few tries to get the technique. (Do not shake the bottle, or several drops will tumble out at once.) Sometimes essential oils are sold in dropper bottles that have special oil-resistant droppers. (Droppers are convenient for you, although they usually add to the cost of the oils.)

If your essential oils don't come in a bottle with either a reducer or a glass dropper, measure small amounts of essential oils with separate droppers (they're sold in drugstores and by some natural-food stores and essential oil suppliers) or a pipette (they're sold by essential oil suppliers). A *pipette* is a long, narrow, plastic tube with a bulb at the top. You squeeze the bulb and then release. This makes the oil go into the tube and then drop out.

If you use a dropper, or especially a pipette, practice first with a little water to get the hang of it before you start transferring your precious essential oils.

Don't contaminate your essential oils by putting a dropper or pipette from one oil into another. If you don't want to have a separate dropper for each oil, you can rinse out all the essential oil with rubbing alcohol. In only a minute or so, the dropper will completely evaporate so that you can put that dropper into another oil. Having two or three droppers allows you time to let one dry while you're using another one.

Unless you're adding essential oils to spice up an already-made product, you also need containers. Bottles and vials are sold at drugstores and many natural-food stores. For fancy gift containers, go to an import store or shop by mail, (see the Appendix). Two more important things that are easy to overlook are a notebook and labels. Keep notes so that you can duplicate a winning success or avoid repeating a complete flop! And label everything so that you can figure out what's what later. I've had a few recipes that I could have made a fortune on if only I'd remembered to write down the ingredients.

The case of mistaken identity: A true story

A few mishaps can come from a combined kitchen and aromatherapy lab like mine. I had better not get started. Of course, there was the facial cream that I made for myself and because all the fancy containers were stored out in my aromatherapy business, I just put it in a clean mayonnaise jar and popped it into the refrigerator. Unfortunately, the jar still had the original label on it. The next day at lunch time, I was writing in my office when I heard loud screams from the kitchen as my family bit into the Dagwood style sandwiches they made with all the trimmings, including what they thought was mayonnaise. At least I assured them that all the ingredients were pure and quite edible, although they didn't agree on the edible part. Rather than revealing any more embarrassing stories, it's enough to say that it's important to do as I say instead of as I do and label everything. Which reminds, there was the time that I added peppermint essential oil to a bottle of distilled water. . . .

Blending scents

An important part of creating aromatherapy products is blending several different essential oils together into a, hopefully, good-smelling and effective combination. You can use just one essential oil at a time, but there are advantages to making a blend. You can do many things with your blend once you have it formulated. (Chapter 4 can help you with ideas on how to put scent into the air.)

Imagine sniffing lemon peel, or a sprig of lavender, or a rose by itself. Nice, of course, but then try to imagine a rose and lavender mixed together with a hint of lemon. The result? A scent so spectacular that you can't get enough of it!

A blend also has the advantage of combining several emotional attributes offered by different fragrances. Some companies now make aromatherapy blends containing several different oils designed to create different moods in your home. You can combine several aromas that all help with an emotional complaint. For example, you can pick up an aromatherapy blend to scent your bedroom to help with your insomnia or an energizing scent that keeps you awake and alert at work. Look for these in herb, natural-food, and gift stores and from sources listed in the Appendix.

Ready, set, blend

If you're feeling adventuresome, put together your own blend. Most people freeze at the thought of concocting their own formula, but it is not difficult. After all, you already have plenty of practice: You've spent your entire life deciding which fragrances you do and do not like.

Start out simple. Try combining two or more scents together to make an aromatherapy blend. (You can find many easy recipes in the Symptom Guide.) As you become more familiar with essential oil scents and properties, you'll find it easier and easier to concoct — and even create — your own aromatherapy combos.

Approach blending the same way you do using an individual scent — decide upon an emotional quality and choose your favorite. It is even okay to combine a scent that increases energy with another scent that is relaxing. This may seem like putting opposites together, but definitely not in aromatherapy. After all, isn't that everyone's ideal state: Being perfectly relaxed yet with boundless amounts of energy?

Tricks of the Trade

To make the best blends, you'll want to rely on a few tricks of the trade. You can find these hints in detail in Chapter 2. Be sure to read the sections "Sniffing 101," "Scent Type," and "Scent Description" because they help you in blending.

Essential oils vary in the intensity of their odor. To make a formula smell good, you want to add small amounts of strong essential oils and larger quantities of the subtle ones. Otherwise, the strong ones will completely overpower the weaker ones. It is far too easy for an especially potent oil such as rosemary to completely overpower the soft scent of an oil such as sandalwood or cedar. When mixing small experimental quantities, 1 drop of a high intensity oil like cinnamon can be way too much. Try adding just a smidgen of oil with the end of a toothpick.

You can easily figure out which essential oils are subtle. I use more of these subtle oils than other oils.

- Cedarwood
- Orange
- Sandalwood

Sniff any of these very strong essential oils right from the vial, and chances are you will draw your face away because they're so strong. I generally use only 1 drop of these oils for every 5 drops of other oils

- Chamomile
- Cinnamon/Rosemary
- Clary sage
- Patchouli
- Ylang ylang

Already, you have the makings of a formula.

A First Formula

8 drops orange

4 drops lavender

1 drop clary sage

Although known for promoting a dreamy relaxation, clary sage has a heady smell. Say that you would prefer something more stimulating. Replace the clary sage with 1 drop cinnamon. For a sensual and sedating blend, then use ylang ylang instead. Cedarwood could turn the blend more woodsy. It's your choice, and the options are almost endless.

There are some even more powerful essential oils. These aren't pungent, just intense. With these, I use only about 1 drop for every 10 drops of other oils.

- ✔ Jasmine
- ✔ Neroli
- ✔ Rose

In blending different aromas, try to follow a few tricks of the trade:

- ✔ **Choose an essential oil that can serve as your main scent in your blend.** Then you need to only add very small amounts of other essential oils to enhance it. What you'll mostly smell is the first scent that you chose with the others serving as background.

- ✔ **Some essential oils have more complicated aromas than others, and they already smell like a blend.** Rose geranium, lavender, jasmine, and bergamot are good examples. Start with one of these and then add another essential oil. It takes only a little of the second essential oil to produce an interesting blend.

- ✔ **Use sharp smelling scents, such as fir, eucalyptus, peppermint, and cinnamon, in small amounts so that they don't overpower the other scents in your blend.**

- ✔ **Use small amounts of ylang ylang because it can overpower the other scents in a blend, and most people find its fragrance overly sweet.**

- ✔ **Rose and jasmine are very expensive essential oils, but fortunately they are also extra-concentrated so that a little goes a long way.** In fact, they are so powerful that you can substitute 1 drop of rose, jasmine, or neroli (orange blossom) essential oil in a recipe that calls for 10 drops of another oil.

✔ **Another trick of the trade is to start with an essential oil that already smells fairly complicated.** An example is geranium, which hints at a combination of herbs, rose, pine, cedar, and lemon. With an oil like this as the start, begin expanding your formula by adding small amounts of other oils, one at a time. Each choice sends your creation in a different direction.

✔ **An interesting way to expand a blend is to choose oils that have similar characteristics.** This performs a delightful trick on the nose as they play off one another. It makes your blend seem more complicated and mysterious because no one can pinpoint exactly what the aroma is. Try combining peppermint and spearmint, lemon and bergamot, or cinnamon and ginger.

Concocting the Simple Stuff

You make aromatherapy products in two parts: diluting and blending. The following sections describe what's important about each one.

Diluting

Essential oils are almost always diluted by mixing them into something. Here are the substances for diluting essential oils. In the aromatherapy trade, they're called *carriers* because they carry the essential oil.

✔ **Vegetable oil:** The most common way to dilute essential oils is into a vegetable oil, which offers many advantages. Vegetable oil's molecules are too large to penetrate the skin. Instead, they smoothly slide over your skin, holding in moisture and protecting dry skin. This makes vegetable oil ideal for body care. If you're not familiar with what vegetable oils are available, check out the sidebar "A slick question: Which vegetable oil to use?" later in this chapter. One oil to avoid is peanut because no matter how much essential oil you add, it smells of peanut butter sandwiches. (Unless you're massaging children — they love it!) Instead of plain oil, you can also use an *herbal oil* (an oil that has herbs infused into it) and then add essential oils to that. Herbally infused oils are available in natural-food stores. (See how to make your own herbal oils later in this chapter.)

✔ **Water:** Even though essential oils and water don't mix well, the two form a good partnership if you want to make a facial spritzer, a household air freshener, or an aromatherapy compress. Distilled water is best to use because it's pure and doesn't contain bacteria or chlorine. Other water-based liquids can replace some or all the water called for in a recipe. An example is aloe vera juice, which is excellent for skin care and helps to heal burns.

✔ **Alcohol:** Rubbing alcohol or vodka mixes with essential oils much better than water. Vodka is more expensive, but is preferred. It contains only pure alcohol and water without any flavors or additives and, compared to rubbing alcohol, it has no smell and is safer. (Rubbing alcohol is poisonous to drink.) *Witch hazel distillate,* which is witch hazel bark and leaves extracted into alcohol, is sometimes used instead. Any alcohol is a mild astringent that is drying, so it's sometimes used for oily skin. It is also useful as a liniment for sore muscles and in any skin product when the greasiness of vegetable oil is a problem — say for those times when you want to apply a pain-reliever to your shoulder, but don't want an oily shirt. (See Chapter 10 for liniment recipes.) When using alcohol, you can make an extra-strength product by buying an herbal tincture instead of plain vodka. Choose herbs that correspond to your project.

✔ **Vinegar:** Only a few aromatherapy products call for vinegar because it's impossible to mask its strong smell even with essential oils. With all the newfangled products available, vinegar has lost the popularity it had for centuries. That's too bad, considering that it improves your complexion and hair. (For vinegar's benefits, go to Chapter 7.) Apple cider is sometimes preferred over distilled vinegar because it contains more minerals and is less likely to be made synthetically.

✔ **Salve or lotion:** If you want a thicker product than oil or alcohol offers, then go for a lotion, cream, or salve, or you may want a hair rinse or shampoo. A shortcut to making these from scratch is to buy a premade, unscented version and then stir in your choice of essential oils. If you buy products that already contain herbs — and they're easy to find — then you get double the medicinal benefits from combining herbs and aromatherapy.

✔ **Herbal oil:** This oil is quite different from an essential oil. It's made by soaking the herbs in warm vegetable oil. Herbal oil is often called an *infused oil* because the herbs are "infused" into an oil base. These oils can replace the plain vegetable oil that is called for in many aromatherapy recipes. The result is a more potent medicine. For example, you can buy or make a vegetable oil or alcohol tincture infused with calendula (used to treat itchy or irritated skin conditions) or of St. John's wort (helps heal nerve pain and inflammation) and then add essential oils.

If you're feeling ambitious, then you can get a book with recipes for making aromatherapy salves and creams from scratch and for preparing your own vegetable oils that have aromatic herbs infused into them, such as my *Aromatherapy* (Crossing Press). To find out more about herbs, check out *Herbal Remedies For Dummies* by Christopher Hobbs, L.Ac., IDG Books Worldwide, Inc., and my *Herbs for Health and Healing,* Rodale Press.

A slick question: Which vegetable oil to use?

Vegetable oil is composed of big, rubbery molecules that make it slide smoothly over your skin, so it's ideal to use in body-care products. When you read the following list, you'll see that not all vegetable oils come from vegetables. In fact, they're far more likely to come from a fruit.

For the technically correct name, you can call them *fixed oils* instead. This is because the oil is fixed in the plant and not easily released compared to an essential oil that moves into the air or on to your hand without any hesitation. (There I go talking science again.) Unlike essential oils, this also means that vegetable oil is too thick to penetrate the skin. These vegetable oils are most often used in aromatherapy:

- **Apricot kernal** is similar in price, color, and texture to almond, with a slightly lighter scent and texture.

- **Avocado** is deep green, rich, and heavy. It's loaded with skin-nourishing nutrients and is recommended for dry skin. It's a little pricey, so it's usually blended with other vegetable oils.

- **Castor** is used mostly to treat skin problems, such as eczema and in castor oil *packs,* which are a special type of compress. It's sold in drugstores and some natural-food stores.

- **Coconut** is very thick, containing twice the heavy fats as lard, and is solid at room temperature. It causes an allergic reaction in sensitive individuals. In case a trace of the solvent is left, coconut oil that is extracted with solvents isn't recommended for use on the skin. (If you're ever in a large southern Mexico market, be sure to visit a coconut oil "factory" where you can see them pressing the delicious-smelling oil with a hand-crank.)

- **Cocoa butter** is derived from cocoa beans. This oil's scent is distinctively chocolate and can overpower the aroma of all but the strongest smelling essential oils. Small amounts thicken skin lotions and creams. It's sold in drugstores and some natural-food stores.

- **Olive** is often preferred for medicinal use because it's rich in healing chlorophyll, can be cold pressed without solvents, and keeps longer without refrigeration than other vegetable oils — for about a year. The strong smell of the dark green virgin oil overpowers other aromas, so a lighter version is used for aromatherapy.

- **Sesame** is a favorite in *Ayurvedic medicine* (a traditional medicine from India). It contains a natural preservative and provides some sun protection. The unrefined oil is rarely used in aromatherapy because it smells so strong.

- **Sweet almond** has a light, sweet scent with a good glide for skin care. It's more expensive than most vegetable oils, and you may need to special order it through a natural-food store because it's not used in cooking.

These following fancy (and I should add more expensive) vegetable oils are popular for use in aromatherapy skin care. Due to their expense, they're often combined with the preceding oils.

- **Grapeseed** is odorless, mildly astringent, and has a light texture and scent, so it's favored in cosmetics, although it's generally solvent-extracted.

(continued)

(continued)

- ✔ **Hazelnut** has a mild fragrance and is so light in texture, it's used in products for oily skin.

- ✔ **Kukui nut** is the thinnest, lightest of these oils and is so nongreasy, it's suitable even for oily skin, although it does have a distinct odor. In its native Hawaii, the nut is used to recondition sun-exposed skin.

- ✔ **Macadamia nut** also has a very light texture, but is slightly heavier than kukui.

- ✔ **Rice bran** has a smooth, nongreasy texture that makes it good for a massage oil or body lotion. It's especially high in vitamin E, so it doesn't spoil rapidly.

- ✔ **Wheat germ** is so thick, you need to dilute it with another vegetable oil. It contains high amounts of vitamins A and E.

Vegetable wax is an oil-like substance found in plants that can be used like vegetable oil. Jojoba, unlike the oils in this sidebar, doesn't turn rancid, so it saves you the worry that your aromatherapy project will spoil. It's expensive, so you may want to save it for products that you want to keep for several months.

Herb oils are included in some high-grade aromatherapy products. These oils are expensive so that is usually reflected in the price of any product that contains them. You can also purchase these oils through mail-order companies that carry aromatherapy supplies (see the Appendix).

- ✔ **Evening primrose:** Along with the herb borage and black currant, this oil is high in *gamma linoleic acid (GLA),* an important fatty acid that helps repair sun-damaged skin and maintain healthy skin and is often used for mature skin.

- ✔ **Rosehip seed:** Another oil high in GLA, this helps regenerative skin, so it's used for stretch marks, burns, scars, and mature skin. The strong fragrance and expense dictate that it's used in small amounts.

Converting measurement

Now you've reached the crucial point. You have your essential oil blend, and you know what base to dilute it in. What you need to know now is how much of the blend to add to your base.

Most aromatherapy applications need the essential oil in a 2 percent dilution. That translates to 2 drops of essential oil for every 98 drops of carrier oil or 10 to 12 drops per ounce of carrier. Essential oils are not all sold by the same system, which can be confusing when you're trying to compare prices or to simply figure out how much you need for your aromatherapy projects. The oils may be sold by the ounce, dram, or milliliters. Likewise, a recipe may be made by the drop, teaspoon, or any of these other measurements. There's even another variable to confuse the issue. The size of a drop varies depending on the size of the dropper opening and the temperature and the thickness of the essential oil. In other words, be prepared for some variations. Table 5-1 helps you decipher all this.

Table 5-1 Measurement Equivalents

Drops	*Teaspoons*	*Ounces*	*Drams*	*Milliliters*
12.5 drops	1/8 teaspoon	1/48 oz.	1/6 dram	about 5/8 ml.
25 drops	1/4 teaspoon	1/24 oz.	1/3 dram	about 1 1/4 ml.
75 drops	3/4 teaspoon	1/8 oz.	1 dram	about 3.7 ml.
100 drops	1 teaspoon	1/6 oz.	1 1/3 dram	about 5 ml.

Beginning blends

In case you want to try your hand at making some essential oil blends, the following blends are simple. In this way, you can see how easily you can create your blends. This book is filled with lots and lots of ideas along with lists of potential essential oils that you can include in your recipes. Here are six simple aromatherapy blends.

Squeaky Clean: Lemon and Eucalyptus

In the kitchen or bathroom, this scent enhances a feeling of cleanliness. Also use it when you need energy or to think faster — as a physical or mental uplift.

Preparation time: *3 minutes*

Yield: *5 drops*

4 drops lemon oil

1 drop eucalyptus oil

Combine all ingredients.

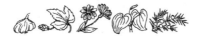

Pep-up Plus: Orange, Cinnamon, and Mint

This combination of spice and mint increases energy, makes you more alert, and also relieves anxiety. While entertaining company, studying, or simply trying to get the housework done, you can appreciate the energizing effects of this blend. Cheerful orange relieves stress, and cinnamon and the mints are perky scents that increase mental awareness and make you feel energized.

Preparation time: 3 minutes

Yield: 7 drops

4 drops orange oil

1 drop cinnamon oil

1 drop peppermint oil

1 drop spearmint oil

Combine all ingredients.

Bliss Blend: Rose, Lavender, and Lemon

Rose essential oil is expensive, so a lot of people do not use it, but if you're in an expensive-but-worth-it mood, try this exquisite blend of fragrances to produce a mellow, yet focused reaction. It's a refreshing, clean scent with a hint of floral.

Preparation time: 3 minutes

Yield: 8 drops

5 drops lavender oil

2 drop lemon oil

1 drop rose oil

Combine all ingredients.

Relax Away: Chamomile, Lavender, and Ylang Ylang

A great way to relax with fragrance — and it works! Use this combination to relax your children (and yourself!) in the evening. Plus, both chamomile and lavender lift your spirits if you're feeling blue.

Preparation time: *3 minutes*

Yield: *7 drops*

5 drops lavender oil   *1 drop ylang ylang oil*

1 drop chamomile oil

Combine all ingredients.

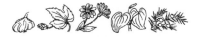

Meditative Mood: Sandalwood and Rose

This is a favorite combination in India where both scents are used to increase a meditative focus and to inspire prayer and contemplation.

Preparation time: *3 minutes*

Yield: *9 drops*

8 drops sandalwood oil   *1 drop rose oil*

Combine all ingredients.

Southwest Holiday: Lime and Juniper

This blend reminds me alternatively of basking in the Arizona sunshine and of vacationing on the coast of Mexico. It's a scent that gets your attention, but then doesn't want you to move too fast.

Preparation time: *3 minutes*

Yield: *7 drops*

5 drops lime oil   *1 drop juniper oil*

1 drop bergamot oil

Combine all ingredients.

Bouffant Bouquet: Rose Geranium, Lavender, and Bergamot

These floral scents blend well together. The combination they produce is an uplifting, relaxing, floral bouquet that makes a good scent for a general living area or for a working space. These scents create a sense of relaxation and emotional balance equally good for company or just for keeping the family happy. These three scents are also antidepressants — in case anyone is feeling down and needs an emotional boost.

Preparation time: 3 minutes

Yield: 5 drops

3 drops lavender oil

1 drop bergamot oil

1 drop rose geranium oil

Combine all ingredients.

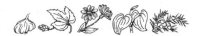

Seven essential oils to get you started

Try these oils when you first start making your recipes:

- ✔ **Chamomile** is a digestive and relaxation aid that also treats allergies, menstrual cramps, depression and inflammation, anxiety, anger, rashes, and dry and problem skin, complexion, and hair.

- ✔ **Geranium** balances the mind and body and helps all complexion and hair types.

- ✔ **Lavender** fights infection, inflammation, insomnia, and pain and relieves depression or anxiety. It's used on all complexion and hair types.

- ✔ **Lemon** (or other citrus) is an antidepressant that kills parasites and is used on oily complexion and hair.

- ✔ **Peppermint** relieves indigestion, sinus congestion, itching, and panic and is a mental stimulant. Small amounts are good for dry skin and hair.

- ✔ **Rosemary** relieves pain, congestion, constipation, and grief and also stimulates circulation and memory. It's used for most complexion and hair types.

- ✔ **Tea tree** fights most types of infection and is used for oily skin and hair.

And here are seven more oils I couldn't live without:

- ✔ Bergamot
- ✔ Cedarwood
- ✔ Clary sage
- ✔ Eucalyptus
- ✔ Marjoram
- ✔ Rose
- ✔ Ylang ylang

Making Your Own Herbal Oils

You can extract essential oils from plants into a vegetable oil base in a simple way. It's a practice that's been done for at least a couple thousand years. The herbs are soaked in warm vegetable oil so that their scent and properties are drawn into the oil base. This soaking creates infused oils because the herbs are infused into it. You can use these oils instead of plain carrier oils in all your aromatherapy preparations for the added healing benefits the herbs provide. You can find them suggested throughout this book — especially herb oils made with St. John's wort or calendula — combined with essential oils as a way to enhance the aromatherapy product's healing value. You can also use this same technique to make fragrant herb oils. This gives you the opportunity to make a body oil from plants such as wisteria, gardenia, and lilacs that are not available as natural essential oils or from plants that are very expensive such as rose or jasmine. (Although expect the scent to be light because a relatively small amount of essential oil is extracted.)

Preparation time: *15 minutes*

Yield: *About 1¼ cups of herb oil*

1 cup dried herbs (or fresh herbs that are wilted)   *about 1½ cups vegetable oil to cover*

1 Coarsely chop the herbs in a blender or with a knife.

2 Place the chopped herbs in a wide mouth jar.

3 Add enough oil to cover the herbs and completely submerge them (see Figure 5-1).

4 Stir the oil with a chopstick or table knife to release any air bubbles.

5 Put the lid on the jar and place it in a warm location, such as outside in the sun (or near a heater or wood stove in the winter).

6 Check the jar every day to make sure that all the herbs remain submerged under the oil. (Some herbs absorb a lot of the oil, so you may need to add more.)

7 After about 3 days in the sun or 1 to 2 days with continuous heat, strain out the herbs.

8 Use this herbal oil as a base and add essential oils to it.

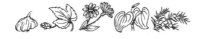

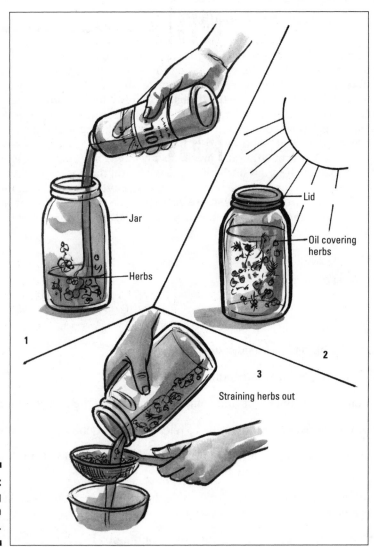

Jar

Herbs

Lid

Oil covering herbs

1

2

3

Straining herbs out

Figure 5-1:
Making your own herbal oils.

Part II
"Inscentives" for Living: Aromatherapy in Your Life

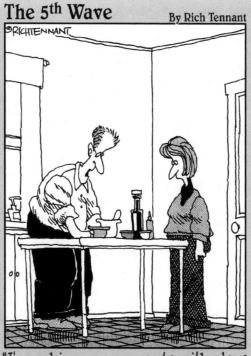

The 5th Wave   By Rich Tennant

"I'm making my own scents with celery seed, almond oil, and rosemary. What we don't use in the bathtub I'll toss with lettuce and serve it for dinner."

In this part

Aromatherapy is versatile stuff. In this part, I look at what you do in your life and how aromatherapy can enhance this activities. I give you scents to take everywhere. There's a chapter for each area of your life provided in Part II. You can take them with you to work, to the gym, on trips, throughout your house, out into your garden, and even into your bedroom to spice up your late evening activities.

If you're feeling super creative and want to try your hand at making a few of your own aromatherapy products, fear not. I explain, in this part, how to put together your own simple creations so that you can play mad scientist. You'll find them very simple so even if you never passed kitchen skills 101, you can whip up all sorts of aromatic combinations for only pennies. Even better, most of my recipes take less than five minutes from start to finish. If you'd rather buy your aromatherapy already made, then that's okay, too. I tell you what to look for so that you get the most for your money.

Chapter 6

Aromatherapy to De-Bug Your Home and Garden

- -

In This Chapter

▶ Driving bugs out of your house with scent

▶ Protecting your clothes from a moth invasion

▶ Making or buying natural insect repellents

▶ Getting rid of lice

▶ Telling insects in your garden to bug off

▶ Dealing with bites and stings

▶ Making simple household disinfectants

- -

> ### Recipes in This Chapter
>
> ▶ Household Spray
> ▶ Sashay Away Moth "Balls"
> ▶ Get Rid of Lice
> ▶ Insect Repellent for You
> ▶ Household Spray
> ▶ Insect Bite Solution
> ▶ Bite, Sting, and Splinter Poultice
> ▶ Enough Already! All-Purpose Garden Spray
> ▶ Fido's Flea Collar
> ▶ Flea Away Pet Shampoo
> ▶ Flea Away House Salt
>
>

*W*hen it comes to bugs, you probably don't think of aromatherapy. Most people don't. After all, aromatherapy is most often considered a therapy to enhance your emotional and physical health or complexion, not something that you'd use out in the garden. Nevertheless, aromatherapy offers plenty of ways to keep annoying insects out of both your garden and your house. What could be a better form of "therapy" than making your home and garden a more pleasant and less stressful place for you to enjoy?

You can use your "scents" on your family and pets and in your house and garden as an alternative to toxic pesticides and repellents. In this chapter, I give you the aromas to use to keep away all sorts of pesky pests.

This chapter contains a few scents that I don't cover elsewhere in this book. That's because the essential oils that have these scents are usually too toxic to use. Some examples are pennyroyal, tansy, and wormwood. However, toxicity is exactly what you need in a bug repellent or bug killer. In the section on pesticides for your garden, I also include catnip, nasturtium, and French marigold even though they're not readily available as essential oils, because you can use the plant itself (which contains the essential oils).

Don't Bug Me: Aromatic Insect Repellents

Insects are nature's aromatherapists. Many of them rely on a very acute sense of smell for the most important things in a bug's life. They use it to locate a mate. (They do so through *pheromones,* the same type of aromatic attractants that get people excited — see Chapter 8.) Equally important, their keen sense of smell directs insects to their food (translate that into you, your pets, your garden, and so on.) Although they're not usually welcomed visitors, many bugs fly miles tracking down a scent.

The time has come to pull in the welcome mat and turn the insect's remarkable sense of smell to your advantage. What aromatherapy has going for it is fragrance, and plenty of it. A strong aroma can create a scent shield to disguise the smells that bugs rely on to locate a food source — your home or garden. Instead, they get hit with a strong waft of pine or citronella. It's not what they're searching for, so little critters go elsewhere. Covering up bug-enticing scents is a good start, but an even better ploy is to use scents that bugs actually hate. That should be enough to send most any bug spinning on its heels in the opposite direction.

Aromatherapy's approach to dealing with unwanted bugs follows the same principles as holistic healing that I discuss in other sections of this book. The first course of action is preventive. Use natural repellents — in this case, aromatic ones — to fend off destructive insects. In that way, they don't even start munching your precious cabbage in your garden or the woolens in your closet. If prevention doesn't sufficiently cut down the insect population, then resort to out-and-out combat. Wipe out the little critters with your aromatherapy arsenal.

Of course, even with all that careful prevention, bugs can sneak through your defense systems at times. If you're their target, and you get bit or stung, aromatherapy again comes to your rescue with remedies to ease your discomfort.

In this chapter, I go over all of the ways in which aromatherapy can help you make your living environment a bugfree zone. My emphasis is on your first line of defense by using aromatherapy repellents. To help easily find the solution that you need, I list the pests that you're most likely to encounter and tell you which scents they like the least.

Note that throughout this chapter, I give you lists of the aromas from which certain insects stay away. All these scents have the people who use them backing their claim. The ones that have also been tested in scientific studies are indicated with an asterisk (*).

In Your House

Your home is a good place to start a bug patrol. After all, it is *your* house or apartment, not a parade ground for ants. It's not a display arena for flies to practice their dives and spins. And, your closets and cupboards are certainly not designed to host feeding frenzies of visiting grain and wool moths.

I use a homemade aromatherapy bug repellent spray to deal with various household pests such as ants and flies. (I provide a recipe later in this section in case you want to make a similar concoction.) I put it in a spray bottle and keep it under my sink ready for action whenever insects start making themselves at home in my house.

I also carry this spray with me on trips, especially if I'm headed to a foreign country with scenic, but rustic, accommodations. There's nothing like a constant parade of bugs through your cabaña to ruin an otherwise perfect holiday. I also find the spray useful to overcome the stale smell of mold in a beachfront rental. (These same essential oils not only hide moldy smells, but eliminate the mold itself.)

Follow these tips to get rid of the most common critters. (The ones that have also been tested in scientific studies have been indicated with an asterisk.)

 ✔ **Ants:** These critters are fairly easy to attack because they travel in regimented lines. Your ants may abhor pine, but I live in a pine forest and watch ants walk over dropped pine needles every day without so much as a little leap, so perhaps my ants are just immune. Anyway, I find that camphor and peppermint work better than pine. Make a spray along their trails, and ants will lose its scent. You can also cut a sponge into small squares, add several drops of essential oil to the pieces, and stick them in the corners of your cupboards or wherever ants find an entrance to your home. (Replace the essential oils every week.) To rid your place of ants, try these essential oils:

   • Camphor

   • Orange*

   • Pine

   • Peppermint

   • Spruce

 ✔ **Flies:** Here's a tough assignment because flies cover lots of territory. Because they fly, they can land anywhere, and you can't very well chase after them with a spray bottle. Keeping flies from coming into the house is difficult unless you scent it so heavily that you won't want to come in either. So, take a hint from yesteryear. In the days before window screens, people hung bunches of anise and bay by the open windows and doors so that flies wouldn't find the place inviting. Concentrate your efforts where flies enter your house and where they are most likely to land — around your windows and doors and on your kitchen counters. Good fly avoiders include

- Anise
- Bay laurel
- Cedarwood
- Cloves
- Eucalyptus
- Orange*

✔ **Cockroaches:** It doesn't take a full invasion of cockroaches in your house before you want them out. Just one of these huge bugs is one too many when you're talking house sharing. Concentrate your repellent action in the dark, damp places where they like to hang out. Try these essential oils:

- Angelica
- Eucalyptus
- Peppermint
- Sage

✔ **Mice:** Okay, I know this isn't a bug, but you'll have to admit that having mice move into your home can really bug you, so I'm including them among household pests. Spraying mint or even placing the fresh or dried leaves of the plant around keep mice away.

- Peppermint
- Spearmint
- Wormwood

Household Spray

Use this spray to discourage pests inside your home. It contains some of the most versatile essential oils. I also use vinegar because the bugs don't care for it at all. It's also cheap, easy to spray, and evaporates without leaving a trace. This recipe is for an all-purpose spray. If you want, alter the ingredients if you've got your sights on a particular bug that you want to attack.

Preparation time: 10 minutes

Yield: 4 ounces

½ teaspoon eucalyptus oil

¼ teaspoon peppermint oil

¼ teaspoon lemon oil

4 ounces vinegar

1 Put all ingredients in a blender and mix.

2 Store in a spray bottle.

3 Shake well before use and spray away!

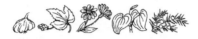

Your clothes closet

The commercial mothballs that ward off wool moths have an unpleasant odor and can discolor the very clothing they protect. Even worse, they contain some very potent chemicals, naphthalene and paradichlorobenzene. As a result, mothballs cause more than 5,000 poisonings a year, according to the American Association of Poison Control Centers.

It's no wonder that insecticides are going natural. The SC Johnson Wax company introduced lavender sachets called Off! Moth Proofer as a safe alternative to moth balls. Other large companies will probably follow suit. You can also make your own sachets for just pennies (see the following recipe). The old tradition of storing woolens in a cedarwood chest is very practical because the scent of the chest is strong enough to deter wool moths. These oils all work well when you're battling moths:

- ✔ Bay laurel
- ✔ Camphor
- ✔ Cedarwood
- ✔ Lavender
- ✔ Patchouli
- ✔ Sage

Sashay Away Moth "Balls"

You can make your own herbal sachets to fend off clothes moths. Toss them in your storage chest or drawers and hang them on ribbons from your clothes hangers. I find that lavender is a very effective moth repellent and smells wonderful, but cedarwood is even better, so I combine the two. Many fabric stores sell small squares of material for quiltmakers. You can buy these ready-to-go squares if you'd rather not cut your own.

Preparation time: *20 minutes*

Yield: *8 moth repellent sachets*

¼ cup lavender flowers

10 drops lavender oil

10 drops cedarwood oil

8 fabric squares, each about 6 inches square that have been cut with pinking shears

8 pieces of string (or ribbon) about 6 inches long

1 Add the essential oils to the lavender flowers.

2 Place the scented lavender in a glass jar for a day or so to give the scents from the essential oils time to permeate them.

3 Lay out the 6 fabric squares with the design (or outside) facing down.

4 Place a heaping teaspoon of the scented lavender on each piece.

5 Bring the edges of the fabric together and tie with the string.

6 Place your "moth balls" in with your woolens.

Your pantry

Grain moths are tiny greyish moths that look like a little stick when they're not flying and otherwise flutter around the pantry searching for cereal and other grains to dine on. I find them especially annoying because they also eat some herbs, mostly roots and seeds. An old tradition that still works as good as it did 200 years ago is to stick a few bay laurel leaves in your grain jars to keep them at "bay."

Whistle while you work

Most essential oils are antibacterial, antifungal, and antiviral, so they disinfect your house to eliminate a much smaller bug: germs. These extra aromatherapy household tips may not make household chores more enjoyable, but they certainly will be more fragrant. If you're too tired to get the housework done, then make sure you're using an essential oil with an energizing scent (or add an extra drop of one to the recipe). If you're feeling depressed because you'd rather be doing anything but these chores, then go for an antidepressant.

Here are ways that you can keep the germ population in your household down and have your home smell good at the same time.

- **Air spray:** An all-purpose disinfectant spray goes a long way to declaring your home a germfree zone. Use it on the floors, countertops, and sinks (and walls if they're painted with glossy paint) in your kitchen and bathrooms. Add ¼ teaspoon eucalyptus and ¼ teaspoon lemon oil to ¼ teaspoon vinegar and ½ cup water.

- **Dishes:** It's likely that your dishwashing detergent already has a citrus scent. If not or if it's very mild, increase its disinfecting ability by adding 15 drops of lemon, lime, or orange to a 10-ounce bottle of detergent. (To keep your hands looking like they never did all those dishes, use the more pricy bergamot oil instead.)

- **Dishwasher:** Add 2 drops lemon or orange oil to the detergent in your dishwasher's soap compartment. This won't do much to scent the dishes themselves, but it works wonders on a smelly dishwasher.

- **Sponges:** Place 3 drops lavender oil on your kitchen sponges and clip them securely in your dishwasher with a clothes pin the next time you wash your dishes.

- **Refuse pails and garbage cans:** Dab a few drops of tea tree or eucalyptus oil on a scrap of paper and throw it in the pail or can.

- **Vacuum cleaner:** Take a small scrap of fabric and place about 10 drops of an essential oil on it. Throw this into the bag of your vacuum cleaner. Even if you have an airtight model so that you can't enjoy the fragrance, it will help to disinfect your vacuum bag.

- **Clothes dryer:** Next time you do the laundry, take a small scrap of fabric that has about 20 to 30 drops of an essential oil on it. It will lend its scent to all the clothes, towels, or sheets, and it certainly makes folding the laundry an aromatic experience!

- **Hand-washed delicate fabrics:** When washing your delicate woolens or lingerie by hand, add 1 to 2 drops lemongrass, petitgrain, or bergamot oil.

On you: Wash those lice right out of your hair

Let's hope that you never have to deal with body lice, but it happens. Just in case, I include a recipe. These oils work somewhat as repellents. However, with lice, as well as their more resilient eggs, it's cause to bring out the killer oils. It takes potent essential oils to do the job, so be very careful that you don't get them into your eyes or burn your scalp. Test a tiny dab on the skin first, especially on children, to make sure that it doesn't burn or cause skin reactions.

Along with the essential oil, you'll need to do some dedicated washing, in hot water, of all the bedding and clothes that were exposed to anyone with lice. Any furniture where heads have laid needs washing or temporarily retirement for about two weeks so that any newly hatched lice will die before they can set up housekeeping again on your head. Also, run a very fine "lice" comb through your hair to remove eggs.

Try these essential oils to battle lice. (I indicate the oils that have been tested in scientific studies with an asterisk.)

- Cinnamon leaf* (not bark, which doesn't contain enough eugenol to be effective)
- Eucalyptus
- Geranium
- Lavender
- Oregano*
- Pennyroyal
- Peppermint*
- Rosemary
- Tea tree
- Thyme* (the type called linalol is gentle enough to use, yet it's still effective)

For a preventive treatment, add 4 drops of one of these essential oils to a mixture of 1 ounce vinegar and 1 ounce water. Use as a hair rinse.

Get Rid of Lice

This is a real killer blend, so use it carefully and be sure to keep it out of your eyes. Testing a tiny dab on the skin first, especially on children, is a good idea to make sure that it does not burn or cause skin reactions. This recipe calls for coating your hair with vegetable oil, which smothers the lice and prevents them from making a mad dash to get away from the essential oils. Be prepared that the oil isn't easy to wash out of your hair. You probably need to shampoo your head a couple times, and even then it will feel a little greasy. (In case it makes you feel better about having greasy hair, the vegetable oil, especially olive oil, actually makes a very good hair-conditioning treatment, especially if your hair tends to be dry or split easily.)

Preparation time: 3 minutes

Yield: 2 ounces antilice treatment

20 drops tea tree

10 drops rosemary

10 drops thyme (because thyme can burn your scalp, use the linalol type which is effective without getting too hot)

5 drops lavender

2 ounces vegetable oil

1 Combine ingredients.

2 Apply the oil to dry hair, cover with a plastic bag or a shower cap, and then wrap your head in a towel. (Comb your hair well before dosing it with oil. Otherwise, you can end up with a tangled mess.)

3 After 1 hour, shampoo your hair without wetting it first to help remove the oil. Rinse and shampoo again. (If your scalp feels irritated before the time is up, go ahead and wash it out right away.)

4 Lice eggs are very resistant, so repeat this treatment in a week and then again in 2 weeks to destroy any newly hatched lice.

Tip: In between treatments, do a preventive hair rinse. You can make this by adding the same number of drops called for in the recipe to 1 cup vinegar. To rinse your hair, shake the vinegar mix well. Then add ¼ cup of it to 1 cup water and use this as your final hair rinse, making sure that you rub it well into your scalp. Lightly rinse with water.

What about insecticides?

The case against using household and garden chemical insecticides and cleaners are the strong chemicals in them. Studies show that some of these chemicals possibly promote cancer and other disorders, such as kidney, spleen, and liver damage. Even being exposed to small amounts over the long term may have health hazards, resulting in nausea, diarrhea, nervous system problems, and skin eruptions. Most of these chemicals are absorbed through your skin and can be inhaled. The products are still on the market because these findings are still unproven, but be especially careful in using household and garden chemicals if you're pregnant.

When you read the labels on household cleaners, don't confuse the names of chemicals with some of the compounds found in essential oils or in the oils themselves. For example, benzene, which is classified by the Federal Drug Administration in the United States as the fifth most hazardous air pollutant, is quite different than the essential oil called benzoin. The powerful chemical germ fighter phenol, which rapidly corrodes skin, is produced from coal tar and is not phenol compounds derived from essential oils.

In the Great Outdoors

My first experience with aromatic bug repellents was impressive, but it wasn't to keep the bugs off me, but out of my garden. I lived in a community where almost every yard had a vegetable garden. My garden had a reputation for being unusual because I tucked so many medicinal and fragrant herbs among the vegetables. I gave my first herb "walks" through my garden for curious neighbors.

My garden soon gained a reputation for more than herbs. Unlike everyone else's garden, it was an oddball in the neighborhood because there were almost no bugs. I could step on a rock and peer over the fence down into my next-door neighbor's garden to see it crawling with wildlife — the unwanted kind! Tomato hornworms, cabbage worms, aphids, and Japanese beetles — they were all there happily munching down the vegetables, but they weren't bothering my vegetables. It didn't take rocket science to figure out that the scent emanating from all my herbs was either too annoying or simply covering up the signals that these pests rely on to seek out food.

On the other hand, at least half of the honey bees in the entire community seemed to be centering their activity around my plants, helping my garden to produce a bumper crop. Many gardens later, I still find this to be true. The abundance of scented herbs that I grow detracts predators to my vegetables but does attract the bees.

This success with keeping bugs out of my garden got me thinking how well some of these same herbs might work to keep bugs off me. My amateur attempts at rubbing various fragrant plants on my arms, legs, and face were fairly successful, but those green streaks left by the smashed plants on my skin made me look like I was decorated with war paint. That's when I started making my own liquid insect repellents. Nowadays, you've got it easy. There are dozens of bug repellents available, not only for you, but for your dogs and cats, too. In this section, I also give you a few recipes in case you want to play mad scientist in your kitchen and create your own concoctions.

On you: Bug out

There's something disconcerting about enjoying the fresh air and the beautiful plants and then to hear the high-pitched whine of a mosquito zeroing in on some patch of exposed skin. It's enough to make you not want to venture past the protection of your screen door. That's where nature's insect repellents come in handy to distance yourself from flying pests such as mosquitoes.

I'll be the first to admit that, when it comes to mosquitoes, aromatherapy bug repellents don't work better than the standard drugstore variety, but they're good alternatives to putting the chemicals found in those repellents on your skin. Considering the potent chemical insecticides that are used in bug repellents, aromatherapy is far safer.

A citronella candle is one way to reduce the number of insects hovering around you without wearing a repellent. Impregnated with citronella, these candles release the scent as they burn. They're available from most camping and household stores and catalogs. (Also, see how to scent your own candles in Chapter 5.)

You can try these essential oils as insect repellents:

- ✔ Cedarwood
- ✔ Citronella
- ✔ Eucalyptus
- ✔ Geranium
- ✔ Pennyroyal
- ✔ Sandalwood

Insect Repellent for You

The good news is that mosquitoes hate the smell of eucalyptus, pennyroyal, and citronella. Unfortunately, so will many of your friends. I like to add a touch of geranium to give the brew a little better aroma. Geranium is a minor bug repellent in itself. Use this flea, mosquito, fly, and tick repellent sparingly because it's potent stuff. Keep it away from your eyes and mouth because it can sting. (Be careful that you don't rub your eyes right after applying the repellent with your fingers.) Also, remember that rubbing alcohol is poisonous to drink. This repellent lasts over a year once you make it. (If you're pregnant, eliminate the citronella and pennyroyal and, even then, use this very sparingly.)

Preparation time: *10 minutes*

Yield: *2 ounces insect repellent*

¼ teaspoon citronella oil	*⅛ teaspoon cedarwood oil*
¼ teaspoon eucalyptus oil	*⅛ teaspoon geranium oil*
⅛ teaspoon pennyroyal oil	*2 ounces vodka or rubbing alcohol*

1 Combine ingredients. Be sure to store it in a glass container because such a strong concentration of essential oils can eat through plastic.

2 Use by dabbing on here and there. Dab wherever mosquitoes tend to hover, such as around your head and ankles.

Bites and stings

If you do get stung or bit, nature fortunately provides as many remedies as she does insects. Use essential oils that reduce inflammation to stop the itching and swelling of bites and stings. It's a good idea to have a bite oil handy. That way, even when you've just been stung and you're in a hurry to slap on a remedy, you can avoid dabbing undiluted essential oil directly on your skin.

The only problem with aromatherapy remedies is that they work so well. You feel so good once the stuff takes effect that you need to remind yourself to restrict your activity for at least 20 minutes to prevent the poisons from circulating through your blood stream. If you tend to have an allergic reaction to that type of sting or bite or show any signs of impaired breathing, faintness, or shock, then get professional help right away instead of depending solely on aromatherapy first aid. (You can also take a half teaspoon of echinacea tincture every 10 minutes to reduce the reaction.)

Insect Bite Solution

A simple dab of essential oil of lavender or tea tree provides relief for a few mosquitoes or other insect bites that don't demand much attention. Chamomile, lavender, helichrysm, or tea tree oils reduce swelling, itching, and inflammation.

Preparation time: 4 minutes

Yield: ½ ounce bottle of bite oil

½ teaspoon lavender oil

½ teaspoon tea tree oil

1 tablespoon vodka or rubbing alcohol

1 Combine ingredients.

2 Store in a bottle with a tight lid. A glass container is best to store this oil, but if you prefer a lightweight, plastic container, choose one made of stiff plastic, which is more resistant to essential oils. It'll last at least a couple years if you store it in a cool, dark place.

3 Dab directly on bite as needed.

Vary It! *I prefer using an herbal tincture such as a tincture of calendula and echinacea of plain oil instead. In that way, I can combine herbs that help relieve an insect bite with aromatherapy.*

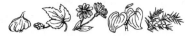

Bite, Sting, and Splinter Poultice

For more severe stings and bites of bees, wasps, ticks, and spiders, combine lavender with echinacea and make into a clay poultice. These ingredients work well together. The clay pulls the poisonous material from the bite or sting to the skin's surface and keeps it from spreading. Echinacea dramatically lessens any allergic response that might occur.

Preparation time: 10 minutes

Yield: About ⅛ cup clay poultice (paste)

1 tablespoon bentonite clay (you can find this clay in a natural-food store.)

1 teaspoon echinacea root tincture

1 tablespoon distilled water

12 drops lavender essential oil

(continued)

1 Add the tincture, water, and lavender oil individually to the clay.

2 Stir the liquid ingredients slowly into the clay until it absorbs the liquid into a consistency of thick paste. (It should be tacky enough to adhere to the skin.)

3 Store in a container with a tight lid so that the mixture does not dry out. Apply directly to bite as needed. If the mixture dries out, stir in enough distilled water to turn it back into a paste and keep it ready for an emergency.

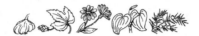

In Your Garden

Whether you have acres of crops, a little patch out back, or even a few cabbages in pots on your balcony, if you grow vegetables or flowers, you certainly have encountered bugs. They may be small, but, as you've surely discovered, bugs have colossal appetites.

Most of these bugs have it all wrong. They seem to think that you're on a mission to provide insects throughout your entire neighborhood with three to 20 square meals a day. You'd almost expect them to rise up and applaud with all of those little feet every time you step into your garden. Of course, that never happens. Instead, they just keep eating nonstop.

If you really want to get on a bug's nerves, then plant herbs that they hate in strategic locations around your garden. The scent of growing herbs is a powerful deterrent, and you get the benefits of having herbs to use and of not having destructive insects around. You can also make a garden spray to use directly on your plants as a natural insect repellent. One way to do this is to prepare it from your garden herbs by tossing a few sprigs of a repellent herb into your blender with enough water to liquefy it into a thin consistency and then straining it through cloth through the sprayer. Another method is to use the essential oils derived from these herbs to make your spray.

Declare your garden a bugfree zone

If you want a truly holistic approach to gardening — similar to what I recommend for your own health — then your best bet is to make your garden as healthy as possible. Insects, as well as plant diseases, tend to attack the least healthy plants. These are the ones that have a weaker "constitution," so they can't fight off predators and disease as easily as they should.

I'm a strong advocate of using organic gardening methods to create strong, vibrant plants. Organic compost is one of the best ways that you can enrich and condition any type of soil. If you're not already familiar with them, find out about using fish emulsion, liquid seaweed, and compost "tea" to help ailing plants.

Table 6-1 lists the fragrant herbs that fend off garden pests. The little research that's been done doesn't always back it up. I indicate with an asterisk which scents science says show promise. The others on the list may work equally as well, but science hasn't got around to testing them yet. For their repellent action, plant these herbs in your garden amongst your other plants and use them to make garden sprays. To make a spray, you can throw either the leaves of a plant or the essential oils themselves into a blender with vinegar and water. (You can find a recipe following this table.)

Table 6-1 Fragrant Herbs to Grow to Make Your Garden Pestfree

Pest	Best Herbs to Grow
Aphids	Cayenne, garlic (coriander, eucalyptus, fennel, garlic, hyssop, and peppermint are slightly less effective)
Asparagus beetle	Basil
Beetles	Eucalyptus, rosemary, geranium
Cabbage looper	Clary sage, dill, eucalyptus, garlic, hyssop, nasturtium, onion, pennyroyal, peppermint, sage, southernwood*, thyme, wormwood
Cabbage maggot	Garlic, sage, wormwood
Carrot fly	Onion, rosemary, sage, wormwood
Codling moth	Garlic, wormwood
Colorado potato beetle	Catnip*, coriander*, eucalyptus, French marigold*, nasturtium*, tansy*
Cucumber beetle	Catnip, nasturtium, rue
Japanese beetle	Garlic, tansy
Mexican bean beetle	Catnip, French marigold*, rosemary, savory
Nematodes	French marigold*
Peach borer	Garlic
Slugs and snails	Fennel, garlic, rosemary
Spider mite	Anise*, coriander, cumin*, oregano*
Squash bug	Catnip*, nasturtium, peppermint, tansy*
Tomato hornworm	Basil, dill, nasturtium, peppermint, thyme, wormwood
Whitefly	Nasturtium*, peppermint, thyme, wormwood

Indian neem tree knocks 'um dead

Neem tree *(Azadirachta indica)* is a tropical tree from India, where the smelly, highly antiseptic leaves are used on skin diseases and placed in strategic areas to discourage insects and now several natural insecticides use extracts from its leaves. Its actions are due partly to the essential oils it contains — and believe me, this is one strong-smelling plant. It kills young aphids, thrips, whiteflies, and the Colorado potato beetle by stopping their development and making it impossible for them to feed and/or digest their food. Although it doesn't instantly wipe out these pests, it's very effective after a few weekly applications. It also repels the Japanese beetle. Even though it's so effective, it doesn't harm most beneficial insects, and it's not toxic to people. Look for garden products that contain it.

The essential oils from a few plants have been developed into natural ingredient pesticides. One new herbal pesticide contains cinnamon oil, which counters many infections in people (see Chapter 11) and wipes out many insect pests and fungal diseases on your garden plants as well.

While most essential oils and fragrant herbs are used to repel insects, some work the other way around and lure pests. This attracts harmful insects away from your other plants. One example — the many species of *Nicotiana,* the tobacco plant, attracts rather than repel tomato hornworms. The scent of both ginger and angelica proved as effective as the standard chemical used in traps to capture the Mediterranean fruit fly, which has become a menace to fruit farmers in southern California and Florida. (The compound in the essential oil that does the trick is one that is found in many other essential oils as well.)

My experience with angelica is that it attracts just about every type of fly imaginable. I tried planting angelica by my doorway once after reading that it was a great fly repellent for your garden, but that book had it backwards. (Don't believe everything you read!)

Enough Already! All-Purpose Garden Spray

This all-purpose spray is made with both essential oils and herbs that contain essential oils. Spray it on your vegetables and flowers. (It works on your herbs, too, although they probably won't need it.)

Preparation time: 15 minutes

Yield: 4 ounces garden spray

5 cloves garlic

1 cup water

½ teaspoon cayenne powder

¼ teaspoon peppermint oil

¼ teaspoon rosemary oil

½ teaspoon liquid dishwashing detergent (biodegradable)

1 Put the garlic, cayenne, and water in a blender and mix.

2 Strain through a fine strainer. (If you don't have a fine enough strainer, then re-strain through a coffee filter. This mixture needs to be able to go through a sprayer when you use it.)

3 Stir in the essential oils and soap.

4 Put the solution in a spray bottle and head out into the garden. Any extra solution keeps for several days if stored in a cool place.

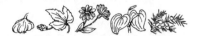

Man's Best Friend: Aromatherapy for Your Pet

No one likes the idea of having fleas in their house or on their pets, and especially on them! However, dosing Fido and Puss with conventional flea powders, soaps, dips, and collars is rough. These flea deterrents contain some of the most potent garden insecticides (usually organophosphates and carbamates). The problem is compounded because dogs, and especially cats, have thin skin that is far more porous than yours. They may have thick coats, but the poisons seep right in. When they groom themselves, they're also likely to ingest them. Flea killers can make them sick, causing nervous system problems, depression or hyperactivity, diarrhea, and vomiting.

In the dog house: Sending fleas fleeing

Not only are fleas uncomfortable, but they irritate your pet's skin and can initiate skin infections. Some fleas even carry a type of tapeworm that the pet can pick up when he licks his coat. And, fleas don't just stay on Fido and Puss. The eggs up residence in your carpets and in dusty corners (sorry to imply that you have any). Then they come out to bite the heck out of your ankles. Although they don't actually kill them, the following scents are guaranteed to make the fleas flee. All of these aromas are also fairly effective at keeping ticks off your pets (and off you).

- ✔ Bay laurel
- ✔ Camphor
- ✔ Chamomile
- ✔ Citronella
- ✔ Clove
- ✔ Eucalyptus
- ✔ Lavender
- ✔ Lemon
- ✔ Pennyroyal

Bee appreciative

If you're a beekeeper, you'll be interested to know about experiments using essential oils to control the parasitic mites that invade bee hives. These mites are a major problem that destroy from 5 percent to a third of the commercial bees in North America, and the wild honeybee population in North America is down about 90 percent. (Although surveys show that most people don't like to have bees around because they can sting, these are important little critters. Many, many plants depend upon bees to fertilize them. One-third to half the food you eat is dependent upon them.)

One method is to place a piece of florist block soaked with thyme, peppermint, eucalyptus, and camphor oils on the top frames inside the hive once a week. In one study, the essential oils almost completely wiped out the notorious *Varroa*

mites in about a month. Other studies focus on using menthol, a component of peppermint, to get rid of another type of mite. Methods such as these sure beat using potent pesticides.

I asked commercial beekeeper Randy Oliver of Golden West Bees for an overview of the essential oil studies. Randy says essential oils produce mixed results in reducing the mite population, but they show promise. He adds that even more important than selecting the right pesticide is selecting the right bees — healthy bees from a mite resistant strain and then keeping them that way. His preventive health approach to beekeeping parallels that of holistic medicine (the orientation toward health that I use throughout this book). That's a good idea if you want to make sure that your world continues to be filled with fragrant flowers.

Fido's Flea Collar

To make your pet a flea collar, use an absorbent string (a flat woven string is a good choice) that is comfortable on your pet's neck. As with any pet's collar, make sure that it's not so tight that it feels as it is choking your pet or so loose that it can get caught on something. This collar is effective as long as the scent remains. The scent disappears in about a week, so take it off and replace with a new one or add another dose of essential oils, following this same recipe.

4 drops eucalyptus oil

4 drops pennyroyal oil

small cotton heavy string, enough to fit around your pet's neck

1 Drop the essential oils along the string and allow it to dry for about 30 minutes.

2 Tie the string comfortably around your pet's neck.

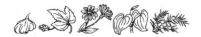

Whatever you do, don't dab essential oil right on your pet because it will go through their skin. They are also smaller than you and can overdose on much less essential oil, so be particularly careful when using these oils for pet care.

For a repellent, use a collar. It's the perfect place for a repellent because fleas like to congregate around a pet's warm and cozy neck. Fleas also like this location because it's impossible for your pet them to nip at them. You can purchase an aromatherapy collar in a natural-food store and in most pet stores. Read the ingredients to make sure that it contains essential oils without any of the toxic chemicals that are usually found in flea collars.

Another place to use flea repellent is in your pet's bed. You can make them a pillow that contains the appropriate herbs and/or essential oils. Or, mist your pet's existing bed and the surrounding area with an aromatherapy spray. (These are good ideas even if you don't have a flea problem to improve the smell of your pet's quarters.) Try a little at first to see your pet's response. Animals are usually attached to their bed and may not care for the same aromas that you do. They prefer more organic smells that you probably consider downright foul. (If you've been around any dog, you know exactly what they sniff when they're out on a walk.) One scent that usually goes over okay with a pet is cedarwood. In fact, you can buy dog beds that are filled with cedarwood chips. If you happen to have a wood shop at home and the floor, you have your own supply of cedarwood chips. (Go ahead and stuff them into a homemade dog pillow and save yourself 60 bucks.)

Orangicide: Killing fleas

Repelling fleas to keep them off your animals is a good idea, but if your pet already has fleas, then the repellent may not be strong enough to make them retreat. In that case, you'll need to outright kill them. You can do this by using one of the citrus oils. They contain a compound that is deadly to fleas. You certainly can't douse your pooch with essential oils, but you can shampoo him or her. The shampoo disperses the essential oils evenly. Several pet shampoos are already available that contain citrus oil (or the active compound in it) to do the deadly deed. You can also make your own antiflea shampoo. (See the following recipe.)

To shampoo your pet, start off by shampooing around his or her neck. (This is especially important if your dog has a ruff with much fur there.) When you douse your dog in water, the fleas start running to your dog's nose, and we both know that this is going to drive your dog crazy and make it difficult for you to shampoo his or her face without getting it in the eyes. (They must have enough of a flea brain to realize that a pet's face is the least likely thing to go under water.) So, I establish a "flea blockade" by first putting the shampoo around the edge of my pet's face and the neck.

So far, I've been referring to washing your dog because it's an activity that's probably already part of your dog's life. Your cat may be a different story. I've had cats that will tolerate a cat shampoo, although barely and constantly reminding me that this is not an appropriate way to treat a cat. Then I've had cats that I can't get near the water even if I'm wearing elbow-high protective gloves. Anyway, the technique works equally well on any furry creature, so I'll let you decide which pets to try.

Besides the essential oil treatment, feeding your pets a wholesome diet that includes brewer's yeast and garlic helps deter fleas. Fleas just aren't so interested in biting into a healthy animal as one that's in poor physical shape and eating poorly.

Flea Away Pet Shampoo

I use orange oil to make Flea Away Pet Shampoo because it not only gets rid of fleas, it kills them. Better yet, it's nontoxic to your dogs and cats or to you. Plus, it's an inexpensive essential oil that is easy to find. That's a combination that you certainly can't beat. Orange essential oil was "discovered" by a researcher at the Coastal Plain Agricultural Experimental Station in Georgia who observed fire ants dying after mechanics dumped a grease containing citrus oil on their ant hill. The researcher tried citrus on flies, which also died, and worked his way up to giving his cat a citrus oil flea bath.

You may not use all this shampoo during one washing. It depends upon how big a dog you have. If you don't use it all, save what's left for next time.

Preparation time: *2 minutes*

Yield: *½ cup shampoo*

1 teaspoon orange oil

½ cup shampoo (any type of dog or people shampoo will do)

1 Mix the oil and shampoo together.

2 Shampoo your dog enough to work up some real lather and massage it around. (Fido deserves something for putting up with a bath, and the massage works the lather around better. If you have some left over, save it for the next flea wash.

3 Rinse your dog thoroughly to remove the shampoo.

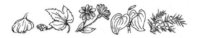

Once you've convinced the fleas to flee, your work isn't over yet. Flea eggs are most likely lying around anywhere that your pet hangs out, and they can stay there a couple of years before hatching. (Only about 20 percent of a household's flea population resides on your dog or cat at any one time.) Fleas are especially fond of warm humid places, so they can rapidly multiply in the summer months. The same day that you give your pet the bath, vacuum the floors and furniture, especially around your pet's favorite hang-outs. Then sprinkle the Flea Away House Salt (see next recipe) behind the furniture and in areas where dust tends to collect. If fleas are bad news around your house, you'll need to do this several times.

The cat's meow

This chapter covers both cats and gardens. Combine the two by planting catnip in your garden for your cats to enjoy. A funny thing about catnip's scent is that it energizes your cat, sometimes to the point of a frenzy, but it relaxes you. It has to do with the difference between your brain and your cat's. In people, the energetic reaction is subdued by the higher parts of our brain. Otherwise, you'd be out there rolling around in the catnip patch with your cat. Be sure to protect the plant while it's young, or your cat may roll a little too hard. Ground cover catnip can grow in a hanging pot, which keeps it out of paw length so that you can distribute the 'nip as an occasional treat, although you may find your cat playing Tarzan in an attempt to get to the pot.

An aromatic reward for your feline companion is a catnip toy. These are sold in pet supply and large grocery stores. Some of the mail-order sources in the Appendix offer them.

Flea Away House Salt

This salt is a repellent that keeps fleas from taking up residence in your house and preventing them from laying their eggs in dark, dusty, unseen, and untrampled areas. Simply sprinkle it on the carpet. Don't worry, the ingredients are harmless and won't trash your carpets. (However, one caution is if your pet's diet is lacking and he is attracted to salt, he may make up for it by licking up your flea powder, and that is both overload of salt and essential oils.)

Even though it contains only two ingredients, this is a well-tested recipe with a great track record because it's been sold for years sold as a fundraiser by the Northern California organization GASP (Group Against Spraying Poisons). The group reports lots of success. The salt absorbs the essential oil and retains the flea-discouraging scents longer.

Preparation time: *2 minutes*

Yield: *1 cup salt*

1 cup table salt

1 teaspoon lavender oil

1 Add the essential oil to the salt drop by drop to evenly distribute it.

2 Lightly sprinkle under your couch or in hidden corners — just the kind of out-of-sight places that fleas like to hide.

3 Store the extra in a glass jar.

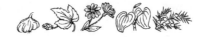

Chapter 7

Mirror, Mirror on the Wall: Aromatherapy for Us All

. . . .

In This Chapter

▶ Determining your skin type

▶ Buying products for your skin and hair

▶ Mastering cosmetic ingredients

▶ Treating your dry or oily skin

▶ Dealing with acne

▶ Caring for your hair

. . . .

> **Recipe in This Chapter**
>
> ▶ Scrub-A-Dub Oatmeal Scrub
>
>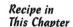

*B*ody-care products are selling big these days, and those that are tagged "aromatherapy" lead the pack. Take a quick tour of the body-care section in your favorite store, and you'll see aromatherapy creams, hair conditioners, complexion soaps, body and massage oils, bath salts, shower gels, and all sorts of items specially designed for your skin and hair.

This impressive success of aromatherapy doesn't surprise me. Aromatherapy benefits your health and beauty in numerous ways. Plus, aromatherapy has scents appeal. Aroma is often as important as anything else that a body-care product offers, and it plays a big role in choosing what you're going to put on your body. It certainly contributes to your enjoyment as you use it. Watch your initial reaction the next time you buy a skin lotion or hair rinse. I bet that the first or second thing you do is to open the lid to discover how it smells. In this chapter, I concentrate on how aromatherapy benefits your skin and hair, but the aromas also affect your moods. (See how in Chapter 1.)

Choosing body-care products can be a lot more complicated than other forms of aromatherapy, much more so than simply sniffing an aroma to heal an emotion or putting a scented cloth on your forehead to relieve your headache. If you feel confused when you encounter shelf after shelf of aromatherapy bottles and jars on your shopping spree, you're not alone. The question of how to choose the proper skin and hair preparations is one that I often hear from my students, customers, and even people who recognize me in the natural-food store and follow me down the aisle juggling a handful of items that they're considering! You may find yourself reaching for a destressing aromatherapy scent to inhale to help you through your decision making process!

Of course, you can always impulse buy and grab the one that smells the best, looks the best, and, if you have time to compare prices, is the cheapest. But, why not get products that really improve the health and beauty of your skin and hair? In this chapter, I take the stress out of shopping by making your task less overwhelming and, I hope, even fun. I divide the types of products that are available into a few categories. Then I help you figure out your own skin and hair type. When you put all of this together, it's a simple step to pick the best body-care products for you. This approach does take some effort, but it is worth it considering that you're talking about caring for your hair and skin.

Taking a Fresh Look at Life with Aromatherapy: Skin Care Products

A reasonable question to ask when you're considering which body-care product is whether you really need to put anything on your complexion. The answer is that it can only help. If you have dry or oily skin, or problems with acne, then what you put on your face can correct these imbalances. Even if you're blessed with normal skin that's not too oily or too dry, you still can benefit from complexion products to keep it that way.

When thinking about what you need for healthy skin, consider where you take your skin. Wind, icy-cold air, dry air, sun exposure, and air pollution are some of things that take a toll on your complexion. So do some less obvious conditions, such as the recycled air in an office, car, or airplane. This is especially true if you happen to sit directly in the line of the air stream. It may feel great on your face, but this is as drying to your skin as spending the day jet-skiing or sailing in a heavy wind.

You don't need lots of stuff on your skin. If you choose the best products for your skin type, then a few items that contain simple ingredients, including essential oils, is all you need. Many products are geared to your face because that's what has to face to world. Even when you're bundled up on a cold winter day, at least some of your face is still exposed and tackling the elements.

Stalking the Shelves of the Body-Care Store

It's hard to believe when you look at the wide assortment of products offered for sale, but only a few types are body-care preparations. However, there are many, many variations on those themes. Take a cream, for example. Instead of one kind, you can find rich night creams, cleansing creams to remove makeup, non-irritating creams for around your eyes, and first-aid creams for damaged skin, but they're all basically cream. Here are the main body-care classifications to help simplify your choices.

- ✔ **Body oil** is vegetable oil-based with essential oils added. It's rubbed on the skin as a massage, body, or bath oil. Because it provides a barrier to keep moisture off the skin, it also makes a good baby oil.

- ✔ **Cream** is a vegetable oil with water added, so it's an ideal moisturizer if you have dry skin. The heaviest and richest cream (containing 40 to 60 percent oil) is reserved for very dry skin.

- ✔ **Lotion** contains more water (50 to 90 percent) than oil, so it's thinner and less oily than cream and so it's better suited for normal to oily skin. It doesn't leave an oily coating and spreads easily over your skin.

- ✔ **Skin toner** is usually a non-oily base, often aloe or witch hazel distillate (sold in drugstores), making it ideal for oily skin. It improves circulation and skin "tone" (thus its name) to give your skin a healthful glow. It sometimes contains vinegar, although the smell makes this a less popular ingredient. (See the sidebar "About using vinegar on your skin and hair," later in this chapter.)

- ✔ **Facial mask** is an astringent, so it increases blood circulation to the skin and gently removes dead, surface cells. It also draws underlying water to your skin's surface. This ever so slightly puffs up your skin, so facial lines seem smaller. However, this illusion has a "Cinderella" effect. The magic wears off in a few hours as water is re-absorbed into your skin and evaporates into the air. You can make a mask from mashed fruit, honey, oil, ground herbs, oats, or yogurt. Whip some yogurt and fruit up in the blender, and you'll have a mask loaded with AHAs (see the sidebar later in this chapter). Adding papaya, pineapple, or ginger root helps soften your skin. Clay is the most drying mask, so don't overdo it and don't use it at all if you have a dry complexion or skin that is sensitive or easily irritated. Leave a facial mask on five to 30 minutes, unless it becomes uncomfortable, and then remove it.

Any type of skin care is most effective when the product lingers on your skin awhile. Timewise, a cream or lotion has much more opportunity to work on your face than a shampoo, hair conditioner, or soap, all of which remain on your skin or hair for only a few seconds before you wash them off.

Super suds: Shampoo and liquid soap

Sodium lauryl sulfate is the current darling of the soap world. It gives most shampoo, shower gels, liquid hand soaps, and toothpastes their suds. A detergent, it has no smell, blends with other ingredients, is not overly alkaline like regular soap, and best of all, produces super suds that everyone loves and expects in a cleanser. It's derived from coconut and sometimes other nut oils, so it sounds quite natural — or is it? Labels on products tell you only about the coconut, not the laboratory chemicals in it and the elaborate process it takes to produce it.

No one can argue that sodium lauryl sulfate is semi-natural, but it's equally accurate to say it's *semisynthetic* (artificially produced). Where a controversy arises is over this compound's safety, and there are plenty of pros and cons. It's fairly gentle, although it slightly irritates skin and can cause eye irritations, rashes, and even allergic reactions. It dries your skin and especially your hair, although most people do use skin lotion and hair conditioner to counter this. Of course, any skin or hair cleanser is usually on your skin for only seconds before being rinsed off, but then again, soaps are one of those everyday experiences.

Hang on to your hat, these are long names, but they're the ones that you'll encounter on the labels you read. And, I'm a firm believer that you should know what it is you put on your body. If you break them down, chemical names are easier to grasp. The *coco* part stands for coconut, *sodium* is salt, and *sucrose* and *glucose* are sugars.

The following are harsh cleaning compounds that use petroleum chemicals. They also may form some chemicals called *nitrosamines,* which are cancer-forming. DEA stands for di-ethanol-amine, and MEA is mono-ethanol amine. They improve the consistency of a product, stop it from separating, and are toxic if inhaled. However, the jury's still out about whether they're a major health problem. These are harsher, but sudsier, in comparison to sodium lauryl sulfate detergents.

- Cocomide DEA
- Cocomide MEA
- Lauramide DEA
- TEA and DEA-lauryl sulfate
- Cocoyl sarosine

Due to controversy, some companies use closely related products derived from coconut that don't suds quite so great, but still clean. When these names are combined with the words hydrolyzed protein, it's an especially mild sudser. These are the gentle detergents:

- Sodium laureth (instead of lauryl) sulfate
- Sodium cetyl sulfate
- Sodium myristoyl sarcosinate
- Potassium cocoate
- Coca betaine
- Sucrose or polyglucose cocoate (very mild, but difficult to formulate into liquid soap)

You face even more choices when it comes to washing your skin and hair. A hundred years ago, it was easy. There were no choices. Everything was washed with plain bar soap: skin, face, hair, floors, and even clothes. Nowadays, things have changed. Skin and hair cleansers come in all sorts of shapes and consistencies, and most of them aren't even soap. Here are the cleansing products for your skin and hair.

✔ **Bar soap** is very alkaline, which helps it removes dirt, but this also makes it harsh, especially on delicate skin and dry skin. Unless you have oily skin, use soap on your face only when you need to remove dirt, grime, or grease. (When you do use bar soap, you can quickly restore your skin back to its natural acidity with a product that contains vinegar. See the sidebar in this chapter about vinegar on your skin and hair.)

✔ **Glycerin soap** is produced during the soap-making process and then removed to make soap more concentrated and clean better. These days, many people prefer the gentle action of glycerin soap. It's translucent and easily molded so that the soap is often brightly colored and formed in interesting shapes.

✔ **Liquid skin soap** is popular because it's dispensed in a pump, which is convenient and more hygienic than a bar soap that is shared by everyone. It usually has a balanced pH so that it isn't overly alkaline. Most liquid soap is made with sodium lauryl sulfate, although this petroleum product is questionable for use on your skin.

✔ **Shampoo** is made with sodium lauryl sulfate, except for a few gentler shampoos that are formulated for babies and sensitive skin (and are often derived from olive and soy oils). Hardly anyone still uses the old-fashioned method of washing hair with soap flakes that have been dissolved in water because this leaves your hair stiff and dull-looking unless it's rinsed with vinegar afterwards.

✔ **Bath gel** is a liquid shower soap made with sodium lauryl sulfate usually diluted, or sometimes another detergent, to produce fewer suds than shampoo.

✔ **Facial sauna** cleanses your skin, removes dead surface cells, opens clogged pores, increases circulation, and moisturizes your face. Do a facial steam twice a week if you have oily or average complexion. (See the sidebar on facial steam if you're not sure how.) If you have dry skin, a facial sauna slightly stimulates more oil production, but don't try it more than once a week or it can be too irritating. Avoid facials altogether if you have very dry or sensitive skin or visible red blood vessels near your skin's surface (called a *couperose complexion*) because heat can worsen these conditions. See the instructions in the sidebar "Giving yourself a facial sauna."

You can also purchase a facial steamer at a large drugstore. They plug in to produce steam that contains a few drops of essential oil. A soft padding on top of a large tube cradles your face so that you can experience the gentle aromatic steam.

✔ **Skin scrub** contains slightly abrasive material, such as ground almond shells (which can be too abrasive), cornmeal, or oatmeal (for a gentle scrub, see the next recipe). As the name implies, scrubs are lightly "scrubbed" on your skin during your shower or bath. They open clogged pores, remove surface skin and excessive oil, and encourage cell growth. Scrubbing dry skin a couple times a week stimulates oil production, but don't scrub daily or you'll expose young skin cells before they are ready to face the world. A scrub is not technically a cleanser, but if you're not covered with dirt, it is all you need to get clean. The following scrub is a good one to try.

Scrub-A-Dub Oatmeal Scrub

This scrub washes your skin when you're not dirty enough to need soap to cut through the grime. As you see, an ingredient list can't get much simpler than this one. You may already have everything you need waiting for you in your kitchen. You can use the scrub as is or make a "soap" bag by tying the corners of a piece of loose-weave cotton fabric (about 8 inches square) into a pouch and using it in place of bar soap.

Preparation time: *5 minutes*

Yield: *About ½ cup scrub*

2 tablespoons oatmeal	*¼ cup distilled water*
1 teaspoon cornmeal (optional)	*5 drops lavender oil*

1 Grind the oatmeal in an electric coffee grinder (clean out the coffee grounds first!) or blender.

2 Drop in the essential oils.

3 To use, add enough water to make a paste.

4 Gently massage your face for two minutes. Use the rest in 2 days or keep it in the refrigerator where it will last about a week.

Vary It! *Use rose water or aloe vera juice, both of which are excellent for your complexion, instead of the water.*

Giving yourself a facial sauna

Steam is a great way to carry essential oils directly to your face.

1. **Add about 8 drops essential oil to steaming water.**

   An alternative method is to pour boiling water over a handful of fragrant herbs to release their essential oils.

2. **Take the pan off the heat and set it where you can comfortably sit next to it.**

3. **Lay a towel over the back of your head, put your face over the steam, and secure the** ends of the towel around the pan to capture the steam (see the figure).

4. **Hold your face about 12 inches from the water with your eyes closed (so that the essential oil doesn't irritate them).**

   Steam for a minute or so and then remove your head and take several breaths of fresh air.

5. **Go back under the towel and repeat a few times.**

   Altogether, steam for five or ten minutes at the most.

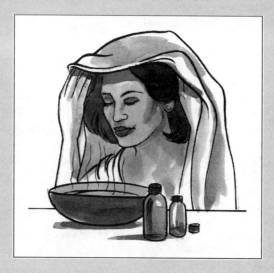

Choosing Aromatherapy Products: Totally A-Maze-ing

Choosing body-care items is hard because they contain an amazing number of ingredients. One list that I saw had more than 400 possible substances! This means that you, as a consumer, not only have to consider the quality and the uses of the essential oils in each formula, but also the numerous other ingredients that may or may not be suited for your skin and hair.

Ideally, ingredients such as vegetable oils, glycerin, lanolin, alcohol, and herbs work with essential oils to enrich your skin and hair. However, that's not all you'll find in the bottle. Body-care products also contain waxes and other stabilizers to prevent all the ingredients from separating. Preservatives may be needed to slow spoilage and additional ingredients provide a desirable color and texture. You don't need compounds like these in homemade aromatherapy products because they don't go through all the shipping, shaking, and long-term shelf-sitting demanded of a commercial product.

Mini-cosmetic glossary

Even if you're science-illiterate, you don't need to let chemistry intimidate you. After all, everything's made of chemicals, including you and me. You can approach chemistry talk just like a foreign language. The reason the names are so long is because the abbreviations for several chemicals are often tied together in a long chain (similar to the way a molecule looks). It makes it easier if you break big chemical names down into syllables, as I've done for you on this list. For example, if you see the ingredient dihydrogenoxide, guess what? It's water: H_2O or di (2)-hydrogen-oxide (oxygen).

The reason I'm explaining this is because I'm a firm believer that you should know what you put on your skin. By law, it's all listed there on the label. If you don't find an ingredient on this list (remember that there are hundreds of them), most natural-food stores have a cosmetic glossary. Here are some strange chemical names of manmade compounds that you'll see most often listed on those aromatherapy products that use them (not all do).

✔ **Benzo-phenone** (di-phenyl-ketone) helps retain scent and color, slows the breakdown of ingredients by ultraviolet rays, and is a sunscreen. *Potential problems:* Hives and skin reactions to sunshine, to name a few.

✔ **Carbomer** is one of the vinyl polymers used to thicken and prevent ingredients from separating.

✔ **Decyl alcohol** prevents a product from foaming and makes the scent last longer. It's found in orange and ambrette seeds, but commercially comes from petroleum.

✔ **Daizo-lidinyl urea** is a pesticide derived from alcohol that is now used as a cosmetic preservative. *Potential problems:* It may release toxic formaldehyde.

✔ **Glyceryl sterate** is produced during soap-making and then used to keep ingredients from separating. Considered safe only in the small amounts used in cosmetics.

✔ **Hyaluronic acid** is a protein in your skin that holds skin cells together.

✔ **Methyl-paraben** is a preservative and germ-fighter. *Potential problems:* Allergic reactions.

✔ **Meth-oxy-cinnamate** is a sunscreen with a fruity fragrance derived from cinnamon. *Potential problems:* Allergic skin rashes.

✔ **Panthenol** is vitamin B-5. It increases luster, moisture retention, and elasticity. It's said to repair and thicken hair.

- **PEG** stands for poly-ethylene glycol, a chemical similar to the ethylene glycol in your car's antifreeze. It's widely used to bind ingredients together into a slick consistency and to soften and protect skin. *Potential problems:* Ingesting a large dose damages your kidneys.

- **Phen-oxy-ethanol** is a preservative, bacteria fighter, and insecticide with a roselike fragrance that helps retain fragrance. It's derived from phenol.

- **Poly-sorbate**, derived from sorbitol (see later in this list), prevents oil and water from separating, controls foaming, and softens skin. *Potential problems:* Some forms cause allergic reactions.

- **Potassium sorbate** is derived from sorbitol (see later in the list) to inhibit molds and yeast and softens skin. *Potential problems:* Very mild skin irritation.

- **Propyl-paraben** kills bacteria and fungi as a popular preservative. *Potential problems:* Skin problems.

- **Sodium chloride** is common table salt that's used in most bath salts and some other products. It's astringent and antiseptic. *Potential problems:* Can be drying

- **Sorbitol** is derived from fruit or seaweed. It has a velvet-smooth feeling and prevents ingredients from separating.

- **Squalene** oil is an expensive antibacterial and scent preserver extracted from olive, wheat germ, and rice bran oils, or shark liver oil with a structure similar to human skin oil.

- **TEA** sounds herbal, but is actually tri-ethanol-amine, which makes cleaners less alkaline.

Usually, these additives are manmade chemicals with long names that don't just rattle off your tongue. A question that I hear often is "What's this really mean?" Not to say that manmade ingredients are inherently bad, but some are better for you than others. Some are downright questionable. The concern is that they're the new kids on the block, and determining how safe they are to use is not always easy.

Watch out for double talk and tricky wording on natural product labels. On one hand, a label will imply an ingredient is coconut when in reality, the finished product is a far cry from the original after being processed in a lab. On the other hand, no one proclaims that a nontoxic preservative like the tongue-twister phen-oxy-ethanol, which is derived from the toxic compound phenol. In either case, you end up with a brand new compound that simply borrowed parts (molecules) from the old one. This manmade process is called *synthesis*, so the end product is a *synthetic*. See the sidebar "Mini-cosmetic glossary" for a list of commonly used compounds.

Making choices: What's best for me?

Life is filled with choices. Choosing your body-care products is no exception. Finding the perfect item is really a process of elimination. Work through the maze of products to narrow down your selection to a few suitable items. Most important: Read those labels. Body-care products must list all the ingredients they contain in order of their quantity, with the most abundant first. (I know a few manufacturers who conveniently leave out or overly simplify the names of chemicals that are in their products, but hopefully most companies are honest.)

Here's what you look for on a label:

- **Essential oils:** Of course, you should see essential oils or fragrant herbs on the label — that's what makes it an aromatherapy product in the first place.

- **Nonsynthetic essential oils:** It's a good sign if the label lists essential oils individually rather then grouping them together as "essential oils" or "fragrance oils." The word fragrance in particular smacks of possible synthetics. In the body-care industry, this term usually denotes artificial essential oils. (Herbs, fragrant or otherwise, should also be listed separately.) Look for any obvious synthetics, such as peach, cherry, lilac, gardenia, and violet flower. If you spot even one synthetic, you may want to dump the entire line from your consideration and move on to another brand. If a company includes synthetics in one product, it is likely that they incorporate them in others. Once your nose discovers a thing or two about scent, you can also sniff out synthetic essential oils. (Find hints on how to do so in Chapter 2.)

- **Familiar names:** Okay, the essential oils seem authentic, but you had better check the rest of the ingredients. Look for names that are recognizable, such as almond oil and lanolin, rather than multisyllable tongue twisters. When the label says something is "derived from," then it is likely to be at least partly synthetic. It doesn't mean that it's bad — just be aware that "derived from coconut oil" is not the same thing as coconut oil. To help you with the label lingo, I list the most common cosmetic ingredients in the sidebar "Mini-cosmetic glossary," and I explain which ones are safe, questionable, or potentially toxic.

You should also consider the following points once you've narrowed down your choices to a few good product lines:

- **The best essential oils for your skin type:** Look for the products that contain the essential oils that are best for your skin and hair type. If you're not sure which type of skin or hair you have, then read on. I tell you how to determine this in the section "Type casting: What's your skin type?" later in this chapter.

✔ **The best type of product for your skin type:** Now you've gone natural with your selection, but you're still holding an armful of creams, toners, conditioners, and lotions. Consider what you need by thinking about what exactly you need. Is it a skin moisturizer for dry skin, a suntan oil to prevent burning, or a toner to reduce acne that's troubling you? Asking yourself what it is that you want to prevent or change concerning your skin or hair should reduce your selection considerably.

✔ **Compare prices:** Only now do you compare the prices. You often do have to pay a little more for pure, natural products. Ironically, it's often that the fewer and simpler the ingredients, the higher the price. However, it's generally worth it if those ingredients include high quality essential oils. Even if your pocketbook is tight, before you put that perfect aromatherapy product back on the shelf because it costs too much, consider how long it will take you to use it. You may not really be stretching your income if you pay an extra $3.50 for a body lotion or shampoo that lasts you a month or two.

Beyond the glitz and glamour: Narrowing your selection

Being picky about where you shop is one way to limit your choices. You may find a few high-quality aromatherapy products on the shelves of department stores and occasionally in drugstores, but your best luck finding the top-of-the-line stuff is in a store that specializes in natural products. Herb, natural cosmetic, natural-food stores, and herbal or aromatherapy mail-order catalogs are good choices. An added bonus is that you're more likely to find clerks who are informed about natural body care.

Even though you've carefully chosen a store that offers natural products, you're bound to find a lot of items with borderline ingredients. No matter what you're told or what you read, cast a skeptical eye toward marketing ploys. After all, what's really important is what is in the bottle, not what's on the outside — or what's in the sales brochure.

Wade through the competition and the claims that "our" product is better than another. One company may brag that their ingredients — including essential oils — are processed in a way that makes them more potent than anyone else's product. Of course, sometimes it's true, but not always. Similar to the candidates in a political election, a product is rarely as good as it claims, and the competitor is seldom all evil. The more exaggerated the claims are that you hear, the more farfetched they may be. No matter what they promise, there's no genie who will pop out of the bottle to grant you a perfect complexion.

Don't let fancy ingredients turn your head, either. The name of the game in marketing is not only to look better, but to be different. The more unique that a product seems, the better the chance that consumers buy it. You'll see products that include exotic herbs, vegetable oils, or essential oils that you've probably never heard or ones that come from obscure places in the world. Sure, some of these items are really all that their label claims, but many times their exceptional properties are really no better than the commonly used lavender or chamomile offered by their competitor. I'm not suggesting that you always stick to the familiar, but be aware that exotic doesn't necessarily imply better (and that it usually does mean that it is more expensive).

Aromatherapy lends itself to some very pretty packaging, and certainly an attractive container and box do stand out. Once again, keep your cool and don't be overly influenced by glitz and glamour. I'll admit that I'm initially as easily swayed by a beautiful bottle as the next consumer, but try to refrain from thinking how nice a pretty bottle could look on your bathroom counter. Instead, concentrate on what it does to your skin or hair.

Go natural, baby

Now that you're holding yourself back from grabbing the blue-faceted bottle with the jeweled lid and the ingredients from Bora Bora, you're ready for some serious investigation. If this sounds as if you should come to the store dressed like private eye Sherlock Holmes and armed with a magnifying glass, it might not be a bad idea. At least the magnifying glass will come in handy when you try to read the tiny print listing the ingredients on the label. I think that it's backwards, but a pretty jar and label stand out, while the ingredients — the most important part — are in tiny, tiny print.

Your assignment is to search for ingredients on the labels that are as pure and natural as possible. Sure, everything is made of chemicals. However, natural ingredients have a much longer track record for efficacy and safety than manmade compounds that are whipped up in a laboratory. I may be old-fashioned, but I feel most comfortable putting chemicals that come directly from nature on my skin and hair rather than newfangled ingredients. My skin care rule is, "Don't leave anything on your skin that you wouldn't put in your mouth."

As you read the labels, you can't help noticing that some companies put more effort than others into having natural products. Of course, it's not easy making a commercial body-care product without fancy ingredients that hold it together and preserve it. Yet, some companies do manage to produce fine products using a fairly simple list of natural ingredients.

About using vinegar on your skin and hair

Here's an example of a new idea that's as old as the hills that has been renamed and converted into one of the latest rages in skin moisturizers, toners, masks, and cleansers: AHAs. This stands *for alpha-hydroxy acids,* which are found in several natural products that have long been used as cosmetics to enhance the complexion. The best known is vinegar.

For most of history, vinegar was used for skin care because it's easy to make, is far less sticky than the other contenders to slap on your skin, and doesn't spoil. However, after a glorious history as a facial toner and hair rinse, vinegar fell from fashion in the 19th century due to its strong smell. (If you're concerned about smelling like pickles afterwards, don't worry — the odor quickly dissipates.) A few vinegar facial products are still produced by herbalists who know vinegar's long-standing reputation. (See the Appendix.)

The reason that these acids, like the ones found in vinegar, are so great is because they moisturize and soften your skin, temporarily smooth out fine lines and enlarged pores, improve texture and discoloration, and maintain your skin's natural acidity. They're suitable for all types of skin and hair and quickly change your skin back to its natural acidity when used to rinse your hair or skin. As if that's not enough, AHAs also help to heal skin infection, psoriasis, eczema, and blemishes. As a result, the concentrated acids are now added to many skin care products, although the pure substance must be greatly diluted or they can irritate your skin.

AHAs are so common you can find them already lurking elsewhere in your kitchen. Yogurt, sour milk, wine, and some fruit juices are also all loaded with these acids. It's no wonder legendary beauties such as Cleopatra bathed in sour milk or wine! Other kitchen sources for AHAs are fruits, sugar, and apples. The purified form used in cosmetics is derived either from these sources, most often sugar, or from petroleum. (My dad, a chemical engineer, used to produce petroleum-derived AHAs in the '40s.) In high concentrations, the purified form is caustic, so you can use it as a facial peel to remove the surface layer of your skin and make your complexion look fresher and younger.

E-scentually Yours: Oils for Skin and Hair

Here's the impressive list of the ways that essential oils heal and beautify your skin and scalp. Don't expect to find each and every one of these properties in all essential oils, but many oils do more than one thing. In addition, some essential oils are stronger in certain properties than others. One may be an amazing antiseptic, while another one works like magic to decrease swelling. (Read more about each oil's properties in the Aroma Guide.)

The acid test

Knowing something about acid and alkaline helps you make decisions about what to use on your skin and hair. These are the opposite ends of a scale that determines a chemical response. They're measured on a pH scale starting with acid at 0 and increasing to extremely alkalinity at 14.

Healthy skin is slightly acid, say around pH 4.5 to 5.5. This allows it to fend off bacterial and fungal infection and to prevent your skin from being tender. When you use an alkaline product — soap is a good example — your skin or hair turns alkaline and then should rapidly return back to its normal acidity. At least that is true in an ideal skin care world. Some people's skin and scalp remains alkaline for quite awhile, making

it susceptible to itching, infection, and rashes. When your hair is too alkaline (with a pH of 9 or more), the hair shafts swell and their outer layer becomes flaky, giving your air a frizzy, fly-away appearance.

You can test the acidity verses the alkalinity of a product using *nitrazine paper* pH test strips that are sold in any drugstore. Follow the directions on the package and apply a little of the product on the strip. Like magic, the strip will turn color, indicating your body-care product's pH. It should be in the pH 4.5 to 7.5 range. That's slightly acid and close to the ideal range of your skin. Hair normally has a pH around 5 so the closer your hair products come to this, the better.

Here's what essential oils do for your skin:

- Penetrate lower skin layers to work on moisturizing and healing. (See Figure 7-1 for a diagram of skin layers.)
- Stimulate and regenerate skin cells, to heal skin damaged by sun, burns, wrinkles, or injury.
- Destroy infectious bacteria, viruses, and fungi, such as those associated with acne and other skin problems.
- Reduce inflammation and puffiness.
- Soothe sensitive or injured skin.
- Regulate over- or underactive oil glands.
- Encourage removal of waste products.
- Contain plant "hormones" (for hormonally related skin problems).
- Treat stress-related skin problems.

TIP

For a truly special product, you can consider not only how an essential oil benefits your skin and hair, but its other properties. For example, choose an essential oil that is good for your skin, relaxes your muscles, and is an antidepressant. (The answer? There are several: Lavender, chamomile, ylang ylang, and rose.)

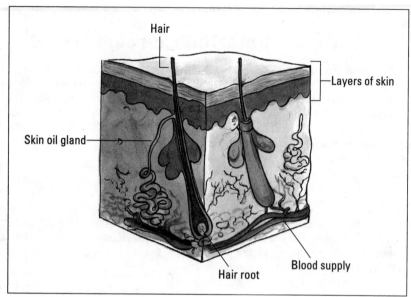

Figure 7-1:
A close-up of the skin layers, hair, and oil glands of your skin.

Type casting: What's your skin type?

To figure out what essential oils and products you need, you need to first determine your skin type. If your complexion is oily, you want to use something that contains essential oils and other ingredients that differ from somebody who has dry skin. Take everything into consideration. Do you tend to get acne and have overly sensitive skin? Are you dealing with a skin problem such as eczema or trying to prevent premature wrinkles? Also consider where you go and what you do. When you're in the sun or wind, maybe sailing or skiing, you need extra protection so that your skin doesn't dry out or burn.

See which categories best describe your complexion. If some places are dry and others oily, you have combination skin — for example, your forehead and around your nose are oily, and the other areas are dry. If so, use two different skin care products, or one specially designed for combination skin.

- ✔ **Dry skin** doesn't produce enough oil, so it tends to be flaky and look dull.

- ✔ **Oily skin** produces too much oil, making it shiny. It may even feel greasy to the touch.

- ✔ **Normal skin** is just right. It isn't too dry or too oily.

If you're wondering what kind of complexion you have, you can try this experiment. Go to bed one night without putting any creams, lotions, or anything on your face. Cut three small strips of paper from a clean brown paper bag. In the morning before you wash or do anything to your face, press a paper on your

---

The inner truth: Hints for skin and hair

No matter what you put on the outside of your skin and hair, it' really what's inside that counts. Having healthy skin and hair depends on your general health — and even more on what you put in your body than what you put on your skin. Healthy skin and scalp need oxygen and nutrients to bring your skin nourishment, and young skin cells are especially heavy feeders. Here are nature's guidelines for maintaining a glowing complexion.

✔ **Eat a balanced diet.** Skin and scalp cells need to be properly fed just like other cells in your body. Regardless of what a product claims, very little of what you put on your skin and scalp provides nutrients. Those come from the food you eat. Eat a wholesome diet and vegetable oils like olive oil that are rich in essential fatty acids. Avoid fried foods, which interfere with your body's oil metabolism.

✔ **Take vitamin C.** Eating a vitamin C-rich diet or taking supplements helps build collagen, your skin's structural framework. Like a trampoline, collagen gives your skin strength and bouyancy. Wrinkles appear when collagen begins to age and lose its integrity.

✔ **Drink water.** Water is nature's moisturizer. It's what gives your skin its plumpness. If you don't drink enough water, your skin and scalp has no resource tank, so it becomes dehydrated. For a graphic comparison, think about the difference between a plum and a prune!

✔ **Avoid stress.** Of course, easier said than done, but stress puts a strain on all of your body and is reflected in your skin and hair. For one thing, stress uses up vitamins B and C, decreasing the amount that is available to your skin and scalp.

✔ **Exercise.** Cells in your skin and scalp depend on good blood circulation to provide a steady supply of nutrients and to carry away waste products. Exercise your muscles to move blood and lymph through your body.

✔ **Get plenty of sleep.** Sleep improves your general health. Your body also uses sleep time to build up your immune system to better fight off infection and disease, including skin, scalp, and hair problems.

---

chin, one on your nose, and the third on your forehead. Keep these on for at least five seconds each. If you have oily skin, you'll see a definite oil stain on the paper strip. Dry skin leaves no oil on the paper at all. Normal skin shows only a slight stain caused by a small amount of oil.

The more you can define your skin, the easier it is to pick out the perfect products for it. In addition to thinking about how dry or oily your skin is, you may also need to take a special condition into consideration. You may find that more than one of the following conditions describes your skin. For example, your dry skin may be mature skin with acne and also sensitive.

✔ **Acned skin** breaks out easily in pimples. In severe cases, this can leave scarring. Use skin care products that are designed to counter the inflammation and infection that often accompanies pimples and blackheads.

✔ **Mature skin** tends to have wrinkles and is thinner and not as plump as younger skin. Use products that keep down irritation and help to rejuvenate your skin cells.

✔ **Skin with enlarged blood vessels** is also called a *couperose complexion*. Avoid heat and essential oils that encourage blood near the surface.

✔ **Sensitive skin** may be sun-damaged or easily flare up with an allergic reaction. Treat it gently with products that reduce sensitivity and inflammation and contain skin healing ingredients.

✔ **Skin problems** such as psoriasis or eczema or a constant infection like ringworm need extra care. Look up these conditions in the Symptom Guide to find out more about how to care for them.

Just like your skin, your hair can be too dry or too oily. It's not actually the hair itself that produces oil, it's your scalp, which is skin, so it's usually the same type as your complexion. If you have dry skin, you probably have a dry scalp. If you're skin is oily, then your scalp is likely also oily. Likewise, they are helped by the same remedies.

Normal skin and hair: Essential oils for everyone's complexion

I am starting off with the most versatile essential oils of all. The following essential oils are good for your skin and hair, whatever the type. They're suitable for hair or skin that is dry, too oily, or a combination. Each one has nearly all of the skin care properties I list in the section "E-scentually Yours: Oils for Skin and Hair," earlier in this chapter. In addition, they're extremely gentle and safe. This great combination of actions makes them the most popular body-care essential oils and the ones that you'll read most often on labels.

✔ Geranium

✔ Jasmine

✔ Lavender

✔ Neroli

✔ Rose

✔ Ylang Ylang

A slick question: Caring for your oily skin and hair

Oily skin has much luster, and may even be shiny from all the oil. Oil reflects light to give it a smooth, silky texture and a healthy looking glow. It protects your skin from drying so that it takes longer to develop wrinkles. However, having oily skin is not always as slick as it looks. It creates coarser texture that is prone to enlarged pores and acne. The real downfall is that the excess oil clogs your pores and then acts like a sponge to collect dirt and skin cells that are shedding that leads to pimples, blackheads, and infection.

If you have oily skin, wash daily with an aromatherapy soap to remove the excess oil. Skin lotion is better than cream because it contains less oil. Some witch hazel and grain alcohol in a skin toner help dry your skin, but don't overdo it; too much drying actually works against you by encouraging your skin to produce more oil. Vinegar is good for oily skin. A hydrosol made from any of the herbs I describe in this section is also good choice. (See Chapter 1 for a description of hydrosols.)

Just like oily skin, oily hair has an attractive shine, but too much makes it look dull, lifeless, and heavy. You need to get to the root of the problem: Roots of your hair where the oil is produced and where it concentrates. Brushing your oily hair from the roots to the tips helps to distribute the oils. Wash it frequently and brush beforehand to make it easier to remove the excess oil. Don't use protein or balsam shampoos because they attract oil.

Here is a list of the essential oils that are best for oily skin and hair.

- Basil
- Cedarwood
- Clary sage
- Cypress
- Eucalyptus
- Helichrysum
- Juniper berry
- Lemon
- Lemongrass
- Myrtle
- Palmarosa
- Patchouli
- Sage

Hair-raising experience

One innovative aromatherapy gadget for your hair is a scent infuser that fits on the end of your blow dryer. This tube holds a small, absorbent disk with a few drops of your choice of an essential oil. It's guaranteed to be a hair-raising experience! The package suggests using essential oils for their mood-changing aromas, but you might as well pick out an essential oil to not only change your mood, but that is good for your hair as well. What pops into my mind is rosemary. It's the most often recommended essential oil for your hair and its scent improves your memory. (While you're at it, you can use your blow dryer to scent your clothing and linens and to calm down your dog as you dry him after his bath.)

- ✔ Sandalwood
- ✔ Tea tree
- ✔ Vetivert

Dry wit: Caring for your dry skin and hair

Dry skin has its advantages because it tends to develop less acne. However, skin normally contains 50 to 75 percent water to stay soft and supple. If it gets too dry, look under a strong magnifier, and you'll see a resemblance to a dry lake bottom in the Sahara desert: A rough, flaky, cracked surface layer of skin with dry areas that slightly curl up on the edges. (See Figure 7-1, earlier in this chapter, for a diagram of skin layers.) The lack of oil in dry skin and hair also makes them look rough and dull because they don't reflect light.

The source of your hair's problem of too little oil is your scalp. Once hair leaves your scalp, it's dead, and it depends upon oil from your scalp to coat it. Underlying skin cells rapidly reproduce into a tightly packed layer that gradually moves upward to replace surface skin as it flakes off. Dry skin has a tendency to shed too quickly, and the underlying skin and scalp are too immature and tender to take on the job and easily become irritated and inflamed. (See Figure 7-1 for a diagram of skin layers.) Hormones determine the amount of oil produced by your skin and scalp, and women tend to have drier skin than men.

If you have dry skin, use cream and lotion to retain and add water to your skin. Stay away from skin products with water-based ingredients, which pull water out of your skin and make it dry out even more. Also avoid skin care products that contain much alcohol because it is very drying. Choose a gentle oatmeal scrub (see the Scrub-A-Dub Oatmeal Scrub recipe, earlier in this chapter) over bar or liquid soaps, which irritate dry skin.

Eleven ways to ruin your hair

Be good to your hair. The best thing that you can do for it besides use natural hair care products is to treat it right. To be very blunt, your hair's dead. Please don't take this personally because it's true for everyone. The good news is that the colors and hairsprays you put on your hair won't adversely affect the rest of your body (except what substances touch your scalp), but the bad news is that because it's not alive, your hair has no resources to recover from mistreatment and build itself up. Here's a list of don'ts that injure hair.

- **Overshampooing:** To be an effective dirt-cutter, shampoo contains compounds that pull away dirt, and the natural oils on your hair along with it. If your hair is already damaged from harsh shampoos, blow-drying, air pollution, or any other things on this list, it's susceptible to the ravages of shampoo.

- **Harsh detergent shampoos:** Since you can't avoid shampooing your hair, at least use a mild shampoo. (You'll find several places that sell shampoo listed in the Appendix.)

- **Brushing hair while wet:** When your hair is wet, it becomes very thin as it stretches to nearly double its length if brushed or pulled. This greatly increases the chances of it breaking.

- **Yanking while brushing:** Even when your hair is dry, it can stretch a little, so don't pull hard with a comb or brush. Also, don't yank your hand as you brush because this encourages hair to snap.

- **Blow-drying.** I don't think that there's a study on this, but I bet blow-drying your hair must equal at least a few hours wind exposure (see the bullet later in this list). If you must dry your hair quickly, at least towel off most of the water first, use a low setting, and leave a little moisture in your hair to dry off on its own.

- **Chlorine:** Swimming in a chlorinated pool or soaking in a hot tub that contains chlorine or a related chemical is bad news for your hair. The effect is similar to using a hair bleach (see the info later in this list). Don't give up these activities, but at least wear a bathing cap while swimming and keep your hair out of the hot tub (whoever cleans the filters will appreciate that also!).

- **Permanents, hair dyes, and bleaches:** Chemicals that change hair color first have to enter your hair's inner structure to strip away the original color when you bleach, lighten, or highlight or dye hair. In both cases, they do this by breaking down your hair's natural protective armor. In short, this partially destroys your hair. That's why bleached blondes have a reputation for having frizzy hair. To color your hair, try a henna blend made with natural herbs, which coats and protects your hair. Henna eventually fades, so the next best thing is a partially natural dye that is sold in some natural-food stores.

- **Lots of sun or wind exposure:** Sunshine and wind have the same damaging effect on your hair that they do on your skin. They excessively dry out your hair. When you're in the sun, wear a hat or scarf, and your hair will thank you by staying in better shape.

- **Air pollution:** Nasty stuff, air pollution, it even gets in your hair. Enough of it can coat your hair and make it seem dirty.

- **Stress:** You just can't get away from the negative effects of stress, even on your head. Stress reduces the nutrients that reach your scalp to feed your hair.

- **Junk food:** No, not on your hair, but what you eat. For the sake of your hair (as well as your skin), stay away from junk food, especially greasy, fried foods.

Dry hair is unmanageable and brittle and easily develops split ends and dandruff with a flyaway look — all because there isn't enough oil in your scalp to coat your hair and hold in moisture. If you have dry hair, only wash it every few days with a mild shampoo that contains moisturizers, some oil, and fatty acids to restore shine to your hair. That way, you won't constantly wash off all the oil or encourage breakage. Protein-rich and balsam shampoos coat your hair to smooth down individual frayed hairs and make your hair look thicker, at least until the protein coat wears off. (High-protein herbs include comfrey and henna.)

For a quick dry hair treatment, rub a couple drops of an essential oil — rosemary or sandalwood are good choices — on your brush or comb before brushing or combing your hair.

The following essential oils are good for your dry skin and hair. They encourage production of your own natural oils in your skin and scalp. Many of these also increase the ability of your skin and scalp to hold in water. Quite a few are anti-inflammatory oils, which are good for dry skin because they reduce skin irritation and puffiness that so often accompany the dryness.

- Carrot seed
- Cedarwood
- Frankincense
- Myrrh
- Palmarosa
- Peppermint (small amounts increase oil production)
- Sandalwood
- Thyme (the variety called linalol)
- Vetivert

In the pink: Sensitive skin

These essential oils reduce inflammation that can accompany dry skin conditions.

- Chamomile
- Helichrysum
- Lavender

Volcanic eruptions: Acned skin

Acne may not present a hazard to your health, but it has the unfortunate habit of impairing your looks. It always strikes at the most untimely moments. Just when you least want your complexion to look like a geological survey map, that's when your skin pores become clogged with oil and infected. A hormonal imbalance takes most of the blame for causing acne. However, holistic practitioners suspect that stress, diet, and toxins in the blood (not effectively filtered out by the liver) contribute to the breakouts.

Essential oils come to your skin's rescue, balancing hormones, reducing stress, and regulating your skin's oil production. This makes aromatherapy the ideal treatment for blemishes, pimples, and other skin eruptions. Shop for something that you can apply directly on the acne. Dermatologists say not to pop pimples, but if you do, wash the spot and use a compress on the spot before and afterward. If you have problems with acne, use the following essential oils to reduce inflammation and infection and rejuvenate your complexion with any skin type.

- ✔ Chamomile
- ✔ Geranium
- ✔ Lavender
- ✔ Sandalwood
- ✔ Tea tree (especially niaouli)

The following oils work well for acne with oily skin:

- ✔ Cedarwood
- ✔ Eucalyptus (especially the variety called "dives" or "broad leaf")
- ✔ Lavender (or Spanish) sage
- ✔ Lemon
- ✔ Tea tree

The following oils work well for acne with dry skin:

- ✔ Clary sage
- ✔ Fennel
- ✔ Frankincense
- ✔ Juniper berry
- ✔ Patchouli
- ✔ Rosemary

Discovering the Secrets of the Ageless: Slowing Wrinkles in Time

As your skin matures, it loses some elasticity and ability to retain water. The dryness and the thinness gradually increases, especially after you turn 40, and mature skin is almost always dry. (To keep water from evaporating, young skin contains natural moisturizing factors that attract and hold in water and oil glands that keep it and your scalp lightly coated.) As you age, gradually adjust the way you care for your complexion. If you're relatively young with dry skin, you may be prone to developing wrinkles early. You can think ahead and treat your skin now with products designed to use on a dry complexion. Here's a list of some things that take their toll on your skin and make it age more quickly.

- **Alcohol consumption** ages your skin. It also takes quite a toll on your liver. (See "Sluggish liver," later in this list.)

- **Fair-skinned** (especially if you have freckles) means that your skin is more vulnerable to the rages of weather, especially sun. It tends to burn more easily and that alone ages your skin. Hereditary might play a role here, too.

- **Dry skin** loses moisture more easily, so it is subject to wrinkling and thus aging sooner than oily skin.

- **Lack of exercise** impairs your general health and usually reduces blood circulation. That means less nutrients and oxygen (which are carried by your blood) make it out to your skin.

- **Poor diet or faulty digestion** restricts the availability of nutrients that are important for your skin's health. Your skin reflects this poor health and eventually shows its age.

- **Radical weight changes** affect skin, which stretches to accommodate the extra bulk and then wrinkles when you lose weight. This also alters how much fat is underlying your skin (see "Thin skin," later in this list). Yoyo dieting impairs your skin's health along with everything else, and usually you're short on sufficient nutrients while you're rapidly losing weight.

- **Sluggish liver** can mean trouble for your skin because you need your liver to store skin-loving vitamins such as vitamin A and to break down substances in your blood that are injurious to skin.

- **Smoking** is the only known activity that adds a couple extra years to you physically. Where it shows most is on your skin.

✔ **Stress** often is a co-factor to create poor health, and skin is no exception. Stress uses up extra nutrients so that they never reach your skin. As I already mentioned, that can mean trouble for your skin's health and age it faster.

✔ **Thin skin** in this case doesn't refer to your emotional state (although that probably does affect your skin). It means that there's not much fatty layer directly under your skin to make it look plump, so it wrinkles easily.

The essential oils suggested for mature skin all help skin cells regenerate and rejuvenate. These oils help to heal the slight skin abrasions that dry, mature skin tends to develop. Here's a list of "anti-aging" essential oils.

✔ Carrot seed

✔ Frankincense

✔ Geranium

✔ Helichrysum

✔ Lavender

✔ Neroli

✔ Rose

✔ Rosemary

Chapter 8

Aromatherapy in the Bedroom

● ●

In This Chapter

▶ Perceiving fragrance in a sexy way

▶ Using sexy scents

▶ Choosing an aromatic turn-on

▶ Understanding perfume and cologne

▶ Discovering women's and men's favorites scents

▶ Fragrancing yourself and your environment

▶ Dining sensually with aromatic foods

● ●

┌─────────────────────┐
Recipes in This Chapter

▶ Scents-ual Touch Massage Oil

▶ A-romantic Whipping Cream

▶ Midnight at the Oasis Balls

▶ Aromatic Love Potion

└─────────────────────┘

*I*f there's one place that fragrance steps into the limelight, it's sex. Aroma offers the ultimate sex appeal. It's a position that it's maintained for at least 3,000 years and doesn't show any sign of giving up. Perfume, cologne, aftershave, pure essential oil — whatever you choose to scent your body, becomes a personal statement about yourself.

And, does it talk! There's no denying that it's downright sexy language complete with all the allure and mystery connected to scent. Like fragrance itself, it says that you're appealing, attractive, alluring, and worth being near, yet mysterious enough to be intriguing. It also implies that you're sexy. Just how sexy depends upon which fragrance you choose.

Just think of the provocative ads that go along with perfumes — naked bodies, clothing torn away, and themes that hint at Parisian nights, tropical isles, unbridled freedom, unspoken dreams, mystery, and glamour. And for the guys, he-man colognes communicate that he is a hunter with brute strength and wild, uninhibited passions, who is running down his prey.

In this chapter, I introduce you to sexy scents from around the world and give you ideas on how to use them. Remember, though, that fragrance can be captivating, sensual, and even downright erotic, but the rest is up to you!

What a Fragrance Says about You: Sex and Smell

You may have noticed this fact already: A fragrance changes depending upon who wears it. That's why it's always a good idea to test scent what you wear as perfume on your skin before you buy it. That's also why you tend to stick to the same fragrance when you find one that really works for you.

This close relationship of your skin's chemistry with scent occurs because you have your own unique, personal odor that is yours alone. Your personalized scent is as individual as your fingerprint. And, it's more important for lovemaking than that sexy-looking sweater you just bought or the way that you comb or color your hair, and maybe even your favorite perfume, cologne, or aftershave.

In fact, your sense of smell is one of the most scents-ual things about you. As much as people in Western cultures try to subdue their personal trademark odor with deodorants and hide it with cologne, perfume, and aftershave, your biological smell holds the key to your sexual allure. It's a way of attracting sexual partners, or at least flirting with them, in a primal sort of way. When sex therapists William Masters and Virginia Johnson suggested that odors influence sexual arousal in the 1960s, they weren't exactly coming up with something new. The word for "kiss" has long been the same word as "smell" in several languages. Eskimos get right to the point by rubbing noses to kiss.

The Scents of Sex

I'm not referring here to body odor or the smell of fear or anxiety that comes with nervous sweating. Personal scent is that musty, subtle, warm smell of a lover's skin — or more accurately, his or her armpit. (Your armpit has it, too, but no one is very aware of their own scent.) I often hear it called *that* scent. Students at my aromatherapy seminars shyly comment that they know what I'm talking about. It's *that* scent that swept them off their feet when they first encountered *that* person. Many describe it as intoxicating.

In a less squeaky-clean era, this personal scent was acknowledged as even more alluring than perfume. Emperor Napoleon of France sent this message to his wife Josephine, "Home in three days, don't wash." The 18th-century German poet Johann Wolfgang Goethe carried his lover's bodice around with him so that he could sniff her fragrance throughout the day in anticipation of the passionate night ahead. In Elizabethan times, a woman gave her lover a "love apple." She peeled the fruit and held it in her armpit until it was saturated with sweat. Thus, he could inhale her fragrance when they were apart. In similar style, young men in the Austrian Tyrol dance with a handkerchief in their armpit and later wave it under the nose of the girl they admire.

Sexy perception of fragrance

History has left an unabashed scent trail concerning fragrance. Those who could afford it in the ancient cultures of the Egyptians, Sumerians, Aztecs, Greeks, Romans, Indian, Chinese, Hebrews, and others made extravagant use of fragrances. Don't kid yourself for a minute. This wasn't just room fresheners to override foul odor or sacred incense to appease the gods. The aromas that they choose are legendary for their use as aphrodisiacs. And, they perfumed everything with sexy scents, their skin and hair, their clothes, their bedding, the wall hanging — you name it, and it was fragranced.

One look at the seductive role of scent as portrayed in the world's great literature, and you'll have no doubt of aromatherapy's lurid past. You might even take a few scentful hints from history. You've probably seen one of the dozens of versions of the *Kama Sutra* (including a pop-up one) that are sold in bookstores. Even though it was written in ancient times, the famous Indian tell-it-like-it-is treatise on love and sex remains a perpetual bestseller. And it refers repeatedly to aromatherapy, as in the following section where it sets the stage for romantic sex.

> "... the outer room, balmy with rich perfumes, should contain a bed ... having garlands and bunches of flowers upon it.... There should also be ... fragrant ointments for the night, as well as flowers and other fragrant substances."

Just to show how sexy fragrance is, the stuffy religious Puritans hated it. During the era when they held power in England, a law was passed preventing women from wearing perfume and any scented accessories. That such laws referred to its sexual allure is evident from a subsequent 1770 parliamentary bill, where a women who seduced someone with the use of scent could be charged with witchcraft. Around the same time, ginger, long used as an aphrodisiac, was out and out banned lest someone get a whiff of it and lose control.

The Austrian armpit approach is certainly more direct than plucking petals off a daisy to see if she loves him or loves him not! Why wait until the two of you become intimate to see if the smell chemistry is really right when you can find out with a simple wave of a hanky? A smell researcher from Duke University, Dr. Susan Shiffman, sums it up nicely, "People who don't like each other's smell don't make it as a couple."

The tiny glands that release this personal scent are scattered all over your body, in your face, nipples, anal and genital regions, and, yes, your armpits. A few are even located in your ears, eyelids, and scalp. What causes all the sniffing excitement are strongly aromatic hormonal substances that these scent glands release. Called *pheromones* (which is a Greek word for "excitement"), they're activated by the *adrenaline,* the hormone that rushes through your body whenever you get excited to fuel your excitement and also make you hyper-alert.

Does sexual attraction make scents?

Pheromones go into swing when you reach puberty, probably triggered partly by the pheromones emitted by the opposite sex. Certainly you can recall when your own teenage hormones came on and quickly accelerated into hyperdrive! (Lack of pheromone excitement may be why adolescence girls in boarding schools tend to begin menstruation later than girls who are in contact with boys.) Women's pheromones can affect the menstrual cycles of other women with whom they live or work so that within three to four months, they menstruate together. Someday, thanks to pheromones, birth control may be only a sniff away. Scientists are currently working on this alternative birth control and also on developing nasal sprays that regulate the menstrual cycle.

Because scent plays such an important role in sex and taste, many elderly people find that they've lost both their appetite for food and for sex. Unfortunately, your ability to perceive smell decreases as you age. By 65, about half the population loses some of their sense of smell. For women, this is especially true of the malelike scent of musk. After menopause or surgical removal of the ovaries, a woman's ability to detect odors declines unless she takes hormones.

I'm sure you get the picture. Pheromones are sexually exciting. Taking advantage of a sure thing, the perfume manufacturer Jovan has created a fragrance that contains minute amounts of a pheromone called andostenone, calling it *Andron.* Banking on the irresistible mix of sex, scent, and imagination, other perfume companies have at least devised provocative names such as Obsession, Poison, Tabu, Touch, White Shoulders, and, to add a little heat to the equation, Fahrenheit for Women. For men, there are scents that exude power: Brut, Tsar, Boss, and Musk, with few secrets here about what's being implied. It's as if the scent will both make you irresistible and overcome all your inhibitions at once, but only because you lost control and are obsessed or subtly poisoned or — reflect on the social implications of this one for a while — the woman is overpowered and dominated. The mystique of fragrance and its intoxicating effect let women get away with things that a "nice" girl won't normally do, really. With this in mind, I can't help smirking at the name of a new men's scent that's called Contradiction.

Not surprisingly, a women's production of pheromones peaks when she is most fertile — during ovulation — luring the male of the species in her direction and announcing her body's acquiescence (even if her mind is having second thoughts!). Her own sense of smell skyrockets to as much as 1,000 times the norm. Pheromones do more than create sexual excitement. Women who have sex with a male partner at least once a week tend to ovulate more often with shorter, more regular menstrual cycles, conceive more easily, and also may have an easier menopause. Ladies, if you want the results, but would rather forgo the man, you get the same benefits sniffing a musklike scent such as that of myrrh. (Everything, that is except for conceiving more easily; musky scents can't do everything. There are some things that you just can't do alone!)

Ways to Spice Up Your Sex Life

Aromatherapy is a spicy subject in more ways than one. Spicy aromas rank high as aphrodisiacs. So do musk, woodsy scents, and vanilla. What all this talk of pheromones leads to is that most famous aphrodisiacs aromas smell somewhat akin to human scents. Here's a selection of some of the world's most famous aphrodisiacs. Use this information at your own risk.

- ✔ **Spicy** scents are apparent in human scent. Sometimes there is a hint of sour or citrus or a woody scent.

- ✔ **Musky** scents like myrrh are reminiscent of personal scents. Research has shown that they resemble the human pheromone androsterone, which is secreted in male sweat — thus the popularity of musk from the sexual scent glands of musk deer, civet cats, and beavers. (By the way, removing their glands means killing the animal, or, at the least, ruining his life.) Musk is used in small amounts. If too intense, it becomes overpowering and animal-like, conveying a message of uncleanliness.

- ✔ **Woodsy** gives another aspect of the human smell. Hormonelike odors are often described "like incense" or "woodlike" like sandalwood. Like musky aromas (see earlier in this list), sandalwood also resembles the human pheromone androsterone.

- ✔ **Vanilla** is the closest scent known to mother's milk. Other sweet scents like benzoin are vanilla-like.

Love potion number 9 (and 10 through 17)

The four scent themes that I describe in the preceding section are well represented in the following list of aphrodisiac aromas. Go ahead. Choose your "poison."

- ✔ **Anise,** which has the smell of licorice, incites sex, according to the ancient Greek herbalist Dioscorides. Fragrance researcher Dr. Alan Hirsch of the Chicago Smell and Taste Treatment and Research Foundation in Chicago, Illinois, says in his studies that the scent of anise was a favorite of both men and women.

✔ **Cardamom** is blended with cinnamon, cloves, nutmeg, black pepper, and carnations (which have a clovelike scent) for a classic Indian and Arab aphrodisiac. Medieval and Renaissance Europeans called it "Fire of Venus" and added it to their love potions. Since Victorian England, Europeans have nibbled on the seed to freshen their breath after dinner to spice up their evenings.

✔ **Cinnamon** entered Western Europe with the Crusaders returning from the East, along with its reputation as an aphrodisiac. Today, it's one of the most popular spices worldwide. Perhaps you know why, considering that it rated high in the studies on sexual scent preferences for both men and women.

✔ **Clove bud** is regarded as a sexual stimulant by the Egyptians, Persians, Arabians, and Europeans. The Hofriyati of the Sudan make a wedding scent for fertility and femininity from clove that also contains sandalwood, musk, and a local fragrant cherry. Women wear the blend to the wedding party so that its scent carries through the air while they dance.

✔ **Coriander** is *the* aphrodisiac of the Middle East, Egypt, and Palestine. It's used in the classic tale, *The Arabian Nights,* as an aphrodisiac. Brought to Europe during the Crusades for use as a love potion, it flavored a popular drink of the Middle Ages called *Hippocras* that was drunk at weddings to inspire love and sex.

✔ **Ginger** was for "burning desire," according to the Persian physician Avicenna. His male impotence recipe mixed it with honey. He then suggested rubbing the mixture on the penis. Ginger's hot stuff, so it's sure to at least get a rise from the guy emotionally. It also benefits the situation by increasing circulation. Women in modern Senegal entice their lovers by wearing ginger in their belts, and in New Guinea, they find men irresistible who rub ginger over their lips, eyes, arms, and chest. Ginger's fragrant flowers, along with other herbs, are also tucked into the men's armbands.

✔ **Jasmine** is called "Queen of the Night" because that's when it releases its fragrance. As a symbol of both sex and love, it's also associated with passions that are released at night. In India, jasmine is used to anoint the body and is placed in bridal wreaths. It's one of the five fragrant flowers used by the Indian god of love, Kama, on his arrows to penetrate the five senses. (On a scientific note, that's exactly what jasmine does. It increases the beta waves in your brain to make you more aware of everything around you.) The fragrance is also used to rekindle fading romance. In the Arabian *Medical Formulary of Al-Kindi,* it's suggested to encourage sex , especially if "the male organ is oiled with [a massage] oil of jasmine at the time of intercourse." He promises that a woman will experience "strong lust" as a result.

✔ **Myrrh** has a musky scent with a chemical structure that is strikingly similar to testosterone. It's worn in the Middle East for both spiritual and sexual inspiration. Since before Biblical times, women have hung small bags of myrrh on a string around their necks so that it falls between their breasts and their body heat can release its scent. In the Old Testament's *Song of Solomon*, you read, "Delicate is the fragrance of your perfume, your name is an oil poured out. . . . My beloved is a sachet of myrrh lying between my breasts."

✔ **Myrtle** was a major ingredient in the 16th-century "Angel Water," used as skin toner, but also drunk by women to increase their sexual attractiveness. It's a potent aphrodisiac in the Middle East and in ancient Greece where it was strewn beside the bridal bed and worn by brides.

✔ **Nutmeg** is favored by the Chinese as aphrodisiac. Although it smells spicy, it actually is a relaxing scent that lowers blood pressure and creates a euphoric feeling, which some describe as intoxicating. In 18th century North America, it was popular in nightcaps; I wonder if they ever considered why.

✔ **Orange blossom (neroli)** is a main ingredient in the popular perfume Poison. Long before this perfume's creation, prostitutes in Madrid, Spain, relied on the scent to seduce their customers. But the flowers are also worn by brides throughout the Mediterranean region for their weddings. It's far more sophisticated than orange or lemon oils, both of which smell a little too clean and fresh for a full aphrodisiac effect — although two lime trees growing next to each other, both in fruit and bloom, are a symbol of open communication in a perfect union.

✔ **Patchouli** is an Indian aphrodisiac with a deep, earthy scent that is said to overcome inhibitions. Its association with wealth and prosperity add to its attraction in India. In the Western world, its association with the counterculture in the 60s, when it was *the* only fragrance to wear, is a turn-off for some who overdosed on it then and a turn-on for others who remember good, and often uninhibited, times.

✔ **Peppermint** is used to overcome frigidity in Arabia, where men also drink it to assure their virility. It's given to stallions and bulls if their sexual prowess wanes. Trobriandmen slip a mint-coconut scented love charm onto the breast of their beloved as she sleeps to inspire erotic dreams of the two of them together. Upon awakening, the dreamer is said to experience an uncontrolled passion. The scent increases stimulating beta waves in your brain.

✔ **Rose** is one of the most important fragrances to inspire love as well as sex in different cultures. It's one of the few scents that still carries the message of an open and receptive heart in the Western world. Cleopatra scented the sails of her barge with rose water to entice Mark Anthony to her bed. (It worked!)

- **Sandalwood** is very close to human personal scent (and the scent that is used in the pig mating pheromone). Ironically, it's often used in under-arm deodorants. It's considered an aphrodisiac throughout the Eastern world. The famous 10th century Arabian physician Avicenna used it to "exhilarate" and "heal passions of the heart." India's ancient text, the *Kama Sutra,* suggests that a man "give her your jasmine garland, lie her back gently, and massage her body with sweet sandalwood oil."

- **Vanilla** is indigenous to the Americas where Native Americans consider it an aphrodisiac and often mix it with chocolate. Tonga Islanders have the same idea about vanilla. They extract the scent into coconut oil and rub the oil on their bodies so that they smell more sexy. The native tribe Kallaway of Boliva uses the vanillalike Balsam of Peru under their arms, and Jivaro women in Peru and Ecuador wear necklaces that include vanilla bean beads for their intoxicating fragrance. A local legend tells of Jivaro men who were irresistibly attracted to a woman covered in these necklaces. (Although the fact that, except for the necklaces, she was quite naked may have contributed.) In the early part of the 20th century, psychoanalyst and sex researcher Havelock Ellis found that workers in a vanilla factory were constantly sexually aroused from being around the scent.

- **Ylang ylang**, a sweet-scenting euphoric sometimes described as intoxi-cating, is used to treat impotency and frigidity. Indonesians take it on their honeymoons.

Maybe not aphrodisacs, but close

Here's an adjunct list of aromas that are classified as mild aphrodisiacs. They're usually mixed with one or more of the more erotic scents.

- **Basil** is used to attract a lover by Italian women who place the potted plant on their doorstep.

- **Black pepper** has a reputation to perk up waning sexual desire.

- **Clary sage** is characterized by euphoria and thus it releases inhibitions, which is not a bad idea when you're using an aphrodisiac.

- **Vetivert** smells like dirt to most people — that is, until small amounts are blended with richer fragrances when it more resembles human scent. It's an important ingredient in Oriental-style fragrances.

Sexy perfumes

Perfumers have relied on combining aphrodisiac scents into enticing blends to make sexy perfumes for ages. Perfume unconsciously reveals what people consciously pretend to hide: sex appeal. Read the list of aphrodisiac scents in this chapter and then look at the line-up of aphrodisiac ingredients they've come up with in this selection of famous perfumes and colognes.

For women:

- ✔ **Obsession:** Vanilla, patchouli, sandalwood, clary sage, cinnamon, benzoin, cedarwood, rosewood, bergamot, and lemon

- ✔ **Opium:** Coriander, clove, myrrh, benzoin, labdanum, and opopanax

- ✔ **Tabu:** Patchouli, benzoin, sandalwood, vanilla, ylang ylang, jasmine, clove, rose, coriander, neroli, cedarwood, and bergamot

- ✔ **Chanel No. 5:** Sandalwood, vanilla, vetivert, ylang ylang, rose, jasmine, neroli, with bergamot, lemon, cedar, and orris

- ✔ **White Shoulders:** Jasmine, rose, clove, sandalwood, benzoin, vetivert, neroli, bergamot tuberose, and orris

For men:

- ✔ **Eternity for Men:** Jasmine, geranium, and orange

- ✔ **Jazz:** Jasmine, rose, geranium, spice, and woods

To appeal to women:

- ✔ **Bill Blass Hot:** Spices with violetlike scent and sandalwood

- ✔ **Brut:** Patchouli, sandalwood, vanilla, vetivert, ylang ylang, jasmine, basil, anise with lavender, geranium, and oakmoss.

Sexy Scents for Men and Women: The Scentual Language of Fragrance

Sex is always a hot topic that attracts the interest of scientists as well as the rest of the population. As a result, you can find plenty of data on sex. Researchers know when people want it, how they do it, and what they think of it along with every intimate detail. From all of this, you can glean tidbits of information about the relationship of sex and scent.

Some of the most fascinating studies are conducted by fragrance researcher, Dr. Alan Hirsch of the Chicago Smell and Taste Treatment and Research Foundation in Chicago, Illinois. You may have already heard of his landmark study on which scents turns men on, especially because it's been freely joked about in the news and on TV talk shows. Much of the amusement revolves around the revealing results that men's ultimate sexy smell is pumpkin pie.

Perhaps the old saying is correct — that the way to a man's heart (and elsewhere) is through his stomach! Hirsch also conducted a similar study to find out what scents turned women on. In both studies, the blood flow in the genitals was measured, while participants sniffed the various scents. (See the details on both of these studies in the following sections.)

What men want

Western men shy away from scenting themselves, unlike their male counterparts in ancient Rome and Greece who favored heavy, clinging floral scents and wouldn't think of going to bed or to war without their fragrant ointments.

Modern men are also more opinionated than women about what they want in a scent. They particularly don't want to smell like flowers, which is consider far too feminine and so presumably is less attractive to women. Perfume companies keep trying anyway to come up with something the guys will wear using woodsy scents such as cedar, juniper, and heather, but with limited success. What men will wear are musky scents — the ones that resemble their own male pheromone androsterone that is secreted in male sweat.

Obviously, these guys haven't read *The Perfumed Garden,* a 14th-century book by the explorer and Arabic translator Richard Burton. (It's available in several translations.) It describes the erotic use of scent to "excite the act of copulation." Not only that, but it explains that "the use of scents has often proved a strong help to man, and assisted him in getting possession of a woman," because "the woman, inhaling the perfumes employed by the man, becomes intoxicated." Maybe fragrance deserves more consideration.

Men have other strong opinions in their smell preferences. The scents that they tend to like women to wear are light fragrances. While women may be dousing themselves with exotic, heavy perfumes, men say that they consider "clean and natural scents" as more free-spirited and uninhibited. They also perceive women who wear these scents in the same way. That's interesting considering that personality tests show extroverted women prefer fresh-scented perfumes, while introverted women go for the spicy Oriental types.

Men find it easier than women to disregard unpleasant fragrances. However, for more than half of the men tested, scents triggered some memory recall of another place and time. Therefore, it only makes "sense" that if you want a man to find you uniquely attractive, don't wear the same perfume worn by his mother, sisters, or especially by a previous lover.

Tales of sex, seduction, and scent

Ancient mythology, the forerunner to modern soap operas and romance novels, is rich with tales of love, sex, and fragrance. The stories about Venus, Roman goddess of love, portray her as perfumed with "pleasant ambrosia." As the story goes, she isn't the least bit shy about flaunting her secret and seductive perfumes on gods and mortals alike and creating all sorts of sexual havoc. Her Greek alter-ego, Aphrodite, indulges in similar aromatic tricks.

Another example of the power that was attributed to fragrance by the ancients is found in Homer's famous Greek epic *The Iliad* and *The Odyssey*, where the goddess Hera uses it to seduce the mighty King Zeus, and Circe, the daughter of the sun god, overcomes the hero Ulysses with fragrance.

Table 8-1 gives the results from the study on men and women's fragrance preferences conducted by Dr. Hirsch that I mention in the beginning of this section. The following scents are the ones to which men are most attracted. Several combinations of these scents were used, and they are the most popular. There were some variations among men according to their age or how often they have sex, but the following list is roughly in the order of how strongly the scents affect men.

Table 8-1	Best Scents, According to Men
Best Scents, in Order of Preference	*Okay scents*
Anise (licoricelike) and cola	Vanilla (especially popular with older men)
Pumpkin pie spice (a cinnamon, clove, and ginger combo)	Orange
Lavender	Musk
Anise (licoricelike) and doughnuts	Buttered popcorn
Cinnamon	
Cola	

Looking over these popular scents in Table 8-1, note that pumpkin pie isn't the only food scents that predominate. The connection may be obvious. Sex and eating are two of the most pleasurable experiences, so interweaving the two is a natural experience. But, it's not just any food. The aromas of some foods — cranberry and chocolate — definitely don't captivate men's fancy. They also don't care for baby powder, even though its scent is similar to the Oriental-type perfumes that are women's favorites. However, none of the scents go so far to actually turn men off.

What women want

In Hirsch's study on what aromas women find sexually stimulating, he discovered some interesting differences in which scents they like among subgroups of women, according to their sexual preferences. Bluntly put, if you're a woman, the scents that you like correspond with what type of sex you enjoy. According to this study, the more inhibited you are, the less you care about fragrance at all. In addition, a greater number of scents turn you off or, at least, leave you cold. On the other hand, if you go for heavy passion, than you also tend to love to indulge in sexy fragrances. Emotionally stable women (according to the psychological testing they went through) have no real aromatic preference. Women who experience many mood changes and are described as "dreamy" tend to prefer flowery scents.

Table 8-2 lists the results from the study. I listed them in order of preference, with the first ones the ones that received the highest ratings.

Table 8-2	Best Scents, According to Women
Best Scents in Order of Preference	*Okay scents*
Anise (the scent of licorice candy)	Baby powder (Oriental perfume scent)
Cucumber (a synthetic fragrance only)	Chocolate
Pumpkin pie spice (a cinnamon, clove, and ginger combo)	Banana
Lavender	Women's perfume

Obviously, like men, women favor spicy scents, such as that of pumpkin pie spice. It's true that many popular perfumes have a spicy theme, such as Tabu and Shalimar. According to other research, women also go for nutty scents such as almond. And then there is banana and cucumber, which conjure up some visual as well as aromatic sexual correlations. (Could it be possible that bananas are considered aphrodisiacs in Egypt and elsewhere because of their shape or because of their smell? Or perhaps a combination of both?)

Of all things erotic, baby powder's high ratings may surprise you. However, the powder's scent is a spicy "oriental perfume," as found in the popular perfumes Obsession, Passion, and Opium. These perfumes combine vanilla, stimulating spices, and woodsy, natural scents — all aphrodisiacs. Speculation in the perfume industry is that women may associate Oriental-type perfumes with comfort and maternal care, especially because they, far more than men, link sexual attraction with nurturing and affection. Another, quite opposite theory is that the scent offers a taste — or I should say a smell — of the exotic.

The Oriental-type perfumes have worldwide appeal, even in places where the use of baby powder on babies isn't a well-established tradition. In New Guinea, the powder is sold as sexy perfume. They wear it as is and also put the powder and coconut oil on grass fronds that they wrap in banana leaves and steam to impregnate the scent into the leaves. Finally, the fragrant grass is tucked into belts and armbands where body heat releases the aroma.

One very curious aspect about Hirsch's study is that no one knows why, but the baby-powder scent ranks very high among women who normally experience an orgasm during sex. However, multi-orgasmic women don't care for it at all. In fact, it actually turned them off, as evidenced by the reduced blood flow to their genitals.

In other research, when Dr. Hirsch asked young women what aromas they found sexy, their association with a scent played a big role in what they liked. These women connect the smell of soap and bubble bath with cleanliness, which they feel is sexy. (This reaction may shed another light on the popularity of baby powder, because it, too, is linked with bathing and cleanliness.) They also like the scent of coconut, which reminds them of suntan lotion and tanned, sexy-looking men. (There might be more going on here, as well, because the smell of coconut is considered an aphrodisiac throughout Polynesia.)

Turn-offs

In his study with women, Dr. Hirsch discovered a category that men didn't have — the complete turn off. These fragrances are listed in order, with the least liked scent first. I doubt that barbecue smoke scent (I envision a cologne named Burned Again?) was high on anyone's list for a man's after-shave to entice a woman. However, the fact that men's cologne appears on this list is curious indeed, especially considering that a survey conducted in Wales found that a majority of women said that men who wear cologne or aftershave are sexier. (Perhaps it was the brand used in this study to which they so strongly objected.)

- Cherry
- Barbecue smoke
- Men's cologne

Some Enchanted Evening: "Scentsual" Seduction

I'll agree with you that a dab of perfume or cologne behind each ear and on the inside of your wrists is a good start. These are *pulse points*. Because the blood vessels are close to the surface of your skin, they heat the scent and help diffuse it. However, you've got some other great hot spots. Just don't overdo it — you don't want to cover up your natural pheromone scent.

Get the Message? Scented Love Notes from Around the World

Throughout the world, from the Amazon to the high-rises of New York and Paris, scent captures people's imagination and stirs their loins, but humans are subject to cultural differences. Beauty — and sensuality — are in the eye, or nose, of the beholder. Not everyone will agree, but African Bushmen say that the sweet scent of rain is the most seductive scent of all. A look at the historical use of aromas and the way that they have been used throughout the world shows that the Western approach is a bit limited and certainly not very creative. There are many ways to get the message across. Borrow ideas from around the world to spice up your sex life.

✔ **For yourself:** Take a hint from Arab women: They first wash and then anoint their whole body with a scented paste made of musk, rose, and saffron. Their hair is often perfumed with jasmine in sesame or walnut oil. On their ears, you'll find a blend of aloewood, saffron, rose, musk, and civet that has a red color. On their neck, they have rose, narcissus, aloewood, ambergris, or musk. Armpits are perfect for sandalwood or ambergris. A tiny drop of aloewood is placed in their nostrils. Of course, such a heady combination is saved for evenings at home. Men wear rose and aloewood behind their ears, on nostrils and beard, and on the palms of their hands.

Try a little scent in your armpit where it can mix with your own personal scent. For women, between the breasts is a classic. If you want, make a trail of scent that leads your partner to new frontiers. Try applying a unique scent to each spot. This is a good way to keep him or her guessing, as well as wanting more.

✔ **Your breath:** For perfumed kisses, chew on an aphrodisiac like clove bud or cinnamon stick, as do people seeking passion throughout the Middle East. Or, use a mint or cinnamon flavored breath mint. Surveys show that most men and women prefer smelling the scent of mint on another's breath. Some men prefer chocolate. Chocolate mints, anyone?

- **Your hair:** Your hair — anywhere on your body — holds scent even better than your skin. Take advantage of this. It's not too hard these days to find shampoos and hair rinses that contains essential oils that have aphrodisiac scents. Some shampoos and rinses are even advertised with this implication, with the ads portraying a woman washing her hair in orgasmic ecstasy. Polynesian women treat their hair with ylang-ylang scented coconut oil while the Chinese traditionally scented their hair and garmets by holding them over incense.

- **Your loins:** Women of Nauruan stand over scented steam in a small tent of woven mats. For this purpose, fragrant plants are placed on a hot rock inside a miniature oven. This cleanses their bodies while giving them a long-lasting perfume. The Barasana males of the Columbian Amazon stick sweet-smelling herbs known to attract women under their G-string.

One way that you can scent your entire body is by having a few drops of essential oils on the rocks. The rocks in your wet or dry sauna, that is. Not ready for a steam bath? How about settling for scented underwear? Tuck a sachet that smells strongly of your favorite aphrodisiac in your underwear drawer. Or, spritz your underwear or lingerie.

- **Your very being:** South Pacific Islanders of Nauru believe that sipping an aromatic drink of scented coconut oil makes the breath and skin unbelievable irresistible. (I'd share the method used to extract fragrance into the milk, but it's a closely guarded secret.) They're thought more irresistible because the scent is emitted from within their body instead of just off the surface of their skin. The Desana of Columbia down strong cups of aromatic herbal teas for the same reason, so that they exude fragrance to attract women (and hunting prey). Mmm . . . must be time for a fragrant meal. See my suggestions in the section "Sharing a Sumptuous Scentual Supper," later in this chapter.

- **Your clothes:** Clothes in Moslem countries are scented by hanging them on a teepee-shaped rack over an incense burner that is filled with similar scents.

Spritz your clothes so that a light scent lingers on them. This technique is best done with clothing that floats, such as scarves and loosely worn shirts and blouses. That way, an aura of scent surrounds you and draws the loved one in closer.

- **Your lover:** You don't have to look very hard to find cultures that believe in scents-ual massage. It a universal thing because there's nothing like an aromatic massage to introduce sex. Of course, this must be done with a massage oil made with essential oils that have aphrodisiac fragrances.

You can buy a blend that is specially designed for this purpose. You can also choose your favorites scent from the list in this chapter. (I include a recipe in this chapter!)

✔ **Your surroundings:** You probably need no introduction to Cleopatra. Even if you don't know her as the most famous Egyptian queen that ever lived, you probably saw her portrayed in one of the Hollywood movies about her life. Cleopatra enveloped herself, her barge, and its sails — in fact, everything imaginable was saturated scent — to entice Mark Anthony to her bed. Granted, you may not go as far as sailing to your prospective lover drenched in perfume in a barge that is carrying slaves who are fanning incense burners to scent its sails. Nevertheless, you'll have to admit that you can scent a lot of things in your surroundings besides yourself.

Scent the curtains, scent the couch, scent the towels. Everything that your lover touches in the environment can have its own soft, aphrodisiac scent. A spray mister filled with scented water does the job quickly. (See the sidebar "Pillow talk" for the perfect technique.) For more ideas on scenting rooms, see Chapters 4 and 6.

✔ **Your bed:** In ancient times, Greek men sprinkled their beds with fragrant powder so that their entire body was scented as the smell was released thorough the night. Louis XIV scented his sheets with jasmine. Greeks and Egyptians would literally cover the bed in rose petals.

If this is too extravagant for your taste (and your pocketbook) or a little too unconventional, then at least scent your sheets. You might as well do the pillows, too. (Forget the blankets; you won't need them with all of that hot passion.) You can either scent your entire linen closets with handfuls of sachets or spritz just the sheets.

✔ **Your food:** King Solomon's garden was said to have been filled with fragrant and edible aphrodisiacs, such as almonds and pomegranates. Two of life's greatest pleasures are eating and making love, so why not combine them? Because taste and smell are so intimately linked — you can't taste without smelling — and food is an obviously sensual pleasure, food scents are definitely "in" when it comes to sex. See the section "Sharing a Sumptuous Scentual Supper" and have a romantic and sensual meal.

Pillow talk

To scent everything, try a spray bottle that contains scented water. Rose and orange water are easy to buy. They're both sold in inexpensive versions at liqueur stores. (They're used to flavor certain alcoholic drinks.) You can also buy higher quality hydrosols in several different scents. (See Chapter 1 to find out more about hydrosols.) The scent dissipates over several hours, so try to do your spritzing around 15 to 30 seconds beforehand.

One important reminder: Make sure that your scented pillow cases and sheets are completely dry before you slide into them so that they won't be clammy.

Scents-ual Touch Massage Oil

Warning! Only use this sensuous blend if you're intending the experience to go beyond a massage.

Preparation time: *5 minutes*

Yield: *2 ounces massage oil*

8 drops ginger

5 drops myrrh

2 drops jasmine

1 drop cardamom

2 ounces vegetable oil

Add the essential oils to the vegetable oil and enjoy!

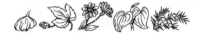

Sharing a Sumptuous Scentual Supper

When it comes to fine, erotic dining, pass on the musk and jasmine and go for the yummy, edible foods. After reading this chapter, you can see that many of the scents considered the most sexy are those of food. That makes it an easy task choosing what's on the menu for your sumptuous scentual supper.

Considering the results from the study conducted by the fragrance researcher Dr. Hirsch (see the section "Sexy Scents for Men and Women: The Scentual Language of Fragrance," earlier in this chapter), you might find that a box of licorice and a pumpkin pie might be more appropriate than candy and roses on your next Valentine's Day, next hot date, or romantic pursuit. Rather than wine, better ply him or her with the licorice-flavored liqueur Ouzo. Because the smell of mint and sometimes chocolate is a favorite to scent your breath, the choice for dessert is obvious: a delicious chocolate mint mousse. Or, while you're at it, how about a rose water rice pudding with cardamom, pomegranate syrup over vanilla ice cream, neroli ice cream over chocolate cake?

After dinner, going to the movies seems like your best choice for a date. It may not matter if the movie has a sexy or romantic theme, just be sure that she gets a box of Good n' Plenty licorice candy and that he gets some buttered popcorn and some orange cola. And, guys, better play it safe and skip the cologne. (Check out the results of what smells women like and don't like in the section "Sexy Scents for Men and Women: The Scentual Language of Fragrance," earlier in this chapter).

The following seasonings are aphrodisiacs that turn any meal into an erotic adventure. The first five on the list are hot spices that are used as mental, physical, and sexual stimulants. The last three, the orange, rose, and vanilla, are calming. You may want to use them all in one meal. That way, your lover will be relaxed, but not too relaxed. You certainly don't want him or her falling asleep.

- Black pepper
- Cardamom
- Cinnamon
- Coriander
- Ginger
- Nutmeg
- Orange blossom (neroli) water
- Rose
- Vanilla

A-romantic Whipping Cream

This sensual delight was invented by herbalist Diana DeLuca for your lover to eat on a rich cake, hot chocolate, or anywhere else that you can imagine.

Preparation time: *6 minutes*

Yield: *1 cup cream*

½ pint whipping cream   *1 to 2 drops essential oil*

1 Whip cream to desired consistency.

2 Add the essential oil and mix well.

3 Add a touch of honey or sugar, if desired.

4 Refrigerate it if you don't use your whipping cream right away. Although it may lose a little of its airiness, the cream will last in the refrigerator at least a couple days, but why wait?

Midnight at the Oasis Balls

This dynamite blend created by herbalist and aromatherapist Mindy Green is something you can make days ahead of time and keep in the refrigerator until the mood strikes you — or your lover.

Preparation time: *15 minutes*

Yield: *12 to 24 balls*

1 cup hulled sesame seeds

2 tablespoons almond butter

2 tablespoons honey

1 tablespoon finely chopped dates

1 teaspoon cardamom powder

1 teaspoon bee pollen

½ teaspoon ginseng powder

½ teaspoon vanilla extract

1 drop rose essential oil

2 tablespoons shredded coconut

2 tablespoons cocoa or carob powder

1 Grind the seeds in an electric coffee grinder or blender.

2 Add the rose oil to the vanilla to dilute it.

3 Mix all ingredients thoroughly and form into balls.

4 Roll in the shredded coconut and cocoa or carob powder.

5 Keep refrigerated.

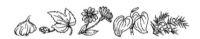

Aromatic Love Potion

Slipping in a few aromantic essential oils and some herbs that are known for their ability to increase libido is one way to enhance a sensual evironment.

Preparation time: *10 minutes*

Yield: *1 quart scented wine*

1 quart red wine

2 tablespoons rose water

1 teaspoon vanilla extract

1 teaspoon ginseng extract (tincture)

1 tablespoon damiana extract (tincture)

3 drops cardamom essential oil

½ teaspoon nutmeg powder

1 Add all the ingredients to the wine.

2 The tastes blend and mellow if you can let this sit for a day or two before drinking it, but this isn't mandatory.

Vary It! *If you don't drink wine, use raspberry or pomegranate juice instead. Pomegranate is a good choice because it has an ancient reputation of being an aphrodisiac. It's a little bitter, so you'll want to either buy a juice blend or add a few tablespoons of honey to sweeten it.*

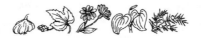

Chapter 9

Aromatherapy on the Job: The Sweet Smell of Success

•••

In This Chapter

▶ Increasing your brain capacity with scents

▶ Taking aromatherapy to work

▶ Improving your memory with fragrance

▶ Keeping your cool

▶ Climbing out of depression aromatically

▶ Relaxing and energizing with scents

▶ Traveling with aromatherapy

•••

*Y*ou live in a fast-paced world that seems to spin faster and faster. Sometimes I wonder how I'm going to get it all done, and I bet you know the feeling. Whatever your job, whatever your lifestyle, your work is probably a big part of your life, and chances are that you work hard. Unfortunately, stress seems an inevitable part of the modern workload. The bad thing is that stress is also a primary culprit in many diseases, and it certainly takes a toll on your peace of mind, as well as your efficiency.

I say that if work is going to occupy so much time, then why not make it a healthier part of our lives? A lot of relaxation techniques are available, but what you need on the job is something that can help you keep working, just with a smile on your face. That alone should do something for your own public relations at work.

Aromatherapy does offer you many ways to deal with the stress and strain of your job. It can help keep you sharp, alert, and on your toes, ready to deal with each new assignment and challenge. It also prevents you from lagging at work, your efficiency dropping, and deadlines piling up. In this chapter, I take advantage of all aromatherapy has to offer to keep you going and to prevent stress. I explain fragrant techniques to reduce tension, anxiety, and memory loss.

Thinking Ahead

Don't expect aromatherapy to answer your dreams by upping your IQ or pushing you into super-drive, enabling you to get twice as much done as ever before. Aromatherapy also doesn't act like a drug. No, you don't experience that head snapping alertness that comes from caffeine pills and other eye-popping drugs, and you won't be doing imitations of Hollywood actor Jim Carrey transforming into the Mask, or Jerry Lewis or Eddie Murphy performing as the Nutty Professor.

Aromatherapy does assist you at your workplace in plenty of ways, mostly through scent alone. It provides you with a boost when you need to wake up or keeps you more relaxed to ride through tension and tight deadlines. Count on it to help your brain power and memory work better. Aromatherapy also helps maintain your attention and energy levels through a long day at the office, yet another meeting, or when you're trying to bounce back from jet lag. In fact, whenever you find dealing with your clients, customers, a boss, or coworkers challenging, then aromatherapy can literally help you change the atmosphere. (For more on the way your brain comprehends aroma, see Chapter 1.) All that's not too bad from smell alone. And, you won't be riding on the rollercoaster of highs and lows experienced when you rely on coffee or drugs to sustain your energy.

If you have a demanding job, you probably need to keep your brain cranked up to your full capacity for eight hours, or maybe longer, every work day. That's easier said than done. Sure, there's always another cup of coffee, but if you're depending upon more than a couple cups a day, you need to consider the health risk. Holistic health practitioners, such as clinical aromatherapists and naturopaths, worry that even a cup a day of the java takes a toll on your adrenal glands. It's at least enough to give you jittery nerves, put you on edge, and make it easier to fall into depression, anxiety, and stress. That's not a good prescription if you're trying to stay on top of your job.

Brainstorm: Bringing Aromatherapy to Work

Sniffing an aroma sounds easy enough, but you may find that introducing aromatherapy on the job is a difficult task. After all, it's scent that I'm suggesting, and you're probably not the only one breathing the air. Your coworkers may or may not take kindly to the idea of having their moods changed by scent. As much as I hate to admit it, some people still consider aromatherapy bizarre and esoteric. That's due to change soon, but until then, there's no reason to be branded the office weirdo.

Even if everyone is in favor of your innovative idea, some fellow employees may turn up their noses at your particular choice in aromas. (In that case, read this chapter and select a different scent that's more universally appealing.) Then again, you may work in a county that has established scentfree work zones to ban the use of perfume and cologne at work in case anyone has chemical sensitivities to fragrance. (Most perfumes and colognes contain plenty of synthetic ingredients that are even more likely than natural ones to cause allergic reactions.) When that's the case, you'll need to be really creative to employ aromatherapy.

On the job scents

Someday, you may come to work and find aromatherapy already filling the place. That may happen in businesses all over the world if they follow the lead of several large Tokyo, Japan, corporations that scent their office buildings with aromatherapy. Throughout the workday, these companies circulate different fragrances through the air-conditioning or heating system at Tokyo's Kajima Construction Company and the Shimizu Construction Company, which developed and patented a computerized ventilation system to distribute the scents.

At Kajima, lemon is the morning wakeup call. This is followed by a midday rose to inspire contented work (or jasmine when the majority of workers are women because that is their preference). Then, after lunch, an invigorating cypress helps employees overcome the afternoon lull. Cypress also fills display areas and the public relation rooms to promote constructive work. Employees even notice that the scented rooms reduce their urge to smoke.

Shimizu disperses peppermint into its offices and conference rooms to increase work efficiency, dispel drowsiness, and lessen mental fatigue. Lavender helps establish a positive mood.

The concept is based on a study in which keyboard workers made far less errors if they sniffed the aromas of lavender, jasmine, and especially lemon, which cut the rate of error in half. It's also supported by the research of Professor Shizuo Torii of the Toho University School of Medicine in Japan on the reaction of brain waves to scents (the brain wave research I mention throughout this chapter). And, it's caught on in places where fast thinking pays off. The Tokyo Stock Exchange is fragranced every afternoon with peppermint to make the brokers feel invigorated and refreshed. Interested? The units cost about $10,000 to $20,000 dollars each.

Aromatherapy does not have to stop at work for these Tokyo workers. During their lunch hour, they can partake in a peppermint refresher at a downtown aromatherapy "bar" called Club Harry's. On the way home from work, they can stop off at one of several atomizer-equipped booths to escape from the stress of commuter traffic. The booths provide a mist of a stimulating scent. Even when they get home, they can relax on _futons_ (a Japanese mattress used for a bed) scented from hanging on futon hangers that emit fragrance. The next morning, they can wake graciously to their scented alarm clocks, instead of the morning news, before they begin yet another scented day at work.

It's not just Japan that's keen on scents on the job. One British firm offers a variety fragrances for companies to pump into the workplace so that employees feel better and are less stressed. They even custom design individual corporate "odor identities" to use like the company logo on stationary and business cards.

If you work in a health-care or educational facility, you're likely to encounter another set of problems when you try aromatherapy, especially if it's recognized as a medicinal therapy. If you need scientific documentation to support your case, see the Appendix in the back of this book to find out how to locate it.

Take a Scent to Work

To make your task in employing aromatherapy easier, here are several suggestions on how to take fragrance to work with you. (See Chapter 4 for details on different ways to fill a room with scent and for some simple recipes.) Choose whatever method seems the most appropriate in your work situation. If you move around on your job, you may need several techniques at your disposal so that you can switch to the best one for each location.

- **Spritz the air:** If you can get away with it, use good aromatherapy-quality essential oils in a spritzer as an "air freshener." Using air fresheners is okay in many workplaces, including most schools. I know several teachers who spritz a chamomile and lavender combo in their elementary school classrooms to keep the kids calm and focused. (Yes, it works!)

- **Plug in an aromatherapy diffuser:** When you don't need to be discreet about introducing aromatherapy into your workplace, an electric aromatherapy diffuser may be ideal to disperse scent. It emits a steady, pure aroma for hours. (I describe several types of diffusers in Chapter 4.) Even though a potpourri-style cooker is much cheaper, the diffuser is often more practical because you don't have to watch over it to keep it filled with water.

- **Sniff an essential oils inhaler:** A far more subtle approach is to stick to personal aromatherapy and not try to improve anyone's mood but your own. Some natural-food stores sell aromatherapy inhalers that contain "mood" blends to affect your emotions. Or, you can make your own "smelling salts" with the recipe in this chapter. Inhalers are convenient because they're small enough to slip into your pocket. Because they look like one of the drugstore inhalers used to clear sinus congestion, you won't seem out of the ordinary when you use it at the office.

- **Carry a scented hanky:** For an even more undetected form of aromatherapy, bring back the era of top hats and carry a handkerchief. Put a couple drops of essential oil on a cloth, and you have the perfect vehicle to carry scent. Every time that you politely cover your nose with your hanky, you'll get an aromatic dose without anyone suspecting that you're really trying to keep your cool or need some energy. This subtle technique works well when traveling on an airplane or train. It doesn't disrupt the person next to you, while you get the benefit of an aromatic lift and get to kill airborne germs.

✔ **Wear as "perfume":** On the risk of being downright sneaky, you can completely avoid red tape at work by wearing pure essential oils as cologne. Health-care workers, especially nurses, who use aromatherapy place a half drop essential oil on their wrist or arms so that the fragrance surrounds their patients as they work on them. (If you want to use sage or rosemary, but they're not your idea of an appealing cologne, then combine the essential oil with your favorite cologne or perfume. Yes, the oil will alter the cologne's fragrance, but hopefully in a pleasing way, *and* you'll get the therapeutic benefits.)

✔ **Use scented hand lotion:** Give yourself a mental or physical pick-me-up during a hard-working day with scented hand lotion. This is opportune when you don't have much time to do anything else at work but rub your hands together. It's also a great idea if you work somewhere you can't put fragrance into the air. Look for a lotion that contains the appropriate essential oils or make your own with the recipe in this chapter.

✔ **Burn incense:** In case you work in an open area, such as a large warehouse, an open garage, or outside (and you don't mind putting up with coworkers cracking '60s jokes and giving you the peace sign), consider burning incense. Its powerful fragrance can scent large areas, and the smoke usually isn't bothersome.

Okay, rub it in

If you're lucky enough to work for a company that brings a massage therapist into your office, take advantage of it. Otherwise, perhaps you can persuade your coworkers to chip in to make it happen. Any stress management consultant can tell you that taking even a short massage break increases your productivity. A massage also makes your body release pain-relieving chemicals (called *endorphins*), which diminish pain similar to the pain-killer drug, morphine.

An office massage uses a portable, padded massage "chair" instead of a massage table. This way, you can stay dressed and can be back at work in 15 minutes flat with your clothes and hair unruffled. Even the massage techniques are designed to assure that they don't knock you out for the next few hours instead of keep you going. This massage doesn't require oil because the practitioner works through your clothes, except for your hands and neck. However, to get extra mileage out of your massage, you can buy a non-oily, alcohol-based liniment and ask that it be massaged on your neck and perhaps your arms, or at least your hands. (Oh, let me tell you that feels so good after a few hours of typing.) Look for one that contains essential oils with brain-stimulating, muscle-relaxing, and circulation-increasing properties. (You know, the ones that I discuss in this chapter.)

Lotion for Emotions

If you can find just a few minutes to spare in your busy schedule, then create your own hand lotion. To save fuss, muss, and time, buy a hand lotion (made with natural ingredients) that is unscented or with very little scent. Some cosmetic, aromatherapy, and natural-food stores sell a "blank" lotion without all the extras so that you can mix in other ingredients. To decide which ones to use, look over the oils listed in this chapter in the sections: "Pepping Up Performance with Peppermint: Stimulants," "A Scenti-Mental Journey: Boosting Memory," "Mind over Matters: Less Stress," "Stay in Control: A Balanced Approach," and "Sleep Tight: Insomnia."

Preparation time: 1 whole minute

Yield: 1 bottle of lotion

4 ounces unscented lotion

20 to 28 drops essential oil

1 Stir the essential oil into the lotion, and it's done! (I told you this was quick!) If you use a blend of several different essential oils, then add 30 drops total (*not* 30 drops of each essential oil). Some essential oils are extra potent, so adjust the amount if you use rose, jasmine, or angelica oils (Use 1 drop for every 8 drops called for in the recipe) or clary sage, chamomile, or ylang ylang oils (use 1 drop for every 5 drops in the recipe).

2 Use as a hand and body lotion whenever you like.

Vary It! *Use 12 drops ginger and 8 drops basil to perk performance. Use 12 drops lemon and 8 drops clove to improve your memory.*

Pepping Up Performance with Peppermint: Stimulants

Sustaining your energy is important if you want to get a job done. One trick to keep ahead is to work in a scented room. According to the research from the psychologists who study scent, aroma considerably improves your mental stamina, concentration, and efficiency. Besides, it makes a much more pleasant environment to work in.

When you get tired or bored, that's when you may find yourself reaching for a cup of coffee or some pills. Your brain waves (those measured through contingent negative variation, or CNV for short) peak sharply in response to stimulants like coffee and stay-awake drugs. At the same time, you can think faster and more clearly. Your brain waves peak the same way when you sniff a stimulating aroma. Granted, scent isn't as powerful of a brain stimulant as a drug or coffee. Nevertheless, the great thing about aromatic stimulants is that they up your brain waves without coffee's or a drug's negative health effects. So, instead of perking coffee, consider the following aromatherapy perks.

- ✔ **Keep attention high:** Scent prevents the sharp drop of sustained attention that typically occurs in anyone after 30 minutes of working. Aromas also keep your mental energy strong by stimulating your body's support system — your autonomic nervous system, which keeps activities such as your breathing and blood pressure on automatic.

- ✔ **No side effects:** Aromatherapy doesn't over-amp your adrenal glands and then leave them flat the way caffeine can. Instead, it does quite the opposite. One way that it does this is to keep your central nervous system calm and stop it from overreacting. This counters rushes of adrenaline that can make you too hyper and nervous. That's a great plus if you're stressed out. Calm essential oils such as lavender oil seem to reduce the nervous system agitation produced by caffeine.

- ✔ **Improve your performance:** Workers in a scented room who spent 40 stressful minutes trying to identify complicated patterns on a computer screen got 88 percent correct answers compared to 65 percent for those working in unscented rooms. The natural fragrances used were peppermint (voted their favorite), benzoin, or cinnamon. In other studies, a room scented with lemon cut computer errors more than half. (Aromatherapists suggest lemon to keep focused and relaxed.)

Using common scents: Brain power

The same essential oils that pep you up and reduce your drowsiness also decrease the likelihood of becoming irritable or of getting headaches. Here are the mind-stimulating scents.

- ✔ Angelica
- ✔ Basil
- ✔ Benzoin
- ✔ Black pepper
- ✔ Cardamom
- ✔ Cinnamon
- ✔ Clove
- ✔ Cypress
- ✔ Ginger

- ✔ Jasmine
- ✔ Peppermint
- ✔ Rosemary
- ✔ Sage

The scents of basil, clove, jasmine, and peppermint oils stimulate your brain waves. So may the other scents on this list, but so far, they're untested. Curiously, the scents of rose, neroli, and ylang ylang oils also stimulate these waves, even though aromatherapists have used them for centuries for quite the opposite reason — to induce relaxation. Obviously, brains are complicated computers that operate in more ways than one, stimulating and relaxing different parts of the brain at the same time. A good example of this dual effect is the relaxing herb catnip. It stimulates your brain's medulla, while calming the "higher" brain responsible for thought processing. In this case, the higher brain wins out with an overall relaxing effect. The same may be true of many essential oils.

Some of these aromas are aphrodisiacs, but don't worry, they won't turn everyone's thoughts to amour — that is, except for jasmine. It's such a potent aphrodisiac, you'd better leave it at home. (For more on this enticing subject, turn to Chapter 8.) How sexy a fragrance seems has a lot to do with the setting and your intention.

Gotta Go-Go-Go Liniment

Here's an example of a recipe to keep you going. It's filled with stimulating fragrances. I've thrown in the bergamot because sticking to just stimulating oils creates an aroma that's just a little too sharp to smell good. It also doubles as a liniment that relaxes overworked muscles.

Preparation time: 4 minutes

Yield: 2 ounces massage oil

9 drops bergamot oil	2 drops peppermint oil
6 drops eucalyptus oil	2 drops ginger oil
3 drops cinnamon oil	2 ounces vegetable oil

1 Combine the oils and stir or shake well.

2 Use for a massage or body oil.

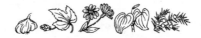

Aroma pick-me-ups

If you're trying to stay alert and awake, sniff any one of the aromas from the list every five minutes or so or fill your office with scent. As with any essential oil, use aromatic pick-me-ups in moderate doses. Some pep-up essential oils can actually turn sedative if you over do them. When you're dealing with chronic exhaustion, try to determine its cause and go to the source of your problem. Refer to the Symptom Guide under Fatigue for more energy hints when you're "burning the candle at both ends."

A Scenti-Mental Journey: Boosting Memory

Your memory is something that you depend upon. Think about it. Without your ability to recall data, you can't find your shoes or watch in the morning, much less remember how to get to work. You use your memory minute by minute. That's why it's downright scary when important facts slip from your mind. You can probably afford to forget where you laid your keys or to pick up bread at the grocery once in a while, but it's a different story when you forget an important phone call that you had to make by two o'clock or the boss turns to you with a question and you *should* know the answer.

Taking a trip down memory lane: Putting scent to use

Aroma helps you remember important facts, places, and names because your sense of smell is closely connected to the areas of your brain that control both your short-term and your long-term memories. These memories governs the this-and-that's of every day life and those of past events. Fortunately, memory is not a one-way street. Information associated with scent is not only stored, but you can also easily retrieve it and fragrance helps you do so. (For more on the brain and its relationship to scent, see Chapter 1.) Here are the primary ways that aroma helps you to remember.

> ✔ **Remember better:** Work in a scented room. You'll notice and retain facts quicker and easier and then file them in your brain where they are easier to relocate. The connection of aroma to your brain's limbic system gives it a direct route to your thought processing and memory. (See Chapter 1 for information on the limbic system.)

✔ **Scent association:** Your recall of past events is much stronger when it's linked to scent rather than sight. You know the experience. You encounter a whiff of a certain perfume or some other fragrance that you haven't smelled for years, and suddenly you're flying back in time to a long-forgotten experience that you associate with that smell. The scent carries everything about that experience: The sights, sounds, and especially your emotional impressions at the time. If you're like most people, you can recall an event that is several months old twice as easily if aroma is involved compared to a visual recollection. As time goes on, your scent memory stays sharp while your visual memory plummets. Years later, you sniff the same thing, and you're instantly journeying down memory lane. Take a hint from students who tried to memorize lists of words. They had better recall later if they sniffed a scent — even something that they didn't like — while doing the assignment and then smelled that scent again when asked to recall the words.

✔ **Stimulate blood circulation:** Take a good sniff of an aromatherapy scent, and you automatically inhale plenty of oxygen. Not bad, considering that the number one reason for a poor memory is not enough oxygen reaching your brain. Too little oxygen makes you feel fuzzy-headed and easily confused. That's just about the last thing you want on the job. (Go to the sidebar "Do inhale" for more on why taking a deep breath sends more oxygen to your brain.)

✔ **Stop "forgetful" chemicals:** Science is just learning how the brain functions and the connection that it has to aromatherapy. One of the ways that sage oil alters your brain chemistry for the better is to stop the activity of an enzyme (called *acerylcholinesterase*) that contributes to memory loss and seems to play a part in Alzheimer's disease. A good thing about sage is that it doesn't disrupt other brain activities, unlike the drug tacrine, which slows degeneration from Alzheimer's but also damages your liver in the process. (Unfortunately, sage isn't strong enough to replace the drug, but researcher hope that scents like this will show them how to make better medicines, probably aromatic ones, for memory loss problems.)

Thanks for the memories

As science investigates aromas that improve your brain power and memory, it keeps proving what herbalists have known all along. In the 17th century, herbalist John Gerard said that sage, "helpeth a weake braine or memory and restoreth them . . . in a short time." The ancient Greeks placed bay laurel wreaths on the heads of their scholars and poets to make sure that their kept their wits sharp. Shakespeare has Ophelia in the last act of *Hamlet* proclaim, "There's rosemary, that's for remembrance."

Have the scents to remember

Use your sense of smell to your advantage by inhaling fragrances that assist your memory recall and stimulate your blood circulation. These same scents do other things as well. They tend to produce more of the brain waves called beta, which help make you alert and attentive. For an added perk, most of these essential oils double as spicy stimulants that help keep you alert — a dynamite combination for mental sharpness. If stress affects your memory, use these essential oils with the calming oils that I recommend in the section "Mind over matters: Less stress." Here are some scents to spark your brain.

- ✔ Basil
- ✔ Bay laurel
- ✔ Bay rum (pimento)
- ✔ Clove
- ✔ Lemon
- ✔ Rosemary
- ✔ Sage

Forget-Me-Not Liniment

You can whip up your own memory blend that also stimulates blood circulation and relaxes any muscle tension you have. Because it has an alcohol base, it's perfect to use for an office "chair" massage. Liniment recipes usually call for rubbing alcohol, but its strong smell interferes with the scent of the aromatherapy oils, so I prefer using vodka instead. (Vodka is a combination of only alcohol and water.) Don't forget: This liniment can get hot, and the heat increases the more you rub it on your skin.

Preparation time: *4 minutes*

Yield: *2 ounces liniment*

8 drops lemon oil

4 drops rosemary oil

2 drops sage oil

1 drop clove oil

2 ounces vodka or rubbing alcohol

(continued)

1 Combine ingredients.

2 Use for massage as often as you can!

Vary It! If you prefer a lotion rather than a liniment, then use any unscented or lightly scent body lotion instead of rubbing alcohol. This lotion is also excellent for massage, and it's not as oily as a typical massage oil.

Mind over Matters: Less Stress

Stress doesn't improve your memory or level of efficiency a bit. On the contrary, it contributes to their slowdown. The problem with stress is that if you endure enough of it for long enough, it short-circuits your brain so that you can't think as fast or as clearly as you should. If you're already under stress at work, having a brain meltdown is probably the last thing that you need.

Working in a stressful environment, straining to get a project done, being bored by monotonous tasks, and being always on the go all increase your body's workload by pushing your adrenal glands on overdrive. You end up working overtime more than you know because you work hard at your job, and then your body also works hard to deal with the physical and emotional effects stress at the same time. It's no surprise that you feel worn out! You also can become drowsy and irritable and develop headaches. If you think that's a bad enough scenario to slow down your work, listen to this. Researchers find that the more stress you experience, the more likely you are to get sick. Then you'll really fall behind at work (not to mention use up your sick days). Ask yourself these questions for a quick check on how well you're dealing with stress.

- ✓ **Fatigue:** Do you feel endlessly tired?

- ✓ **Insomnia:** Do you have sleep disturbances, such as waking up often at night or in the early morning, and you're unable to get back to sleep? Do you have vivid dreams that are accompanied by restless sleep?

- ✓ **Headaches:** Are you starting to have migraine or tension headaches that seem related to your work?

- ✓ **Digestive upsets:** Do you experience heartburn, a loss of appetite, indigestion, constipation, or diarrhea?

- ✓ **Circulation problems:** Do you ever have heart palpitations, an irregular heartbeat, high blood pressure, or get out of breath easily?

- ✓ **Emotional responses:** Do you sometimes feel nervous or hostile, overreact emotionally, or frequently want to cry? Do you feel an increasing amount of depression?

Do inhale

There's something to say for the increased inhalation that automatically happens when you sniff an essential oil. Taking deep breaths slows your breathing down, and that makes you feel less anxious and stressed. Breathing sends more oxygen to help your brain and also to your muscles to help them function properly and relax easier.

Watch out for those midday yawns. They are your body's attempt to convince you to breath more air, and they signal that your brain is longing for more oxygen. Working at a desk, especially if you're on a computer, puts extra strain on your neck and can interfere with your need for oxygen. The tight muscles that result constrict your blood vessels and all of the oxygen-rich blood traveling to your brain. In a vicious cycle, the neck tension impairs your brain activity. That slows down your work pace and makes you stressed. To top it off, the longer work hours increase your neck tension.

> ✔ **Sexual problems:** Do you have problems with sexual desire, impotence or infertility?
>
> ✔ **Muscle cramps:** Do you find yourself clenching your jaw, or is your jaw or neck extra tight or sore?
>
> ✔ **Sweating:** Are you sweating for no obvious reason, or do you often have a very dry mouth or feel exceptionally thirsty?

If you answer yes to even one of these questions, you may already have a stress problem. If you answer yes to several of these questions, you had better keep reading. You're probably overstressed.

It makes good scents: Aromas for stress relief

Your body's various responses to stress are linked to the hypothalamus in your brain. This part of your brain controls many functions in your body. Since the hypothalamus is part of your limbic system which processes smell, aromatherapy goes direct to ease your stress (see Chapter 1).

Relaxing fragrances — the ones that help you deal better with stress — tend to produce slower frequency brain waves (delta waves), and they also prompt some theta waves. Both delta and theta waves bring out your quiet and meditative side. Many of these relaxing aromas also increase another type of brain's waves, the alpha waves. These are the ones that make you feel centered and focused. You may not need it, but these scents additionally have antidepressant properties just to smell them. (There's more on depression and anxiety later in this chapter in the section "Stay in Control: A Balanced Approach.") The aromas of lavender, bergamot, marjoram, sandalwood, lemon, chamomile, and valerian, in that order, produce sedating brain wave patterns in your brain, according to CNV testing.

- ✔ Bergamot
- ✔ Chamomile
- ✔ Lavender
- ✔ Lemon
- ✔ Melissa (lemon balm)
- ✔ Marjoram
- ✔ Neroli (orange blossom)
- ✔ Petitgrain
- ✔ Rose
- ✔ Sandalwood
- ✔ Valerian

Are we having fun yet? Adrenal exhaustion

If you push your adrenal glands to the limit with stress, they stop functioning properly. Stress impairs the ability of your adrenal glands to operate and makes you more easily stressed. In the early stages of problems, adrenal glands often go overboard when responding to even small amounts of stress. Eventually, they hit the hammock in exhaustion, and you end up with "tired" glands. They don't respond enough, leaving you feeling drained and unable to get excited about much of anything: work, family, sex, vacation . . . it all becomes a blur.

The adrenal glands seem to respond best to certain scents. Try the following essential oils as fragrances that you sniff and especially in a massage oil — along with a massage, if possible! (Massage is one of the best stress-reducing techniques to use with aromatherapy.) Look for aromatherapy blends that combine these essential oils with other anti-stress oils.

- ✔ Clary sage
- ✔ Spruce
- ✔ Pine (especially the species called *syvestris*)

Stress Less Massage Oil

This massage oil reduces stress and keeps you relaxed, but still alert enough to get your job done.

Preparation time: 2 minutes

Yield: 2 ounces massage oil

8 drops lavender

4 drops geranium

2 drops clary sage

2 drops spruce

2 ounces almond (or other vegetable) oil

1 Add the essential oils to the vegetable oil.

2 Mix everything together well and use as a massage or body oil.

Vary It! *If you want, use this same blend to scent the air. Mix the essential oils together without the almond oil to make yourself a Stress Less blend. Use this with any of the methods I suggest in Chapter 5. You can find instructions for the appropriate number of drops to use for each method in that chapter.*

Stay in Control: A Balanced Approach

Anxiety wears many different faces. One way that it manifests is the nervousness that you may feel when giving a presentation, going for a job interview, or perhaps when flying. A little anxiety is rarely a problem. Feeling a few butterflies in your stomach and getting energized from the burst of adrenaline that often comes with anxiousness may even improve your performance. However, if your anxiety level reaches the point where it turns your hands clammy from sweat and your mouth becomes so dry that you can barely speak, it's not going to help you a bit. If you feel anxious throughout the day, you probably have difficulty concentrating, and then you can't sleep well at night. Anxiety can also make you too fearful or preoccupied with problems at work and blow the smallest upsets way out of proportion. Some people become so anxious that they have panic attacks in certain situations in which they become immobilized with fear and anxiousness.

Keeping your focus isn't just about staying mentally stimulated or how much you can relax. Get too hyper or go down too far, and you can't keep your mind focused. For optimum brain power, you also need to be emotionally stable. Stress exaggerates anxiety, and anxiety or frustration at work can also lead to anger. This can be tough at work because — no surprises here — most people don't like to be around someone who's angry. However, unresolved anger that you can't readily express only creates more stress. No matter how hard you try to concentrate on your work to avoid it, feelings of doubt, anger, mistrust, or fear can creep into your consciousness to take their toll.

Keeping your cool

I know that this all sounds pretty grim, but aromatherapy does offer gentle assistance to help you rebuild your emotional equilibrium. Just inhaling the scents of lavender and sandalwood increases the alpha waves in your brain. These waves decrease all the miscellaneous, idle chatter that runs through your mind and encourages your mind to relax. These two aromas have a long history of creating meditative states. Other alpha wave essential oils are eucalyptus, pine, and fir, which are stimulants, so they offer an extra element of increased attention when you sniff them. Blood pressure rates jump when you're nervous, but just sniffing the scents of marjoram, orange, or geranium drops your pressure two to five points (both the systolic and diastolic rates). That's not significant enough of a drop if you suffer from high blood pressure, but it does indicate a lowered level.

Reduce anxiety

Researchers studying aromatherapy's effects on emotions find that it eases feelings of apprehension, loneliness, and rejection. Some scents make people even feel less embarrassed, and even happier. One study asked participants, "What kind of person makes you angry?" Once everyone became sufficiently riled up, pleasant scents calmed them down better than the folks who didn't have anything to sniff.

The New York subway doesn't usually exemplify great etiquette. It's push and shove all the way to get to your destination on time. However, researchers discovered that when cars are scented with pleasant food aromas, passengers in them push each other much less and act genuinely more content than usual.

Even a new patent is on a product that brings aromatherapy into the workplace. The combination of neroli, valerian, and nutmeg is rubbed into the skin or inhaled, and it's designed to relieve anxiety and stress and also to reduce blood pressure. At least one study describes the scent of lavender as one that creates an inner sense of peace.

- ✔ Chamomile
- ✔ Clary sage
- ✔ Fir
- ✔ Geranium
- ✔ Juniper
- ✔ Marjoram
- ✔ Melissa (lemon balm)
- ✔ Neroli (orange blossom)
- ✔ Nutmeg
- ✔ Orange
- ✔ Petitgrain
- ✔ Rose

Geranium and valerian are both stimulating and sedative to your brain (according to contingent negative variation patterns that I mention previously in this chapter under "Pepping Up Performance with Peppermint: Stimulants.") This duality simply indicates that these scents have a "balancing" action. They go up or down depending upon the needs of an individual. Herbs that do this very thing are known as *adaptagens* because they "adapt" to your personal needs, and they also teach your body to "adapt" well in different physical surroundings and emotional circumstances. With aromatherapy, these scents are useful for a variety of emotional problems. Many people find valerian's scent objectionable (it's described as resembling dirty socks), but the roselike fragrance of geranium is generally well liked. The scent of geranium creates harmonious situations that cause you to feel better about yourself and others when you sniff it.

One apple a day may keep more than the doctor away — it can fend off nervousness. Apple is one the scents that make people less anxious, especially when mixed with cinnamon and clove. The next time that you have to speak before a group, try eating an apple beforehand. And, if you have a chance, sprinkle a little cinnamon on it. (This scent is only available as a synthetic.)

Climb out of depression

If you have a tendency to get depressed, or if you're just feeling down once in a while, then you can turn to the following aromatherapy antidepressants.

- ✔ Angelica
- ✔ Bergamot
- ✔ Cardamom
- ✔ Chamomile
- ✔ Cinnamon
- ✔ Clary sage
- ✔ Clove

- ✔ Cypress
- ✔ Lavender
- ✔ Lemon verbena
- ✔ Lemon
- ✔ Melissa (lemon balm)
- ✔ Orange
- ✔ Orange blossom (neroli)
- ✔ Petitgrain
- ✔ Rose
- ✔ Ylang-ylang

Smelling Salts

You can make your own anxiety-relieving smelling salts.

Preparation time: *4 minutes*

Yield: *1 tablespoon smelling salts*

3 drops bergamot

2 drops geranium

1 drop neroli (or 3 drops petitgrain)

1 tablespoon rock salt (or other coarse salt)

1 Combine ingredients.

2 Carry in a closed container and sniff as needed.

Vary It! *Add the same essential oils (in the same amount) to 4 ounces vegetable oil to create a massage oil. If you can't get a massage, then add a couple teaspoons of this massage oil to your bath water and enjoy!*

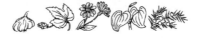

Un-nerving experience

Choose any aromatherapy method, such as a light bulb ring, potpourri, or an aromatherapy diffuser, to dispense scents to relieve anxiety into the air (see Chapter 5). If you're on the go a lot, carry them with you in an aromatherapy inhaler (easy to buy) or as smelling salts that you make yourself (easy to make).

If you're already taking antidepressive or anti-anxiety drugs, it's safe for you to use aromatherapy with them. Severe anxiety points to imbalances in brain chemistry. Because this is a physical problem, besides trying a few aromatherapy techniques, also ask your doctor and other health caregivers for suggestions on how to help your body cope. If anxiety causes heart palpitations or chest pains or makes you feel dizzy, then select a scent from the "Mind over Matters: Less Stress" section in this chapter. Good examples are ylang ylang, sandalwood, frankincense, and marjoram.

You can take your state of mind either up or down using fragrance. You can also combine scents that relax and stimulate. Don't worry about creating aroma warfare by mixing two opposing scents. Aromatherapy doesn't work that way. What could be better than being highly focused and relaxed at the same time? After all, isn't this what everyone wants — to have every muscle in your body completely relaxed, but to be alert and focused at the same time?

Tips for Business Trips

Flying through time zones can disrupt your body rhythms so that you can experience fatigue, dizziness, nausea, depression, and pressure in your head after the flight. It may take you a day or so to adjust, probably time you don't have to spare if you're there on business.

London's Heathrow International Terminal offers an "After-Flight Regulator" set of aromatherapy blends developed by English aromatherapist Daniele Ryman to help you overcome jet lag. It is also conveniently offered at some of the area's hotels.

Virgin Atlantic Airlines and Air New Zealand provide their first class and business passengers with an aromatherapy kit to combat jet lag, also developed by Ryman. A relaxing floral scent appropriately called "Asleep" goes into your bath water or is used with your shower so you sleep off your jet lag. Just so no one gets confused, the other formula is clearly labeled "Awake." It's stimulating peppermint to make you alert and positive without feeling groggy when you finally get to that important meeting.

Personally, I don't find a lot of time to take a bath when I'm busy packing and preparing for a business trip and certainly not while I'm on it. That is, at least until the work is done and by then, so is the jet lag! I prefer to carry my aromatherapy around everywhere in a spray bottle. Using a hydrosol in the bottle is especially nice. (What's that, you may ask? Turn to Chapter 1 to find out more about them.)

I don't think I could fly anymore without having my trusty aromatherapy spray in my carry-on. It counters the stuffy cabin's recycled and overly dry air, not to mention being totally refreshing. Once when I was traveling across the U. S. on a long plane trip from San Francisco to Boston, my spray kept misting on the businessman next to me. He was sound asleep, so I figured he wouldn't know the difference. When we landed, he kept commenting on how unusually refreshed he felt and then said, "It must be sitting next to you." (No, I didn't tell him my secret.)

Arrival Revival

If you don't plan on flying New Zealand Air in the near future, then make your own aromatic spray. Both essential oils in this recipe are excellent for making you relaxed, yet focused — a perfect combination for the frequent flyer. (You might consider carrying this scent on board in your carry-on when you fly to assure that you have a mellow flight.)

Preparation time: *5 seconds*

Yield: *A delightful aromatherapy spritzer!*

12 drops lavender oil

5 drops geranium oil

3 drops rose

2 ounces distilled water

1 Add the essential oils to the water in a spray bottle.

2 Shake gently each time before spraying.

Vary It! *If you're in need of a wake-up call, then replace the geranium in this recipe with peppermint oil. If it's not convenient to spritz, go ahead and make either blend without the water and rub a drop of it on your wrist to sniff while on your way running off to your conference or meeting.*

TIP

In addition to aromatherapy, drink plenty of water and eat lightly before and during your flight. When traveling across three or more time zones, start readjusting your sleep patterns a couple nights before your trip. If you're traveling or commuting in your car, or your job just involves a lot of driving, then take aromatherapy with you. Flip to Chapter 4 for ideas to scent a car.

Travel Companion: Eye Relax

While you're either traveling or at work, here is a quick and easy way to relax your tired eyes and brain. As an added bonus, it helps get rid of early morning puffy eyes to keep you looking bright-eyed and alert.

Preparation time: *5 minutes*

Yield: *2 eye bags*

½ cup water

2 tea bags (chamomile or regular black tea)

1 Bring a half cup water to a boil.

2 Pour the boiling water over 2 tea bags of chamomile or regular black tea, steep for a few minutes, and then let cool enough so that they don't burn your eyelids.

3 Squeeze the excess water from the tea bags and place 1 bag over each of your closed eyes. If handy, also place a small, folded cloth over the tea bags to hold them in place and block out light.

4 Relax with the tea bags over your eyes for at least 3 three minutes.

Home at Last: Having the Scents to Unwind

It's all too easy to bring the problems of work home with you. Just as aromatherapy gets you through the day, it can also help you to unwind when you finally get home.

Use it to help you be more focused with your friends or family, even when you're tired. Maybe after a long day at the office, you want to be alert enough to go over your child's school report or to take in that late night movie without falling asleep. Aromatherapy can ease tension at home as easily as it can at work. My aromatherapy suggestions for jet lag (see the preceding section) and relaxation work just as well while you're on a family vacation as taking a business trip.

Hot/Cold Pack

One of my favorite ways to unwind with fragrance is with a bean bag pillow. These small pillows come in various shapes and are not really filled with beans, but rather with flaxseed, rye grain, or some other whole grain. The magic comes when you heat them in your microwave oven or pop one into the freezer to chill. The heat or cold stays for at least an hour or longer depending upon the pillow's design.

I have a pack that wraps around my shoulders, but I've got my eye on a lumbar pack and I've even seen slippers. After a long day punching computer keys, I like to fall asleep with a narrow pillow under my neck or shoulder. And that's the beauty of these bags. There's no water to spill on your couch or bed as with a hot water bottle. Unlike a heating pad, you don't have to worry about falling asleep and forgetting to turn it off and you can lay right on top of the bag, even mush it into any convenient shape you choose. (Look in the Appendix for places to purchase these pillows.)

Throwing a (foot) ball: Bathing your feet

One aromatherapy treatment that feels really great at the end of the day is a foot soak. If your job has you on your feet a lot, you'll find that this bath offers blessed relief to sore, tired, worn-out feet. The hot water relaxes your feet and encourages the essential oils to penetrate into your feet. And, in case you've had one of those overly cerebral day at the office, there's nothing like it to focus your attention on your feet instead of your head! A foot bath can be real ball for your feet and is perfectly safe so it's something that you can do every day. Don't argue that you don't have the time. The bath only takes a couple of minutes to prepare, and you can stick your feet in it while you watch TV or talk on the phone. If you work at home as I do, you can even place a foot bath under your desk. In case your feet tend to get chilled at work or coming home during the winter, a foot bath gets your blood flowing to warm up your feet, as well as the rest of you. Because it improves the circulation in your legs, a foot bath should lessen the likelihood of you developing varicose veins from too much standing or hemorrhoids from too much sitting. If you've already developed one of these conditions, then use a foot bath as one of your therapies.

Soak Those Pups Foot Bath

One way to make a foot bath is to soak your feet in a strong herbal tea (which pulls out the essential oils). However, essential oils are faster and easier. The oils that you choose determine if you relax, wake up, or think better. Feel free to replace the essential oils in this recipe with other oils.

Preparation time: 2 minutes

Yield: 1 foot bath

1 to 2 quarts water

5 drops tea tree oil

5 drops sage oil

2 drops peppermint oil

1 Heat the water or use hot water from the tap that is just cool enough to stick your feet in.

2 Fill a container that is big enough for both feet with the warm water.

3 Add the essential oils to the water and stir to distribute them.

4 Soak your feet for at least 15 minutes — and relax!

Vary It! Adding ¼ cup Epsom — a common type of salt that's sold in all grocery and drug stores to relax sore muscles — are a good addition if your feet are sore or just plain "dog tired."

Vary It Some More! When making any type of foot bath, you can also add a drop of your own choice of essential oil for whatever emotional impact you need. See the Aroma Guide for some ideas.

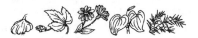

Sleep Tight: Insomnia

Travel can make havoc with your sleep schedule, especially if you're on the move a lot, and even more so if you're crossing time zones. Lack of sleep leaves you feeling tired the next day. If you don't get adequate sleep for weeks or months, you easily develop symptoms of sleep deprivation such as dizziness, confusion, agitation, and depression. If you travel for business as I do, then you really need a good night's sleep to do your best the next day.

The effects of some fragrances are comparable to sedative drugs. Some of the smell receptors in your brain are the same ones that activate the sedative drugs Valium and Librium. That means fragrances have a direct route to relax and put you to sleep. Napping in scented room lulls elderly patients to sleep as effectively as the drugs designed to treat insomnia. And, once they do nod off, fragrance makes their sleep much less restless.

Here are the aromas that send you to dreamland.

- ✔ Bergamot
- ✔ Chamomile
- ✔ Citronella
- ✔ Clary sage
- ✔ Frankincense
- ✔ Geranium
- ✔ Lavender
- ✔ Melissa (lemon balm)
- ✔ Mandarin
- ✔ Neroli
- ✔ Rose
- ✔ Sandalwood
- ✔ Tangerine

Essential oil of citronella is not typically suggested to increase sleep. However, one study found that the essential oil improves sleep for both healthy people and those who have a sleep disorder or nervous condition that keeps them up at night. In fact, it works better than taking repeated doses of hops extract, a well-known herbal sedative. (See the Sleep Pillow recipe, later in this chapter.) I've tried citronella, and it works. Add about 4 drops of the essential oil to a warm bath.

Nightly Night Blend

This is a versatile blend for you to use to scent your room or your bed sheets. (Chapter 4 tells you how.)

Preparation time: *4 minutes*

Yield: *About 4 applications*

6 drops bergamot oil

3 drops geranium oil

2 drops chamomile oil

1 drop frankincense oil

1 drop rose oil

Combine the oils together and use in any of the suggested applications to scent a room.

Vary It! *You can easily turn this same blend into a massage or body lotion. Add the essential oil mix to 2 ounces vegetable oil or an unscented body lotion.*

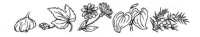

Sweet Dreams Sleep Pillow

Sleep pillows are a European tradition. Scented sleep pillows work amazingly well to knock you out at night. I travel a lot, so I carry one with me. No matter where I'm sleeping, my pillow always smells like home. By now, just the association of the scent with sleep is enough to send me off to dreamland. You don't need to lug around a regular bed-sized pillow. A miniature version is fine. The herb hops is as much responsible for invoking sleep as the lavender. Many people scoff at the idea — it just seems too easy — but when sensors tested the air above a hops-filled pillow, they detected three essential oil compounds in the hops. (The Japanese researchers who conducted this study said that herbal pillows "facilitate falling asleep or to minimize stressful situations. . . .") The chamomile helps make you sleepy and is said to ensure good dreams.

Preparation time: *20 minutes*

Yield: *One 7 square-inch sleep pillow*

2 pieces of cloth about 8 inches square

¼ cup hops flowers (strobiles), dried

⅛ cup chamomile flowers, dried

⅛ cup lavender flowers, dried

15 drops lavender essential oil

1 Make a small pillow by sewing the 2 pieces of cloth together on 3 sides, leaving 1 end open.

2 Blend the herbs together. Then sprinkle the lavender oil on the herbs and stir them to distribute it.

3 Spoon the herbs into the pillow through the open end and then sew up that side.

4 Put this little pillow under your regular sleeping pillow or tuck it inside your pillowcase.

(continued)

Tip: The scent pillow lasts for many months. When it starts to get faint, crush it a little to release more of the scent. Eventually, when it no longer has much scent at all, add a couple drops of lavender to the pillow's corner and place the pillow in a plastic bag for several days. This allows the scent to permeate throughout the pillow. Re-scent as needed.

Vary It! If you like, add a tablespoon of dried basil leaves to your sleep pillow before in that basil's fragrance prevents nightmares and agitated sleep. To dream more, add a tablespoon of the dried leaves of mugwort to the mix, but be aware that it will indeed produce more dreams, and you may not get much sleep! Want to remember your dreams? Then add a tablespoon of rosemary dreams. (Remember, rosemary — that's for remembrance!)

Mental clari-tea

For more suggestions and simple recipes, look up these headings in The Symptom Guide: High Blood Pressure, Carpal Tunnel Syndrome and Repetitive Strain Injuries, Depression, Eye Inflammation and Stress, Fatigue, Forgetfulness, Headaches, Insomnia, Muscle and Back Pain, Nervousness, and last, but not least, Stress. Aromatherapy helps you deal with fatigue, depression and anxiety, but for a permanent solution, seek a holistic approach.

If you notice that your mental performance lags behind its usual level, then there's even more natural help than your "good scents." Herbs such as ginkgo leaf, gotu kola leaf, ginseng root, and Siberian ginseng root improve your brain power and memory. Herbal antidepressants such as a tincture or pills of St. John's wort leaf and flower, help to ease depression. (Have a knowledgeable health professional help you select antidepressive herbs if you're already on medication to treat depression.) Relaxation techniques, counseling, a wholesome diet, and exercise are all good ideas. Also, try to get enough sleep and — you probably get the idea by now — reduce stress in your life as much as possible. Read the previous section on Stress on how aromatherapy can help you do so.

Chapter 10

Aromatherapy at the Gym

· ·

In This Chapter

▶ Improving your performance with better circulation

▶ Making a massage oil to up your circulation

▶ Increasing your stamina with aromatherapy

▶ Getting a sports massage

▶ Decreasing inflammation with aromatic oil

▶ Getting a mini-warmup with a liniment

· ·

*Y*ou may have already joined the current fitness craze. In the last couple decades, millions of people have adapted fitness as a way of life, as they bounce, run, flex, prance, and pant their way to better health. If you're a regular at the gym and wouldn't think of missing your aerobics or swimming class or batting balls, pumping iron, or doing any physical exercise on a regular basis, then you've caught the fitness bug.

Unlike other bugs that I discuss in this book, this one is a good one to catch. If you're committed, it may as well be to something healthy. Vigorous, yet sensible exercise certainly fits that bill. Along with all the panting and grunting and sweating from a good workout, any even-paced, regular exercise does all sorts of good things for your health. You improve the functioning of your cardiovascular system (it comprises your heart and blood circulation), you tone your body, and you keep your weight down. For bonus points, you also feel on top of the world after a workout. This emotional uplift is partly due from your sense of accomplishment and just the fact that you got your blood circulating. However, exercise also affects your brain in very positive ways. It can lift you out of the ho-hum doldrums and even help counter depression.

It's almost too good to be true. You can dance, swim, hike, play ball, or participate in any number of enjoyable physical events and end up being healthier in both body and mind. Yet with all that muscle action comes the probability that sometimes you'll push yourself a little too hard and a little too far. The outcome is sore muscles. As an even more serious consequence (if you torque this or that in the wrong direction), you can end up with sprain or a strain. Any of these result in pain — something that you'll surely like to avoid — but if you're a serious athlete, it can mean worse consequences in lost training time.

In this chapter, I show you how to go for the gold by avoiding getting off track from your sport's fever with down time due to a pulled muscle or fatigue.

Getting Off to a Good Start: Aromatherapy's Basic Training

It doesn't matter if you're pumping iron at the gym or pumping pedals on a bike, aromatherapy is an important addition to your workout regime. Even if you're pounding a hammer rather than the track or doing any job that works your muscles hard, aromatherapy helps you keep in shape to get the job done. It not only can ease already hurting muscles and minor sports or work-related injuries, it also helps prevent them from getting sore in the first place.

Go for the gold: Early Olympic athletes

The Ancient Greek athletes knew what they stood to gain from aromatherapy to help them win: Enhanced performance and ability. These highly regarded athletes were treated to a special sports massage that included scented massage oils. A different massage oil was specially formulated for each part of their body. Mint was rubbed on their arms, thyme on their knees, almond oil on their hands and feet, and cinnamon and rose in palm oil for their chest and the jaw. Even their hair and eyebrows were given special treatment with marjoram.

In India, athletes also received the red carpet treatment. A 12th-century text describes a daily bath ritual that was recommended to improve athletic performance. After bathing, the athlete was massaged with fragrant oils. The suggested essential oils were jasmine, clove, pine, cardamom, basil, coriander — all discussed in this book — along with the less familiar saffron, agarwood, champaca, pandanus, and costus essential oils in a sesame oil base.

A modern version of this Indian treatment, the "Invincible Athletes" program, adapts India's ancient Ayurvedic medicine, along with aromatherapy, to develop a sports program for professional runners, skiers, bodybuilders, and cyclists. One devotee is the triathlete Colleen Cannon, who credits the program with helping her to rank in the top three female triathletes and to win the U. S. women's best short-course.

Whether you're a dedicated decathlete or a weekend warrior, your athletic capability relies on several factors. Four things are especially important for your performance, and it's a matter of team spirit because they all need to work together for you to reach your highest physical potential. Fortunately, aromatherapy covers all four of these:

- ✔ Muscle strength
- ✔ Endurance
- ✔ Concentration
- ✔ Stamina

Oils to improve circulation

In the long run, essential oils improve your athletic performance by increasing blood circulation. (By the way, these essential oils help improve your circulation even if your version of enjoying athletic competitions is from the bleachers or sitting in front of the TV.) Here are essential oils that are sure to get your blood moving and give your performance a kick start.

- ✔ Cypress
- ✔ Eucalyptus
- ✔ Fennel
- ✔ Geranium
- ✔ Ginger
- ✔ Juniper
- ✔ Lemongrass
- ✔ Rosemary

Shape up: Move that blood

Having good blood circulation has a lot to do with staying in physical shape. Your blood runs a constant course that brings the oxygen for energy to your individual cells from your lungs. Your blood also runs nutrients for fuel from your digestive organs to your cells. It's vital for you as an athlete to have good blood circulation to bring your muscles the generous supply of these goodies that they require to keep them pumping.

The essential oils listed in the section "Hot stuff: Oils for liniments," later in this chapter, increase circulation. Because these oils are hot stuff, use these oils very "gingerly" and well diluted in a massage oil. Unlike the other circulation oils listed in this section, they are for use just on your sore muscles, not over your entire body. Hot oils are also not recommended for use in your bath.

Oils to improve blood vessels

Here's a second list of essential oils that also are good for your blood system. They aren't quite as powerful in increasing circulation as the first set of oils, but they have something else going for them. They improve the integrity of your blood vessels. As your blood pumps faster and with more force, your blood vessels stay strong and flexible.

- Bergamot
- Cedarwood
- Chamomile
- Frankincense
- Grapefruit
- Lemon

Two of the most effective ways to improve circulation and to ease stiff muscles are to get a relaxing massage or to take a hot bath — with essential oils, of course. For a bath, add 3 to 6 drops of circulation-stimulating essential oils to the hot water. For a massage, buy a massage oil that contains some of the essential oils that I suggest or make your own using the following recipe.

Massage Oil for Circulation

Here's a recipe that I like. If you don't get the massage, don't despair — you can at least take advantage of this oil by rubbing it on your arms and legs.

Preparation time: *5 minutes*

Yield: *2 ounces massage oil or lotion*

10 drops lemon

6 drops geranium

4 drops rosemary

2 ounces vegetable oil or lotion

1 Combine all the oils.

2 Use as a body massage oil.

Hydrotherapy

The term *hydrotherapy* refers to the therapeutic use of water *(hydro* means water). It's an excellent way to get your circulation moving and helps to relax stiff muscles as well. To try out hydrotherapy, you need to expose your body to the extremes of hot and cold by alternating back and forth between the two. You can do this by going into a sauna, a hot tub, or a bathtub of hot water. Then come out of the heat to hose or rinse yourself down with cold water every five or ten minutes. This may sound brutal, but ohhhh . . . it feels so good once it's over, and it certainly does get your blood moving! (So much so, that if you do have heart problems, you should pass on doing this therapy.)

To add aromatherapy to your hydrotherapy regime, add essential oils that I recommend to stimulate circulation. You'll need about ten drops to put on the hot "rocks" in your sauna or to add to a two to four-person hot tub. (Unlike vegetable oils, the components in essential oils are too small to gum up your hot tub — but make sure that you're using only pure essential oil with no additives.) To be on the safe side, go easy at first by adding a few initial drops to make sure that the essential oil you add isn't going to be too intense. It shouldn't sting your eyes or skin.

Stay on Track: Stamina

Stamina is what keeps you going so that you can make that goal, play that last round, or ski one more slope before you quit. It's one of the important aspects of your physical performance.

Several essential oils help you maintain your physical endurance and stamina and keep you focused at the same time. What is even more impressive is that they help you stay on track through their scent alone. That means you can carry an essential oil or even a sprig of the plant itself with you to sniff during training or a workout. (You can buy aromatherapy inhalers that contain scents that are designed to increase your stamina.) Not surprisingly, most of these essential oils for sport's stamina are the same ones that increase mental focus and your attention span. (Turn to Chapter 9 for more information on these particular oils or to make your own smelling salts.)

Rub a dub: Sports massage

Exercising past your conditioning ends up being painful, but it never hurts to plan ahead for a massage. The sooner that you get your massage to work out the stiffness or inflammation, the better. If you work at a desk during the week and then you lift weights all afternoon Sunday or you sign up for that 40-mile, weekend bike ride or run that marathon, chances are that you'll be plenty sore Sunday night. If you've been in full training, but need to push yourself to build up more, then you'll probably feel it the next day. If you're expecting to be sore, then think ahead and schedule a massage for Sunday evening. This is especially smart if you're planning to go to work Monday morning.

I asked Josh Levy what you can expect from a sports massage. Josh is a sports massage specialist and an instructor at Phillip's School of Massage in Nevada City, California. Josh says that a sports massage involves many techniques, and he doesn't stick to one method. It depends on what shape you're in — or more likely how out of shape you are. If you're sore from overextending yourself or your muscles are cramping, then a deep massage is what you need. This squeezes out the stuff, called *lactic acid,* that builds up in your muscles when you work them and lingers around creating soreness and stiffness. However, you don't always need to go to a specialist. A good Swedish-style massage typically goes deep enough. The rubbing and muscle kneading of either Swedish or sports massage relies on using much massage oil. If your massage practitioner isn't already using a muscle-relaxing massage oil, show him or her my suggestions in this chapter for essential oils or buy a suitable massage oil and ask that it be used on you.

If you pull a muscle or ligament, or pinch a nerve, go to a sports massage specialist to straighten you out, literally. A sports massage practitioner then works around, not directly on the injury (although they may place an ice pack there) to release the areas that usually tighten up around an injury. If he or she knows their aromatherapy, you can also expect an anti-inflammatory preparation. A sports massage practitioner also can assist you if you're in regular training.

Unfortunately, aromatherapy hasn't caught on in the gym yet. But just imagine; someday you may walk into the gym and smell cinnamon and peppermint to increase your stamina instead of everyone else's sweat. For now, when you're working out at home, you can fill the room with one (or a blend) of these stimulating, stay-on-track fragrances. (See my suggestions for doing this in Chapter 4.) Here are the aromas to increase your stamina.

- ✔ Angelica
- ✔ Basil
- ✔ Benzoin
- ✔ Black pepper
- ✔ Cardamom
- ✔ Cinnamon

> ✔ Clove
>
> ✔ Cypress
>
> ✔ Ginger
>
> ✔ Peppermint
>
> ✔ Pine
>
> ✔ Sage

Essential oils do keep you more alert, but some herbs can offer you even more stamina without taking dangerous steroids. Check out the benefits of herbs such as ginseng.

Stamina isn't just about keeping your focus, maintaining a good blood flow, and having energized muscles. It has to do with how quickly your muscles recover from the stress of exercise. This is especially true when you push yourself beyond your muscle's limitations in an effort to build up more muscle strength or to finish in first place. What makes your muscles feel stiff more than anything is the buildup of lactic acid. You can help avoid this from happening by getting oxygen to your muscles (see how to in the section "Oils to improve circulation," earlier in this chapter). Aromatherapists find that a massage oil containing lemongrass essential oil is especially good to counter lactic acid buildup.

Fire or Ice? The Hot and Cold of It

Judging that fine line between full performance and injury is difficult, but try to be realistic about how far you can push yourself. If you do physically overextend your body, you have two treatment choices: hot or cold. That translates to one of two products: An aromatherapy liniment or an aromatherapy anti-inflammatory. Although the actions of both preparations are due to the essential oils they contain, the difference between them is like night and day.

> ✔ **Liniment for sore muscles:** Rub a liniment on your skin, and it brings blood to the underlying area and, as a result, makes the area very warm. This heats up sore muscles and relaxes them. It also warms up your muscles before you exercise. (But don't use a liniment on an area that is swollen because it will only make it worse.)
>
> ✔ **Anti-inflammatory for swollen injuries:** An anti-inflammatory has exactly the opposite effect of a liniment. You can apply it to sore muscles, but it's more often used on sprains, strains, or muscle cramps. These injuries are more severe, and more painful, than simply having sore muscles. They almost always involve at least some swelling, making an anti-inflammatory suitable.

A swell idea: Reducing inflammation

Inflammation, otherwise known as swelling, results when fluid from surrounding tissues seeps into the damaged area. It typically happens when you pull or tear a tendon, ligament, or muscle — all the things so common with sports. If the injury is discolored with the blue, red, or purple of a bruise, then you also have blood from broken blood vessels seeping in. (The blood makes the area extra warm to the touch.)

All this added fluid is what causes swelling. With the swelling comes congestion that restricts proper blood flow. You need that flow to bring nutrients and oxygen to your cells and to remove toxins to hasten repair. In addition, all the swelling pushes on your nerves and makes your injury hurt like crazy.

Either a sprain or a strain can happen when you exert your body past the strength of your muscles or joints. A sprain occurs at your joints when the fibrous tissues called ligaments are stretched too much. A strain happens when your muscles, or the tendons that hold them in place, are pulled or torn. Confusing the two is easy because both cause rapid swelling, heat, and pain and restrict your ability to move. Often a sprain and sometimes a strain becomes bruised and discolored. Sound confusing? Don't worry, they both get the same treatment.

Oils that reduce swelling

The benefits of reducing swelling are obvious, and two of the best ways to do so are ice (see the section "Injured warrior") and anti-inflammatory essential oils. The following essential oils reduce swelling and thus restore blood flow and diminish your pain.

- ✔ Chamomile, German
- ✔ Geranium
- ✔ Helichrysum
- ✔ Juniper
- ✔ Lavender
- ✔ Marjoram
- ✔ Rose

I'll have to admit that pain does win some points. It alerts you to the fact that an injury has occurred and makes you want to deal with it — if for no other reason but to reduce your discomfort. The pain and swelling also work together to keep you from moving that area. This is one way your body can "talk" you into lying off exercise long enough to give your injury time to heal. A problem with using an aromatherapy anti-inflammatory is that it reduces swelling too well. Your injury often feels so good that you have to remind yourself not to move the injured area or to keep it stationary with a sport brace.

Take good care of sport's injuries so that they don't cause future problems. A simple strain or sprain seldom needs a physician's care, unless your joint feels loose or unstable or your injury is extremely swollen or painful. However, an untended ankle sprain, which is the most common athletic injury, can plague you for years and sometimes your entire life. If you're not sure how serious your injury is, then go ahead and use your aromatherapy first aid. But also see your doctor, especially if there's any chance that a bone is broken.

Injured warrior

If you have a sprain or a strain, get into action right away to reduce the swelling. This relieves the pain and stops further injury. Remember RICE: Rest, ice, compression, and elevation.

- **Rest:** Try to move the injured area as little as possible so that you don't increase the irritation

- **Ice:** Use ice, or at least the coldest thing around. Then, here's the aromatherapy part you've been waiting for. Before applying the ice, rub on an anti-inflammatory preparation. Any oil or alcohol-based product that contains the appropriate essential oils I mention in the preceding section will work. (There's also a recipe in this section for a Strain and Sprain Compress.) Then apply the ice. After about 20 minutes, remove the ice, rest the area for 15 minutes, and then put on more ice. Repeat this for a few rounds, or as long as it takes to reduce the swelling.

- **Compress:** Press lightly on the injury to further reduce the swelling or bind with a compression bandage.

- **Elevate:** Comfortably support the injured area so that it rests higher than your heart (if possible) and doesn't move. The height drains excessive fluid away from the hurt.

Ice Is Nice: Herbal Cubes

Ice is the coolest thing going to treat all sorts of sports- (or work-) related injuries, including sprains, strains, and bruises.

Preparation time: *10 minutes*

Yield: *About 6 herbal ice cubes*

3 teaspoons chamomile flowers   1½ cups water

3 teaspoons lavender flowers

(continued)

iling water over the herbs and let them steep in a covered pan about 15 minutes. (This extracts the essential oils out into the water.)

2 Strain out the herbs.

3 When the tea is cool, pour it into medium-sized ice cube trays.

4 Place the filled trays in the freezer.

5 When frozen, pop the cubes out of the tray and place them in a sealed plastic bag or a container. Store these in your freezer. Mark them well so that your family doesn't confuse them for homemade popsicles! (Trust me, this can happen.)

6 Pull a frozen herbal cube out of the freezer whenever an accident calls for it. Don't use them in the plastic bag as you might other ice cubes, but directly on the skin so that it can receive all the healing benefits of the herbs.

Sprain and Strain Compress

A compress offers a fast way to get both anti-inflammatory essential oils and cold on to a sports-related injury. If ice cubes are available, you can slip them inside the folded cloth of this compress to make it colder and even more effective. You can repeat fresh applications of this compress as often as needed until both the swelling and the pain diminish.

Preparation time: *2 minutes*

Yield: *2 compresses*

6 drops German chamomile oil or lavender oil   *about ½ cup cold water*

1 Combine the water and oil.

2 Swish a cloth in the solution so that it's absorbed.

3 Lightly wring out the cloth, fold it, and apply over the injured area.

> ***Vary It!*** *If you have it on hand, add 1 teaspoon extract (tincture) arnica or St. John's wort extract (tincture) to the recipe to make an extra-strength preparation.*

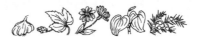

St. John's Sprain and Strain Oil

St. John's wort and arnica are two well-known herbs that work as anti-inflammatories. When you get hurt, you want to do everything that's possible to heal quickly. I like to combine the best of both worlds, herbalism and aromatherapy. The result is a double-strength formula that is so effective, it seems to work like magic.

Preparation time: 5 minutes

Yield: 2 ounces oil

2 ounces St. John's wort oil or arnica oil

12 drops lavender essential oil

8 drops marjoram essential oil

2 drops chamomile essential oil

1 Combine the ingredients.

2 Apply liberally to the skin over the injury, as often as needed.

Vary It! *If you can't come up with either St. John's wort oil or arnica oil, then you can resort to using plain vegetable oil.*

Warming up to aromatherapy: Liniments

A liniment is an old-fashioned idea that is ideal for today's fitness-crazed society. If you're a sports enthusiast or work out at the gym, you're probably already familiar with liniments such as the Chinese Tiger Balm or a drugstore version that alleviates muscle pain.

The idea behind a liniment is that it heats the area just like a hot pack. Both a liniment and hot pack work in the same way by drawing blood to the area to warm it up. The heat then relaxes your tight and sore muscles with a "deep" heat as your blood circulates through your muscles.

It turns out that liniments are more than an afterthought. Fitness experts now suggest that it's far better to apply a liniment before exercising, not afterwards. If you're into sports or working out, you already know how important it is to warm your muscles up before participating in any strenuous physical activity. A warm muscle can stretch and tighten much better than a cold one. This puts far less pressure not only on the muscle itself, but also on your ligaments and tendons. When a cold or tight muscle can't stretch properly, it puts a tremendous pull on these connective fibers. They're not designed to do major stretching — that's the muscle's job — so if the muscle is cold, they're subject to being torn. As a result, warmups cut down tremendously on sports injuries.

A liniment acts somewhat like warm-up stretches. Dr. Frank G. Shellock, a research scientist at Cedars-Sinai Medical Center in Los Angeles, California, found that applying a liniment relaxes cold muscles so that they are able to stretch better. I won't suggest that any athlete, or even the occasional jogger, should forego warmups in favor of a liniment, but you do get a lot more out of stretching when you combine it with a liniment. If you do skimp on doing a real warmup — and many people do — then at least let a liniment help you get more mileage out of whatever you do.

Hot stuff: Oils for liniments

A liniment contains hot oils, such as cinnamon and clove, that are diluted into either an oil or alcohol base. This is then rubbed on your skin over the muscles that you plan to use the most.

- ✔ Bay laurel
- ✔ Bay rum (pimento)
- ✔ Black pepper
- ✔ Cinnamon
- ✔ Clove bud
- ✔ Ginger
- ✔ Juniper
- ✔ Peppermint
- ✔ Thyme

These hot oils have the potential to be irritating. Be careful not to accidentally rub your eyes or mouth after applying a liniment and wash your hands well after applying it. Remember, the idea is to warm the skin, not burn it. Not only are these essential oils extra strong, but a liniment needs a higher concentration of essential oils than a massage oil so that it heats up. Because it contains so much hot essential oils, a liniment is designed for what I call "spot" therapy. Unlike a general massage oil, it's rubbed only on the spots where it's needed and not over your entire body.

Easin' muscles

Besides the hot-stuff essential oils, many liniments also contain muscle-relaxing essential oils. In this way, while a liniment warms a muscle to ease its tension, it also directly relaxes it. These muscle-relaxing essential oils are the most often used.

- ✔ Lavender
- ✔ Marjoram
- ✔ Rosemary

Tricks of the trade

A liniment relieves pain by increasing heat. This requires creating a sensation of lots of heat, but it must be done without burning your skin. Liniments accomplish this by playing several tricks on the brain.

✔ **Liniment Trick #1:** Pain creates a reinforcing loop between the muscle and brain; your muscle is crying with pain, and your brain agrees. (It's like a mother who tells her crying child how much a scrape must hurt, and then the child cries all the louder.) All of this focus on pain makes it hard for a tightened muscle to relax. However, as the heat from the essential oils increases, the brain starts getting nervous. It's forced to worry less about the muscle and concentrate on what appears to be the real emergency: Your skin is burning. Of course, you and I know that your skin is not really burning, but your brain doesn't. This gives your muscle a chance to relax. It increases blood flow to the underlying area by three to four times.

✔ **Liniment Trick #2:** A liniment has yet another trick up its sleeve to make it seem so much hotter than it really is. The trick is to include at least one of the following essential oils in the liniment formula.

- Peppermint

- Camphor

Both these oils increase the sensation of heat without really increasing the heat. They do so by sending hot and cold nerve impulses to your brain. When the brain receives these confusing, alternating messages of hot and cold, the contrast between the two makes the heat appear to be more intense than it really is. As in trick #1, your brain is so worried about the possibility that your skin is burning, it hardly has time to care about a sore muscle. I prefer using peppermint over camphor, which is potentially toxic. You don't need to avoid buying a liniment just because it contains camphor (many of them do), but go easy when you use those products.

Here's an easy way to understand how peppermint can be hot and cold at the same time. Put a peppermint candy on your tongue and suck air in through your mouth. You'll feel the slight burning sensation produced by peppermint on your tongue and the refreshingly coolness of it in the air you are breathing in. The sensation is icy-hot.

✔ **Liniment Trick #3:** You can increase the warming action of a liniment even more by rubbing your skin after applying the liniment. The more that you rub, the hotter it gets.

Heat Treat Liniment

Liniments come in many different types, and all are made with essential oils. You can buy them at drugstores or in natural-food stores (if you prefer one with better quality ingredients). Here's also a liniment that you can make at home. Remember that rubbing alcohol is poisonous, so be sure to mark the container appropriately and don't use it on broken skin or use vodka instead.

Preparation time: *5 minutes*

Yield: *2 ounces oil*

8 drops eucalyptus oil	*4 drops cinnamon oil*
8 drops peppermint oil	*4 drops clove oil*
8 drops rosemary oil	*2 ounces rubbing alcohol or vodka*

1 Combine ingredients in a bottle with a tight lid.

2 Shake or stir a few times a day for 3 days to disperse essential oils in the alcohol. Shake the mixture before using.

Vary It! *You can replace the alcohol with vegetable oil to produce an oily liniment that holds in heat-relieving pain better, although you've got to put up with the greasiness.*

Of course, any illness can hamper your activity level, but that's especially true if you have problems with fatigue, muscle pain and backaches, arthritis or rheumatism, menstrual cramps, nerve pain, or just plain stress. If these problems are impairing your level of physical performance, then look up your condition in the Symptom Guide. If you're having trouble with a lack of energy, then also look in Chapter 9. To read more about how pain works, see Chapter 11. There's also a section in the Symptom Guide that covers athlete's foot. Along with good circulation, you need strong lungs to get all that oxygen you inhale into your blood in the first place. It you suffer from asthma or another lung conditions, look in the Symptom Guide for ways that aromatherapy can help you.

Chapter 11

Getting Well with Smell

● ●

In This Chapter

▶ Treating your simple health problems

▶ Understanding medicinal properties of essential oils

▶ Deciding when to choose an aromatherapy treatment

▶ Using antiseptic essential oils on infections

▶ Soothing your pain and swelling

▶ Conquering indigestion

▶ Using essential oils for strong immunity

▶ Using aromatherapy safely

Recipes in This Chapter

▶ Happy Belly Tea

▶ Chai Tea

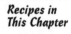

● ●

*F*eeling a little queasy? Have a splitting headache? Then, you've come to the right place. This chapter covers medical aromatherapy. It gives you information that you need to treat all sorts of minor health problems.

Simple Cures for Simple Woes

Aromatherapy is versatile enough to treat many common ailments. These are the simple complaints that you already take care of yourself without consulting your doctor. But, instead of using an over-the-counter drug to ease a cold, headache, indigestion, or bee sting, you can turn to aromatherapy as a natural alternative. After all, that's what aroma*therapy* is — a healing therapy. The *aroma* part of the word refers to the aromatic plants that are used in this therapy.

Aromatherapy does offer plenty of benefits over conventional drugs for many of your everyday woes. In some cases, it's even a better choice than medicinal herbs to heal minor health problems. Granted, aromatherapy isn't the answer to all health concerns — you need to look beyond aromatherapy to deal with heart, kidney problems, diabetes, or any number of other serious disorders. In cases such as these, aromatherapy can still be used, but as an adjunct remedy that helps relieve some of the symptoms to make you feel more comfortable.

Essential oils are the aromatic molecules in fragrant plants that both make them fragrant and give them many medicinal properties. Read this list of the advantages of aromatherapy for healing, and you'll surely agree with me that essential oils are custom-made for healing.

- **Are inexpensive:** A little essential oil goes a long way, making aromatherapy products reasonably priced. Compared to over-the-counter drugs, they're downright cheap.

- **Are compact to carry:** If you want to travel with your aromatherapy remedies, it's easy. A few small, lightweight items are all you need, especially when you consider that many essential oils do double-duty by treating more than one condition.

- **Work with, not against, you:** The complex chemistry of essential oils means that they work with your body and its healing process. Like the closely related herbal therapy, the emphasis in aromatherapy is to assist your body in operating better and eliminating the cause of your disease — not just to get rid of your symptoms. This deep healing is holistic medicine's specialty. That way, you don't come down with a related disorder a few weeks or years from now. Essential oils wipe out an infection (but not the cells harboring it) and stop injuries, such as burns, from releasing toxins into the surrounding healthy tissue. They tend to not kill good bacteria, only the bad dudes, and do not create a resistance to bad bacteria as do many drugs. Simply put, aromatherapy promotes your health. This is a different story from many drugs, which are as destructive as they are constructive. Sure, sometimes you need to pull out the big guns, but drugs can act like an artillery, destroying healthy cells in their path as they kill the invaders.

- **Go directly to affliction:** Essential oils penetrate your skin to sink into underlying tissue. Many times, this is an advantage over ingesting an herb. Any medicine that you swallow must travel through your digestive tract before it reaches your blood system. At that point, it's distributed throughout your entire body. Instead of using such an indirect route, essential oils take the express way to target the source of your problem. You simply rub a diluted essential oil on your skin over a painful or infected area, and they're absorbed right where they're most needed.

- **Work quickly:** Because essential oils don't take the time to pass through your digestive tract, they offer another advantage. They reach their destination in your body quickly and go to work almost immediately. So, you don't need to wait around for relief. Because essential oils encourage injured cells to heal, you recover more quickly.

- **Can be used with drugs:** In most cases, you can use essential oils along with pharmaceutical drugs. There's not much risk of reducing the action of your medicines or of making them extra potent — as sometimes happens when you combine drugs with each other. One reason is that the oil is absorbed directly into tissues, so only tiny amounts reach your bloodstream. Also, drug interaction is less likely with the conditions for which aromatherapy is most used, such as indigestion, skin problems, and infections — although, when in doubt, check with an herbalist or aromatherapist. (See the sidebar in Chapter 3 for more information.)

- ✓ **Leave quickly:** Your body eliminates essential oils within several hours, so no residue remains. At first glance, it may seem an advantage for medicine to linger in your body, but this can make it accumulate and produce an overdose.

- ✓ **Have few side effects:** If you stick to store-bought or homemade products that contain safe essential oils, as most aromatherapy products do, you're rarely bothered by unwanted side effects unlike over-the-counter drugs.

Getting Serious: Treating Chronic Problems

There are all too many examples of long-range (chronic) health problems — the kind that can continue to plague you year after year. Conditions such as eczema, PMS, asthma, arthritis, and headaches have physicians scratching their heads trying to figure out a cure. So many times, it's just when you think that you finally have it licked that the problem comes back in full vengeance.

At least many chronic conditions come with one plus. When medical science doesn't offer you much hope, you're free to try alternative medicines such as aromatherapy. Plenty of people are happily helped by aromatherapy after years of unsuccessfully trying the medical route. However, you need patience, especially if you've had an affliction for several years or more. If you don't see any change after a month or so of aromatherapy treatments, you may be literally barking up the wrong tree (or some other plant). If that's the case, then alter your remedy. You might try seeking a clinical aromatherapist or herbalist (most herbalists know plenty about aromatherapy) to help you.

In your search for alternative medicine to treat a chronic condition, you can start with aromatherapy, but don't stop there. As good as aromatherapy is for healing, it can't do everything. Use herbal medicine in conjunction with it. As both an herbalist and aromatherapist, I use whatever remedies are most appropriate. Many times that means combining the dynamic duo of aromatherapy and herbalism. Together, they're more effective than either one alone, especially for treating chronic problems. To work holistically on your health problems with herbs, diet, and lifestyle, turn to the Symptom Guide and look up your condition. (If you want more information, check out *Alternative Medicine For Dummies* by James Dillard, M.D., D.C., C.Ac., and Terra Ziporyn, Ph.D., and *Herbal Remedies For Dummies* by Christopher Hobbs, both published by IDG Books Worldwide, Inc., and *Herbs for Health and Healing,* by me, Kathi Keville.)

Seven Ways to Use Aromatherapy Medicinally

Now that aromatherapy is so popular, you'll have no trouble finding the medicinal products. Some of these contain pure essential oils, while other products incorporate fragrant herbs. (They still count as aromatherapy because the essential oils draw out of the herbs during the preparation.) The best one for your condition depends upon what you're treating. Here are seven common ways that you can use essential oils medicinally.

- ✔ **As an oil**, such as a vegetable oil like grapeseed or olive oil or a waxlike jojoba, with healing essential oil added to it to rub on your skin. Fancy versions include salves, lotions, and creams. *For a body or massage oil or lotion, use about 6 to 8 drops of essential oil per ounce.*

- ✔ **As a bath oil** containing skin-healing essential oils to use when you bathe. For a similar remedy, you can add a few drops of essential oil to your bath water or to a foot or hand bath. *For bathing, use 3 to 6 drops essential oil per tub, depending upon the strength of the oil and the size of your bathtub. You can also prepare a foot or hand soak with 5 drops essential oil in a basin of either hot or cool water.*

- ✔ **As a tincture** (which is in alcohol and water) or sometimes a vinegar that is rubbed on your skin. It often comes as a liniment for sore muscles and joints or a wound antiseptic. Essential oils in diluted vinegar make a good hair rinse. *A liniment contains a high concentration of essential oils, around 24 drops (or about ¼ teaspoon) per ounce of tincture or rubbing alcohol. It is designed to be used only on the painful muscle or joint and not for overall massage.*

- ✔ **As an aloe-based preparation** that contains medicinal essential oils to dab or spray on skin problems, especially burns or poison oak. *Typically, 10 to 15 drops of essential! oil is used per ounce, and the resulting remedy is applied on the injured area.*

- ✔ **With an inhalant,** inhale the steam from simmering water that contains essential oils or a nasal inhaler to bring essential oils into your sinuses and lungs. *To make an inhalant, it takes about 3 to 5 drops of essential oil in a pint to a quart of steaming water.*

- ✔ **As essential oils diluted in water** for use as skin washes, mouthwashes, hair rinses, air fresheners, body sprays, and douches. *The dilution of essential oil in water varies with the different applications, but it's generally around 5 drops essential oil for a mouthwash, 10 drops per ounce for a body spray, and 15 to 20 drops per ounce for a room freshener.*

- ✔ **As a compress** to hold essential oils over an injured area or headache. (A *compress* is a folded cloth that is soaked in a combination of water and essential oils and placed over the problem area.) *You need about 5 drops essential oil in a cup or two of water to make a compress.*

Whatever type of preparation you choose, repeating the application every few hours keeps a constant level of essential oils in your body. This is especially true with an acute (temporary) condition that you want to knock out quickly. For long-range disorders, a typical prescription is twice daily, but this varies with different afflictions.

Essential Facts: Using Essential Oils

You probably want to know how essential oils work. It's all in their chemistry. An essential oil is made up of an assortment of different substances, each with their own healing properties. Put together different combinations of these substances, and you've got an entire bag of tricks for healing. (You can find more essential oil chemistry in Chapter 1.)

Although essential oils are all slightly different, each one is simply a variation of the same theme. It's not unlike going to the coffee shop where you're confronted with an array of flavored muffins. They vary depending upon which extra ingredients they contain, but they're all very much muffins. Likewise, an essential oil contains many ingredients, but it still shares much in common with other essential oils. Their basic structure identifies them as essential oils. This similarity also gives them many of the same healing properties.

Aromatherapy is no stranger to researchers. They've been studying the properties of essential oils for years. So far, these oils have proved themselves strong medicine. It's no surprise to me, but the healing properties of plants used by herbalists for centuries to treat infection and pain contain active essential oils.

Four areas of healing

When I consider how essential oils work as healers, four major categories stand out. Although not every oil has all four aspects, they're found in the majority of oils. These functions aren't the only ones performed by essential oils. (For example, many essential oils increase blood circulation, eliminate lung and sinus congestion, and alter hormones.) Yet, in the following four arenas, essential oils are workhorses. That's good news when you consider how many disorders are covered in these four arenas. You'll notice in reading this chapter that some essential oils, being the versatile healers that they are, cover more than one of these aspects. Essential oils:

- **Kill microorganisms:** Target bacteria, viruses, fungi, and parasites.
- **Relieve pain:** Relieve your pain by reducing inflammation, relaxing sore muscles directly or through heat, dulling the pain response, and reducing inflammation.

✔ **Tone digestion:** Aid digestion by improving your appetite and digestion process, relieving nausea, eliminating gas, increasing digestive enzymes, and relaxing intestinal muscles. Some oils also stimulate digestive juices. In addition, the scent-relaxing essential oils help relieve nervous indigestion.

✔ **Repair cells and stimulate immunity:** Enhance your immune system so that it better fends off and eliminates disease. Clean up disease, infection, and waste from cells through your lymph system and the production of white blood cells. Many essential oils encourage skin cells to heal and keep skin toned in several ways, including regulating its oil production. (See Chapter 7 for more on caring for your skin with aromatherapy.)

For more on the specific essential oils to use for these conditions, along with aromatherapy recipes, look up your specific problem in the Symptom Guide.

About the essential oils in this chapter

You'll notice in reading this chapter that it's divided into the four primary conditions that are treatable with essential oils. In each section, I give you a list of suitable essential oils to treat that condition. This gives you plenty of options. You know which oils to look for on the labels during your next aromatherapy shopping spree. The lists also help you design your own aromatherapy products. In deciding which oils to include on these lists, I looked at the results of many scientific studies and compared and compiled the findings. I also considered the results that I've seen in my 30 years of practicing aromatherapy, along with observations from other aromatherapists. I left out essential oils that I consider too toxic for you to use and those that are difficult to find.

Dr. Science says, "It works!"

The prestigious American Association for the Advancement of Science looked at the research from major U. S. universities and concluded that aromatherapy has genuine health benefits. They think that the studies done so far show much promise and that more investigation is needed to discover more about how aromatherapy can be used in medicine.

Doc, it's like this. . . .

I find the complexity of designing an aromatherapy formula an interesting and fun challenge. It means choosing the best essential oils to treat both the medical condition and the individual. Sometimes it's just one oil; other times, a blend of oils works the best. Then I need to decide what is the best mode of application. Nevertheless, the most fun comes at the end when I see the positive results from using aromatherapy. If you feel creative and want to try your hand at making formulas but you need a jump-start, find out more about an essential oil by looking up its properties in the Aroma Guide. I also give you simple formulas in the Symptom Guide.

Here's an imaginary scenario to custom-design an aromatherapy blend. Say that you need a germ-fighter to treat an uncomfortable lung infection. It began as a flu, but has now developed into a bacterial infection. You'd like to use something that is well suited for your lungs, but that also relieves your pain. Because your asthma's acting up, you need to avoid any essential oils that aggravate it and wouldn't mind having something to treat the asthma itself. In addition, you need to reduce the stress that made your asthma flare up in the first place.

(Answer: One essential oil, lavender, answers all these requirements. A good way to use it is to steam with it several times daily. For the aromatherapy answers to other health-related problems, refer to the Symptom Guide.)

Don't Bug Me: Natural Antibiotics

Germs are all around. You co-exist with all sorts of microscopic creatures, some beneficial for your health and some not-so-good. Not to sound paranoid, but germs lurk everywhere, just waiting for someone to cough in your face, or for you to cut your finger or to down some less-than-fresh morsel of food. You've probably encountered your share of invasive attack organisms, so you're no stranger to the misery of a cold, an infected wound, or a bout of food poisoning.

To test an essential oil's ability to conquer infection, researchers mix the infectious darlings with the essential oil in their laboratory. Then they peer through a microscope to see whether the oil destroys or at least restricts the microbes. Almost all essential oils do counter infection to some degree. They attack bacteria, fungus, and viruses with amazing effectiveness because they easily enter tissues and cells that harbor infection. And, they most often kindly leave the beneficial organisms alone. At the same time, essential oils make the environment (that's your body) healthier and thus a less hospitable home for them to hang out.

Here are the three types of infection that I address one by one.

- ✔ Bacterial
- ✔ Viral
- ✔ Fungal

Germ warfare: Treating bacterial infection

Bacteria grow in colonies. It wouldn't be so bad if they could be content with a small homestead, but no, give a bacteria an inch and it wants to take over the world, or at least your body. If a bacterial infection that crops up in one place gets a strong enough hold, then it has its sights on more territory. Many bacterial infections aren't highly contagious, but with a little effort, they'll even move to someone else and give them the infection.

That's why essential oils are so important for treating infection. They destroy harmful bacteria, but they don't stop there. Some oils also interrupt the growth cycle of bacteria and starve them by restricting their ability to use oxygen and other sources of energy. A big advantage of essential oils is that, due to their complex chemistry, bacteria don't develop a resistance to oils as they can with antibiotics.

You may not realize it, but you're probably already using essential oils to destroy bacteria. If your dishwashing soap contains lemon oil, it's in there for more than just its pleasant scent — it's a strong germ-fighter. As you can guess from its name, the ability of PineSol (and similar cleaning fluids) to wipe out bacteria is pine oil. You may have aromatic memories from when you were little of your mother rubbing a vapor balm on your chest when you had a chest infection. Perhaps you've rubbed it on your own kids. The antibacteria compounds in vapor rubs come from eucalyptus, thyme, and mint. One popular mouthwash, which won the American Dental Association award for the most effective over-the-counter plaque-fighter, is a mix of thyme, eucalyptus, and mint to kill the germs that are responsible for bad breath, tooth decay, and gum disease. An aromatic cream that is made with essential oils has been around for years, killing the bacteria that accompanies acne.

Good antibacterial killer oils

Here's a list of the most powerful antibacterial essential oils. These are killer oils that knock out common intestinal, skin, and lung infections, including staph, strep, and pneumonia. The test results on these oils are certainly impressive. Thyme oil proved as potent as standard antibiotic drugs!

- Bay laurel
- Cinnamon
- Clove bud
- Garlic
- Oregano
- Savory
- Thyme

The preceding essential oils are strong antiseptics, but the problem is that they're also potent skin irritants. You can use them, but do so carefully and always when greatly diluted. Rather than risk burning your skin with thyme oil, use a salve that contains it. Because using these oils safely is tricky, one alternative is to use the herbs themselves. (The whole herb, from which an oil is extracted, contains the essential oil.)

Killer oils, gentler versions

This next list of bacteria fighters tends not to be quite as strong as the killer oils, but they're still powerful. That makes these essential oils much more popular to use in skin medicines because they won't burn so easily. Instead, these oils produce the opposite effect by reducing swelling and irritation. This is especially true of lavender, helichrysum, marjoram, and geranium. (Also see the section "Reducing swelling" in this chapter.) The essential oils with asterisks seem to be the most potent ones, at least according to the studies.

- Bay rum (pimento)
- Benzoin
- Cardamom
- Eucalyptus*
- Frankincense
- Geranium
- Helichrysum*
- Lavender*
- Lemon*
- Lemongrass
- Marjoram*
- Myrrh*
- Myrtle*
- Pine*

- ✔ Rose*
- ✔ Sage*
- ✔ Sandalwood
- ✔ Tea tree* (including the niaouli type)
- ✔ Vetivert

Doing it: Aromatherapy for bacterial infections

Examples of infections that are treatable with essential oils are those of the skin, bladder, bowel, ear, gum, sinus, skin, and throat. Look up your problem in the Symptom Guide for details on how to treat it and for some simple recipes. If you have a skin infection, look for a salve or tincture that contains antiseptic essential oils or herbs. (The process of making a salve or tincture pulls essential oils from the herbs into the product.) An antibacterial spray has the advantage of treating an injured area without touching it, and you can spritz it into the air as a room disinfectant or spray it on countertops and floors as a disinfectant. Spraying lemon essential oil into the air increases its antiseptic properties because compounds *(terpenes)* in the oil combine with oxygen. In case you have an infection harboring in underlying tissue, rub on a massage or body oil that contains antibacterial essential oils, and they'll go through your skin.

Inspecting infection: Treating Viruses

Viruses are tricky and elusive little critters and not very polite. They take up residence and reproduce without invitation. Another thing about viral infections: They love travel and will gladly take a trip to reside with someone else with whom you're in close contact. And, many viruses aren't inhibited at all about space travel, so they go propelling through the air in search of new terrain to invade. The infections that they cause include colds, flu, herpes, shingles, mumps, chicken pox, and even warts.

One unpleasant thing about viruses is that they use your cells as a host, even to the point of manipulating the DNA and RNA, which provide instructions for cell operations. This makes viruses especially difficult to eradicate without harming your own cells. Medical science can't touch most viral infections — even the common cold. If you've ever gone to your doctor for a bad cold, he or she may prescribe antibiotics, but that's only in case you develop a bacterial infection as a result of the virus weakening your system. You get nothing for the cold virus itself. Only recently have drugs been devised to fight viral diseases such as herpes and the HIV virus that causes AIDS, but the drugs' effectiveness leaves something to be desired.

Gut reaction

Humans may have evolved a taste for spicy foods because the spices that flavor them kill the microbes that make food spoil, thinks Dr. Paul Sherman, an evolutionary biologist at Cornell University, New York. He looked at 4,164 traditional recipes from 36 countries and found that the hotter the climate — and the faster food turns bad — the spicier the food. Cool climates, on the other hand, lean more toward less antiseptic flavorings, such as celery seed and caraway seed. When he tested 43 spices, onion, garlic, oregano, and allspice (due to their essential oil content) knocked out all 30 different kinds of bacteria. Cumin, cinnamon, cloves, and cayenne hot peppers did in three-quarters of the bacteria.

In another study, the essential oils of bay, cinnamon, thyme, and clove were strongest out of 21 essential oils tested in destroying common sources of food poisoning: _E. coli, Salmonella, Staphylococcus,_ and _Listeria._ Nutmeg oil also proved particularly effective against _Listeria._ Bay and thyme oil destroyed the most common bacterial cause of diarrhea, _Campylocbacter,_ which was also the most resistant bacteria.

Kansas State University found that adding garlic to salami or cloves to tainted hamburgers almost completely destroys _E. coli,_ again due to the essential oils they contain. The runners-ups against _E. coli_ were cinnamon, oregano, and sage. Marjoram destroys salmonella food poisoning.

You'll notice that many antibacterial essential oils are extracted from kitchen spices. Eating these herbs is especially appropriate considering that puts them in direct contact with the digestive tract infections they are so good at destroying. So, instead of trying to deal with oregano essential oil, sprinkle oregano on your pizza for a medicinal dose.

Good antiviral oils

Aromatherapy includes many essential oils that treat viral infections. Many antiviral oils do double time and also kill bacteria. That's good news if you have both types of infections or you're not sure which bug you've got. This full coverage also helps ward off a bacterial infection from invading on the heels of a viral flu or cold. The essential oils with asterisks seem to be the most potent antivirals, at least according to the studies.

- ✔ Bay*
- ✔ Bergamot*
- ✔ Black pepper (be careful when using this potent oil)
- ✔ Cardamom
- ✔ Cinnamon bark (be careful when using this potent oil)
- ✔ Clove bud (be careful when using this potent oil)
- ✔ Eucalyptus*
- ✔ Garlic*

- Geranium*
- Holy basil
- Hyssop, the type decumbens*
- Juniper*
- Lavender*
- Melissa (lemon balm)*
- Lemongrass
- Lemon*
- Marjoram
- Myrrh
- Oregano* (be careful when using this potent oil)
- Rose
- Rosemary*
- Sage*
- Tea tree*
- Thyme* (the type called linalol is the safest)

Doing It: Aromatherapy for viral infections

For herpes or other skin infections caused by a virus, use a salve, lip balm, or oil that contains appropriate essential oils. Several herpes products are available. Add a few drops of an antiviral essential oil to steaming water and inhale the aromatic steam into your sinuses and lungs to flush out a cold or flu virus. (Don't try this with hot essential oils, such as oregano, black pepper, cinnamon, or garlic — they can burn!) You can also rub on a massage or body oil that contains essential oils. For more tips on dealing with viruses, look up specific viral infections in the Symptom Guide.

Fungus among us: Treating fungal infection

Once a fungal infection takes hold, it has a tendency to spread like crazy. And, that's only the beginning of the bad news. These infections are quite social, spreading themselves from one person to another. A fungus also has the irritating habit of itching like crazy. You know that already if you've ever had ringworm, one of the most common fungal skin infections. It includes athlete's foot and the graphically named "jock rot," which shows up unabashedly on a man's crotch. The athletic association with this infection comes from the fact that funguses — ringworm among them — thrive in a warm, moist environment, and athletes get hot and sweat a lot. Moreover, athletic sports gear that includes tight, look-at-these-muscles pants and triple-layered-for-high-performance shoes is a friend to fungus because it holds in the sweat.

Another fungus that gets around is *candida* (actually a yeastlike fungus, which is also attracted to warm, moist places). It's already found in most people's digestive tract, where it probably plays a minor role in the digestive process. It's when candida gets out of hand and multiplies like crazy that it causes you problems: indigestion, fatigue, and sometimes fuzzy thinking. Candida also thrives in the inside of your mouth (where it is called *thrush* and creates patchy spots), the vagina (where it is called a *yeast infection*), and your toenails and fingernails, which it discolors and cracks.

Good antifungal oils

After reading these descriptions of the problems caused by funguses (see the preceding section), you'll be happy to know that a long list of essential oils fight these infections. The essential oils with asterisks seem to be the most potent ones, at least according to the studies.

- ✔ Basil (the type called holy basil is especially potent)*
- ✔ Bergamot*
- ✔ Black pepper (be careful when using this potent oil)
- ✔ Caraway
- ✔ Cinnamon* (be careful when using this potent oil)
- ✔ Clove bud* (be careful when using this potent oil)
- ✔ Coriander
- ✔ Cumin
- ✔ Garlic*
- ✔ Geranium*
- ✔ Lavender
- ✔ Lemon
- ✔ Melissa (lemon balm)
- ✔ Lemon eucalyptus*
- ✔ Lemongrass*
- ✔ Marjoram
- ✔ Myrrh
- ✔ Oregano* (be careful when using this potent oil)
- ✔ Peppermint*
- ✔ Sandalwood

✔ Tea tree*

✔ Thyme* (be careful when using this potent oil)

Doing it: Aromatherapy for fungal infections

A product that contains vinegar or powder with essential oils in it is an effective way to treat skin and nail infections that are caused by a fungus. Both the powder and vinegar are very drying, so they discourage further growth. You can also soak your nails in a foot or hand bath containing a few drops of an essential oil. Swab the inside of your mouth with essential oil diluted in vegetable oil if you have thrush. To treat candida, add essential oils to douche water for a vaginal infection. If you want to make your own recipes, look up your problem in the Symptom Guide. (Go easy with hot essential oils such as black pepper, cinnamon, clove bud, or peppermint because they can burn your skin, especially if a fungal infection makes it raw and tender. Never use these oils to treat a vaginal infection.)

Nip Pain in the Bud: Six Ways to End Pain

More than anything else, it's the discomfort of pain that sends you searching for a cure to any disease. At least in that sense, pain is good because it alerts you to physical problems in your body of which you otherwise may not be aware. Even when you do know that something's wrong, you have to admit that if it doesn't hurt, it's darn easy to put off dealing with it.

Okay, maybe you're not ready to embrace your pain, but you certainly must be ready to get rid of it. If you experience minor pain, essential oils usually help, sometimes as effectively as over-the-counter drugs. The oils are also far safer to use and, used properly, don't carry the same risks of damaging your liver. But don't expect these aromatic pain relievers to alleviate severe pain the way a prescription drug can. Serious pain is one of the times to be real grateful for advanced *allopathic* (standard) medicine. You certainly wouldn't want to go into surgery with a handkerchief of lavender and camphor over your nose as was done in the good ol' days.

There are plenty of times that aromatherapy is the answer to easing your pain. Essential oils do this in six different ways. I list these six categories in the following sections, along with the essential oils that go along with each one. Having lots of choices is especially useful if you want to take pain-relieving essential oils for an extended time because you'll get better results if you switch to a different blend of oils every week. In some way, your body's pain sensors seem to become accustomed to essential oils and eventually don't respond as well to them. You see that some versatile essential oils are on more than one list. The essential oils with asterisks seem to be the most potent.

Numb it

One way to dull pain is to go direct and numb your nerve endings. That's how the following essential oils work.

- ✔ Clove bud* (be careful when using this potent oil)
- ✔ Frankincense
- ✔ Chamomile (especially German)
- ✔ Helichrysum
- ✔ Lavender
- ✔ Lemongrass

Reduce swelling

You may not find inflammation a hot subject unless you have an infected cut or a bruise, but decreasing swelling is one of essential oils' most important qualities. That's because swelling causes most of the pain you experience. If you get headaches, menstrual cramps, or bruises, repetitive strain injury, sore throat, insect bite, or almost any type of infection, they all involve inflammation that pins down your nerves, and that pressure causes pain. These are the anti-inflammatory pain relievers.

- ✔ Chamomile, German*
- ✔ Geranium*
- ✔ Helichrysum*
- ✔ Juniper
- ✔ Lavender*
- ✔ Marjoram*
- ✔ Myrrh
- ✔ Rose*
- ✔ Tea tree

Heat and penetrate pain

Essential oils that produce heat relieve your pain by bringing blood to the painful area to warm it up and let your muscles, connective tissue, and nerves relax. The heat also provides deep, penetrating relief. Be sure to use these hot oils "gingerly" in small, well-diluted amounts, or they can burn your skin. Don't use them at all on a "hot" injury, such as a burn or a swelling.

(Instead use the essential oils that are suggested in the section on lessening swelling, earlier in this chapter.) They'll only increase the inflammation. Here are essential oils that are both heating and penetrating.

- ✔ Bay laurel
- ✔ Bay rum (pimento)
- ✔ Black pepper
- ✔ Cinnamon
- ✔ Clove bud
- ✔ Ginger
- ✔ Juniper
- ✔ Peppermint
- ✔ Thyme

The following oils are penetrating, but not heating.

- ✔ Marjoram
- ✔ Rosemary
- ✔ Sage

Stop pain in your brain

Pain can happen anywhere in your body, but it takes your brain to register that it's happening. Essential oils can go right to the top of the command to tell your brain to pretend that the pain isn't there. Lemongrass and ginger oils act similar to the sedative opiate drugs that are derived from opium to act on the brain without affecting your central nervous system. Lemongrass oil depresses the higher, cerebral cortex, part of your brain (and its cough center) so that the pain sensations don't get registered. Frankincense oil also reduces pain sensations in your brain, and probably other essential oils work in a similar fashion. There are likely other essential oils that also halt brain pain that haven't yet been studied. These are the ones that I know about so far.

- ✔ Frankincense
- ✔ Ginger
- ✔ Lemongrass

Short circuit pain-causing substances

Certain essential oils slow the action of pain-causing substances. The following are examples of essential oils that go through different routes. Cayenne oil lessens nerve pain by decreasing the amount of "substance P" in your body. That P stands for pain because it carries pain messages from nerve endings in your skin to your central nervous system. Cayenne oil's active compound (capsaicin) gives substantial pain relief to three-quarters of the people who try it. Yes, yes, this is hot stuff, but the burning sensation quickly goes away, and so does the pain of herpes, shingles, diabetic neuropathy, psoriasis, and post-surgery. You can buy over-the-counter skin creams in any drugstore. On the other hand, birch (which often masks as wintergreen when sold because the two smell so much alike) is an aspirinlike pain reliever. In fact, it contains the same compound as aspirin, making it useful to ease a headache, menstrual cramps, arthritic pain, and simple aches and pains. One way it does so is by slowing down the hormonelike prostaglandin$_2$ that's responsible for causing muscles to cramp and some types of headaches. Ginger works in a similar way to ease muscle contractions and arthritic pain. Both birch and ginger are good to relieve muscle cramps like menstrual pain, also painful joints, and some headaches. The essential oils that dampen pain-causing substances are

- ✔ Birch (be careful when using this potent oil)
- ✔ Cayenne (be careful when using this potent oil)
- ✔ Ginger

Relax and sedate it

These essential oils aren't exactly pain relievers, but they do relax sore and stiff muscles and, as a result, they lessen your pain. They also relax your mind through their scent alone. That's a convenient combination because you automatically smell their aromas as you use them. (Also look up the scents that reduce stress in Chapter 9.) Here's a list of the relaxing essential oils.

- ✔ Chamomile* (especially Roman)
- ✔ Clary sage
- ✔ Helichrysum
- ✔ Lavender*
- ✔ Lemon
- ✔ Lemon eucalyptus
- ✔ Lemon verbena

> ✓ Marjoram*
>
> ✓ Melissa (lemon balm)*
>
> ✓ Myrtle
>
> ✓ Petitgrain

Doing it: Aromatherapy for pain

One of the most relaxing ways to relieve pain is with a massage using an aromatherapy oil or liniment containing pain-relieving essential oils. Massage is especially good for that slow, aching pain caused by long-term, chronic disorders. (The massage itself not only relaxes you, but it subdues pain.) It's thought to slow down the release of substance P (see the preceding section) by stimulating substances (called *enkephallins*) that work like natural opiates.

It's not nearly as enjoyable, but an alternative to massage is to rub a pain-relieving massage or body oil or a liniment on yourself. Another method is to place a compress over the area that hurts. For individual suggestions, look up the following disorders that involve pain in the Symptom Guide: Arthritis and rheumatism, sprains, strains, bruises, burns, canker sores, headache, herpes, repetitive strain injury, sore throat and laryngitis, teething, nerve pain, or inflamed breast, eyes, or bladder, gum, and ear infections, or stomach, intestinal, muscle, and menstrual cramps, hives, insect bites, fluid retention, and bladder, ear, gum, lung, and sinus infections.

Musta Been Something I Ate: Indigestion

Aromatherapy gets to work at the first stage of digestion, as the scent signals your brain that food is on its way. Simply sniffing pasta sauce, baking bread, or anything tasty sends your stomach grumbling in anticipation. The smell alone begins a chain-reaction throughout your digestive tract. (Just think how bland a meal tastes when you have a stuffy nose, and you can't smell anything!) Almost immediately, digestive juices to digest food are released in your mouth, stomach, and small intestine.

Good digestive oils

Aromatic digestive herbs are often described as stimulants, but most of them are really pretty laidback. Their function is to relax your intestinal muscles. This slower pace gives your food more time to help prevent gas from developing and stop cramping. Peppermint, the all-time star digestive oil, relaxes your intestinal muscles within 30 minutes and prevents nausea. (Just don't overdo it; too much peppermint can *cause* nausea.)

The aroma from any of these essential oils aids your appetite and digestion. Most of them also help you overcome nausea, often by blocking the signal in your brain that tells you to vomit. Cardamom, lavender, rosemary, and juniper oils do this. To soothe burning irritation in your stomach, look to melissa (lemon balm), lemon, or fennel. Cinnamon increases the action of enzymes to break down food and rosemary aids in its assimilation. These essential oils not only help cure indigestion, but they address the source of the problems by destroying bacterial, viral, or fungal infections that can harbor there in your digestive tract. (Refer to the lists of essential oils in those sections of this chapter, and you can see that there are many matches.)

- Anise
- Basil
- Cardamom
- Chamomile
- Cinnamon (be careful when using this potent oil)
- Clove bud (be careful when using this potent oil)
- Coriander
- Dill
- Fennel
- Ginger
- Juniper berry
- Melissa (lemon balm)
- Lemongrass
- Lemon
- Oregano
- Peppermint
- Rosemary
- Sandalwood
- Thyme

Doing it: Aromatherapy for indigestion

To treat digestive woes such as poor appetite, headaches related to poor digestion, heartburn, and plain ol' belly upsets, use an aromatherapy massage or body oil that contains the essential oils I mention in this section. Massage the oil over uncomfortable areas of your abdomen. (The massage often helps with digestive distress as much as the oil.)

Improving your digestion can be as effortless as adding the herb or spice itself to your food. Culinary spices and tea are good ways to get the medicine where it's needed in safe, but effective, doses. That's easy to do because most of the essential oils on this list come from culinary herbs. You can also drink most of these herbs, especially peppermint, cardamom, thyme, melissa (lemon balm), and chamomile, as tea. (The essential oils in these herbs are extracted into the hot water.) Essential oils that reduce stress, such as lavender and melissa (lemon balm), can improve your digestion whenever you're under stress. Tension restricts digestive juice, constricts muscles, and probably contributes to disorders such as colitis, stomach ulcers, and irritable bowel syndrome. You can find some simple recipes for specific digestive problems in the Symptom Guide.

Happy Belly Tea

The directions for making a tea with any of these herbs are the same. If you're feeling creative, you can blend several of the herbs to make a total of 2 teaspoons. Then follow the same instructions. Here's one of my favorite herb blends. It makes a delightful tea, either hot or cold.

Preparation time: *12 minutes*

Yield*: 2 cups*

2 cups boiling water	*½ teaspoon chamomile flowers*
1 teaspoon melissa (lemon balm) or lemongrass leaves	*½ teaspoon peppermint leaves*

1 Pour the water over the chopped herb in a pan or pot.

2 Cover and let sit about 10 minutes.

3 Strain out the herbs and drink your tea. Keep any leftover tea in the refrigerator for a couple days.

Vary It! *Replace the herb in this recipe with any one (or a combination of several) of the herbs listed in the section "Aromatherapy for indigestion," earlier in this chapter. Some of my other favorites for herb tea are cinnamon, ginger, melissa (lemon balm), and lemongrass.*

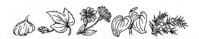

Chai Tea

If you're in a spicy mood and you want to improve your digestion, try the East Indian drink chai. Coffee shops throughout North America are starting to offer it. You can also make your own. Chai tea often contains black tea for the pick-me-up that the caffeine in it offers, but here's a version without the tea (which isn't easy to digest).

Preparation time: *20 minutes*

Yield: *2 cups*

3 cups water

2 teaspoons freshly grated ginger

2 two-inch-long cinnamon sticks, broken into small pieces

¼ teaspoon whole cloves

⅛ teaspoon whole peppercorns

5 cardamom pods

½ cup milk (or substitute soy, rice, or almond milk)

1 pinch nutmeg powder

honey to taste (optional)

1 In a medium saucepan, combine the water, ginger, cinnamon sticks, cloves, peppercorns, and cardamom pods.

2 Cover and simmer for 10 minutes on low heat.

3 Add the milk and heat on low for an additional 5 minutes.

4 Strain into mugs, sprinkle nutmeg powder on top, and sweeten with honey, if desired. Store any leftover tea in the refrigerator. It will keep a couple days.

> ***Vary It!*** *If you need that caffeine buzz, go for the green. Green tea offers more health benefits than the black. To the preceding blend, add ½ teaspoon green tea when you add the milk in Step 3). Then continue with the recipe. Try this blend as a substitute if you're trying to cut down on coffee. (Then also add an additional ½ cup more boiling water to the beginning of this recipe.)*

> ***Vary It Another Way!*** *Rather than use a sweetener like honey or sugar, I prefer to use a sweet herb called stevia. Add ½ teaspoon stevia leaves when you add the milk. (Then also add an additional ½ cup more boiling water to the beginning of this recipe.)*

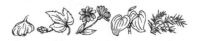

Seek Immunity: Immune System and Cell Repair

If your immune system goes out of whack, it can be trouble. Having a healthy immune system is your insurance against coming down with any illness, short or long term, minor or serious. Conditions that can get you if your immune system is weak include the common cold, viral disease, allergies, fungal and bacterial infections, cancer, and psoriasis — you name it, and it's your immune system's responsibility to protect you from contracting it.

Your immune system is actually a complex group of several smaller systems that must keep in communication and coordinated. If communication breaks down and the system gets confused, it can view normal substances in your body as invaders and then wage an all-out attack. This creates an allergic reaction as seen in hay fever, asthma, and food allergies. In some cases, an immune system responds by fighting against its own body. Examples of such autoimmune disorders are lupus, some infertility, and probably rheumatoid arthritis and diabetes. Quite possibly chronic hepatitis, atopic dermatitis, and degenerative disorders with no other known cause are also included.

Be on an immune alert if you tend to get sick often or are tired most of the time. These are clues that it's time to build up your immune system. Actually, it doesn't hurt to try to be healthy all of the time. View essential oils as preventive medicine that not only help to get you well, but keep you from getting sick in the first place.

The essential oils that are good for your immune system probably work much like immune herbs by teaching your body how to operate better rather than simply handing out temporary instructions. Your body's response to enhanced immune action is a little harder to identify than something like pain or an infection, but essential oils can play an important role in the health of your immune system. How they work exactly to aid your immune system is not always clear, because the immune system is complicated and there is still much for scientists to learn about its functions and also the way essential oils relate to it. There are probably more oils that work on your immune system, but here are three lists of the ones that do show an ability to increase your natural immunity to disease.

General immunity stimulants

This first category of essential oils is vague because so is the understanding of how they work. What is known is that these oils increase various actions of the immune system.

- Bay laurel
- Cinnamon (be careful when using this potent oil)
- Eucalyptus
- Frankincense
- Oregano (be careful when using this potent oil)
- Sage

White blood cell stimulants

While they're busy revving up your immune system, many essential oils also conveniently fight infection at the same time. A number of essential oils enhance immunity by increasing the production of white blood cells. These are the cells that patrol your body, cleaning and literally gobbling up foreign invaders. In addition, some essential oils detoxify the substance in insect bites and stings so that you don't react so strongly. At least some of these oils undoubtedly perform other, still unknown, jobs that are associated with immunity. These essential oils work with the body to fight infection and heal itself.

- Bergamot
- Chamomile
- Lavender
- Lemon
- Myrrh
- Pine
- Sandalwood
- Tea tree
- Thyme (be careful when using this potent oil)
- Vetivert

Hastening healing

Here's another list of essential oils that work in conjunction with your immune system to heal individual cells. These oils repair skin damage and encourage new cell growth, which results in faster healing. Their ability to protect tissue lessens the further destruction of injured or infected skin and tissue. The regenerative properties of these oils also improve your skin's general condition and appearance, so you find them widely used in body products and cosmetics. You can read more about them in Chapter 7.

- ✔ Carrotseed
- ✔ Frankincense
- ✔ Helichrysum
- ✔ Lavender
- ✔ Rose
- ✔ Rose geranium
- ✔ Sandalwood

Eliminate metabolic waste

Your lymphatic system is the garbage collector of your body. Somebody's got to do it. The job falls to the lymphatic fluid that floats through tissues to clean out waste debris that is produced as a result of natural metabolic functions. The garbage collection sites are the lymph nodes, which are located throughout your body. They filter out any toxicity to keep your blood clean. The main lymph nodes are in your throat, groin, breasts, and armpits. These hot spots swell up and get sore as they collect debris if you develop an infection near that area. Here are essential oils that help the lymph eliminate waste from your body.

- ✔ Bay laurel
- ✔ Grapefruit
- ✔ Juniper
- ✔ Lemon

Doing it: Aromatherapy for immunity

If you have a chronic disorder or you have a tendency to get sick, your immune system probably needs attention. Look up the specific problems that relate to your immune system in the Symptom Guide to find some simple recipes. Problems that you'll find that are related to immunity include allergies such as asthma, dermatitis and psoriasis, fatigue, hives, insect bites, poison oak and ivy rashes, lung congestion, uterine problems, bowel disorders, as well as all the infections listed in this chapter under viruses, bacteria, and fungi, and most of the disorders under pain and immune system problems in general. In other words, almost every disorder in that section revolves around having a healthy immune system.

A massage using the appropriate essential oils is a good way to use the oils, especially when it is a lymphatic massage that encourages the flow of lymph. Natural immunity is lowered by emotional or physical stress, poor diet (such as too many sweets), smoking, and too much alcohol. Even "good" stress, like a vacation or getting married, can lower your immune response. This means that, as with so many other physical problems, you should turn to the anti-stress essential oils I cover in Chapter 9 if stress is a part of your life.

Play it safe

Before you start using aromatherapy as medicine, I want to talk safety. You can never be too careful when it comes to your health, so follow these general rules for safety. (Also read the section on the safe use of essential oils in Chapter 3 before you dive into medical aromatherapy.)

✔ **Only turn to aromatherapy if you're certain that you know what's wrong with you and it's something you feel confident treating on your own.** Consider this first rule your golden one. When you have a health problem that normally sends you to a doctor — either conventional or holistic — then by all means go. I know some sad stories about individuals who didn't get a proper diagnosis and thought they were dealing with a relatively simple infection when they really had a staph infection in their blood system or had cancer. (No one died, but they're still sad stories.) My rule here: If you have any doubts about what you're doing when your health is at stake, then don't take chances by trying aromatherapy alone. Seek a correct medical diagnosis before starting any self-treatment.

✔ **Don't wait for a medical situation to get out of hand.** There's always a chance when you're taking care of yourself that you're using the wrong remedy or treating the wrong condition. When you're dealing with minor first aid — say a burn or a sprain that isn't bad enough to send you to your doctor — then expect your aromatherapy treatment to help relieve your pain and start the healing process right

away. Your condition should show signs of healing within the next day. The same is true if you've come down with a cold or flu. A seemingly minor infection can spread and rapidly worsen if not properly treated, so if you get sicker, re-evaluate that trip to your physician, acupuncturist, aromatherapist, herbalist, or somebody! How long you wait depends upon how much of an emergency you're facing, so listen to your common sense.

✔ **Always dilute!** An occasional exception to this rule is when you're using very gentle essential oils. For example, at times it's most convenient to dab a half drop of lavender essential oil on each temple to ease your headache or when you place a drop of tea tree essential oil directly on an insect bite or a herpes outbreak. However, putting a pure essential oil straight on your body generally isn't wise. They're just too concentrated. One little drop easily equals the amount of essential oil that you drink in a couple cups of herb tea. No one would think of downing 24 cups of tea at one sitting, although I've heard of people slathering themselves with the equivalent amount of essential oil.

✔ **Use essential oils safely.** Even relatively safe herbs that are fairly harmless in herb form, such as thyme, oregano, and wintergreen, turn into a potent medicine as a pure essential oil and must be used carefully. Undiluted, oils such as these burn your skin and the inside of your mouth. It's not just burning your skin that's at stake, but stress

(continued)

(continued)

to your liver and kidneys. (Read Chapter 3 for details on essential oils safety and a list of potentially toxic oils.) Using a plant that contains essential oils in its herb form to make tea, as with chamomile or peppermint, or to season your food is easier and safer than diluting pure essential oil to ingest it. You can safely sprinkle herbs such as thyme and oregano on your food and in doing so gain a medicinal dose of their essential oils.

✔ **Don't eat 'um.** Ingesting essential oils is not a good idea. That's because they're so concentrated. Most aromatherapists in North America, the United Kingdom, Australia, and Japan prefer sticking to the external use of essential oils. Taking essential oils internally is a more common practice in France, but

this is typically after you visit a professional aromatherapist who carefully prescribes the exact amount of a diluted oil and length of time to take it. Otherwise, you could all too easily take an overdose. The oil itself is also carefully selected so that it is pure and unadulterated and prepared in a pharmacy. The safest and most effective method in aromatherapy is to take low doses. Remember that more is not better when it comes to aromatherapy.

✔ **Try, try, again.** If the first remedy you try doesn't work, then experiment. You may find that you respond better to one oil than another that has nearly the same properties.

Part III
The Part of Tens

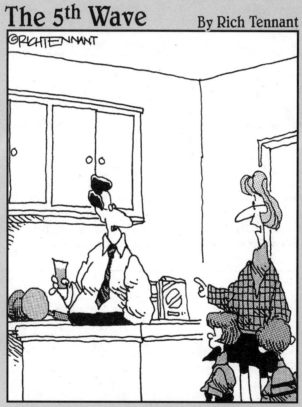

The 5th Wave   By Rich Tennant

©RICHTENNANT

"Hand me that mallet and a box of chocolate chip cookies. The kids want to make up aroma sachets for their bedrooms."

In this part

Here, I give you some extra tips on ways that you can incorporate aromatherapy into your life. Once you're excited about aromatherapy, it's contagious (in a good way!). You'll have fun with your family or friends taking an afternoon off to go on a scented adventure. And, I wouldn't want to neglect your garden and the fragrant plants you can grow in it. I provide you with all the tools you need so that you can proudly display your green thumb while showing off your fragrance garden.

Chapter 12

Ten Ways to Add Fragrance to Your Life

. . . .

In This Chapter

▶ Going places to find aromatic experiences

▶ Traveling to fragrance gardens

▶ Taking a luxurious bath

. . . .

*Y*ou can find dozens of ways that you can incorporate aromatherapy into your life as you read this book without even stepping out your front door. In this chapter, I give you ten or so ways to have aromatic experiences by venturing a little further. Whenever I travel anywhere to conduct a seminar, my first question is whether there is a botanical garden, an herb farm or shop, or some other aromatic place to visit while I'm there. By now, I've seen the United States by following my nose.

I'm sure that you'll also discover that the world is indeed filled with fragrance. Each one of these ideas is a particularly nice experience to either share with a friend or explore on your own. Be adventuresome, and you can really go places with aromatherapy!

Plant Your Own Fragrant Herb Garden

Growing your own herbs for use in aromatherapy not only gives you a good supply of aromatic material, it also makes your home and its surroundings more beautiful and fragrant. (See the details on cultivating aromatic herbs in Chapter 13.) You can find plants to buy at plant nurseries, herb farms that are open to the public, and often at farmer's markets. If you're looking for unusual herbs not offered at these places, then see the Appendix in this book for ways you can track down mail-order companies that carry a large selection of plants or seeds.

Get an Aromatherapy Facial

Take the time to give yourself a real treat. Men, as well as women, enjoy a facial and benefit from how it conditions your skin. Check your local Yellow Pages for someone who offers aromatherapy facials. You can ask beauty salons and spas for recommendations. If you can't splurge right now on getting a professional facial, then hook up with a friend and give each other facials using the aromatherapy products and the techniques that I describe in Chapter 7.

Get a Massage with an Aromatherapy Massage Oil

Most massage practitioners use an oil or lotion when they give a massage, and it's usually one that is scented. For the ultimate experience, seek out a practitioner that is trained not only in using different essential oils for their aromatherapy effects, but also in different aromatherapy techniques and you're in for a treat. Also consider getting an Ayurvedic massage, which uses several types of aromatic oils and is an aromatic experience that you won't forget. (You can find recipes for making your own massage oils in Chapters 9 and 10.)

Take an Aromatherapy Class

As the popularity of aromatherapy grows, so does the number of educational possibilities. Aromatherapy classes and seminars are certainly an aromatic experience in themselves! I provide a list in the Appendix to help you find these courses. Some courses offer certificates to show that you completed the course, although at this time, no recognized certificates of aromatherapy actually provide you with a license to practice. Still, learning about aromatherapy in a classroom setting really brings it to life because you can sniff the oils as they're discussed. Often, an instructor guides you through creating your own blends, and you may get to see a demonstration of distilling essential oils.

Visit a Fragrance Garden

Most major cities have a botanical garden, and these gardens usually include a fragrance garden. The fragrance gardens at the Los Angeles County Arboretum in Arcadia and Strybing Arboretum in Golden Gate Park in San Francisco both have fragrance gardens that are purposely set into a raised bed on a hillside, placing the fragrant plants at your fingertips and at nose level. Both of the these gardens are designed with the low vision visitor in mind. The L.A. garden even provides signs that identify each plant in Braille.

If you're not sure where you can find a botanical garden near you, then look in the phonebook under public gardens. You can often find a small public botanical garden associated with a university. Even if you don't, the botany department can usually point you in the right direction. Local plant nurseries should know the whereabouts of various gardens, and you can also track down the local chapter of the Herb Society of America to help you out. You'll almost always find a public garden in a major city in the United States. This is also true in many other countries throughout the world. Other places to try are herb farms that are open to visitors. They're likely to have many fragrant plants in their garden, even if they don't devote an area specifically to fragrant plants.

Here are places that you can find fragrant herb gardens.

- **Arboretum of Los Angeles,** Arcadia, CA, 626-821-3222
- **Cleveland Botanical Garden,** Cleveland, OH, 216-721-1600
- **Denver Botanical Garden**, Denver, CO, 303-331-4000
- **New York Botanical Garden,** Bronx, NY, 718-817-8700
- **North Carolina Botanical Garden,** University of North Carolina, Chapel Hill, NC, 919-962-0522
- **Strybing Arboretum,** Golden Gate Park, San Francisco, CA, 415-661-1316
- **U.S. National Arboretum,** Washington, D.C., 212-245-2726

Take an Aromatherapy Tour

Special tours are occasionally organized to visit aromatherapy hot spots, such as the lavender fields and essential oil distilleries of Grasse, France. The Appendix can help you find out about such opportunities. International aromatherapy conferences often have tours of local highlights related to the subject either before or after the conference so that you can see the aromatic sights of the area.

Take an Aromatic Bath, Ah!

Here's one fragrant experience to try at home or for when you finally get away and have the time to luxuriate. An aromatic bath is a great way to relax and takes approximately 40 minutes — but please, take as long as you like! Follow these steps for a great, relaxing bath experience.

1. **Arrange your bathing supplies: thick scented towel, warm robe, slippers.**

2. **Put on soothing music.**

3. **Light incense or place a few drops of your favorite essential oil in a potpourri cooker.**

4. **Draw a hot bath.**

5. **Add half a cup of scented bath salts to the water.**

6. **Make a soothing cup of chamomile tea and drink it while the tub fills.**

7. **Light a candle and turn off the lights.**

   Optional: Add 1 drop of an exotic essential oil like rose or jasmine.

8. **Step into your bath and relax for 30 minutes with no thoughts of the outside world.**

9. **Emerge and dry off.**

10. **Dust with a fragrant powder or apply a moisturizing cream to your entire body.**

11. **Wrap up in your warm robe and carry the candle to the bedroom.**

12. **Place a fragrant dream pillow under your bed pillow and slip into scented sheets and enjoy fragrant dreams and a restful sleep.**

    (See Chapter 9 for directions on making a dream pillow.)

Chapter 13

Ten Herbs to Grow for Fragrance

Many of the essential oils that I discuss in this book come from fragrant herbs that you can grow yourself. You can use the herbs that you grow to cook and to make the many different aromatherapy products that I describe throughout this book. Herbs are a cinch to cultivate. Even if you don't think that you have a green thumb, you'll probably be surprised how easy it is to grow herbs. They're much less demanding than vegetables or flowers. If you do already have a flower or vegetable garden or plot, then it's a simple matter to tuck in a few fragrant herbs. If not, you can grow a good selection of herbs in a few square feet of ground or in a planter.

I've grown herbs for more than 30 years and find that they perfume the air around my house. They also adorn the landscaping with their color and interesting variety of textures in their leaves. Yet another benefit is the assortment of butterflies — and in some cases hummingbirds — that come to visit them. If you'd like to make aromatherapy creations from your herb garden, it's easy to do. See the recipe in Chapter 5 for making herbal oils.

Here are ten of the fragrant herbs that I find especially easy to grow in a small area or in containers. In the following ten sections, I give you the basics that you need to cultivate each one. I tell you if the herb plant is an *annual* (lives for only one season), a *perennial* (lives for many years), or a *biennial* (lives for two years and doesn't flower until the second one). I also say how much sun it needs, the best soil conditions, how big it will get, and some special tips in case you want to grow your herbs in containers. (For the aromatherapy uses of these herbs, look them up in the Aroma Guide.)

Cultivation Tips for All Ten Herbs

First, here's some cultivation tips for all ten herbs.

- ✓ When deciding where to plant the herb in your garden, consider how tall it grows so that you can place taller herbs behind the shorter ones.

- ✓ Check how wide the herb grows to determine how far apart to plant each one. Divide the plant's width in half and then add a couple of inches for breathing room. (A 14-inch wide herb needs to be planted at least 9 [7 + 2] inches from its neighbor.)

- ✓ All these particular herbs prefer neutral to slightly alkaline soils (with a pH around 6 up to 8). Avoid using peat pots or potting soil mixes that contain a lot of peat moss, which are far too acid.

- ✓ These herbs appreciate regular watering, either from rain or a sprinkler. I find that a drip system on a battery-run timer makes growing herbs really easy. All that's left for you to do is to clear away any weeds around the base of the plant and harvest!

- ✓ With the exception of peppermint, none of these herbs like to have their roots constantly wet, so water them deeply a few times a week instead of keeping their soil constantly moist.

Even if you don't have any garden space at all, you can still grow herbs in planter boxes or pots. Container plants need only a little extra care to keep them looking vibrant. In most cases, you'll need at least a gallon-sized container that has a few holes in the bottom to assure good drainage. (Large pots are sized by the gallon, as if you're buying milk. Small pots are sized by the number of inches across the top.) The windowsill kits that sell herbs in cute 2- to 3-inch pots are fine for baby plants, but any self-respecting herb plant will soon grow out of it. If a pot gets too tight with roots — a situation that gardeners describe as *root bound* — then it's hard for the plant to get enough water or nutrients out of the soil. You can prevent this situation by keeping your container herbs cut back since the more leaves, the more roots that a plant needs. One good point about constantly harvesting your herb plants is this encourages you to use them. Also, feed container plants a couple times a year with an organic liquid fertilizer, such as fish emulsion. (Be forewarned that this fertilizer smells.)

Basil

Bushy basil grows so rapidly it fills in empty spots in your garden and forms an attractive, low border along a pathway. Or, follow the example of the Italians, Morrocans, and Greeks and set pots of basil on a sunny porch or windowsill to repel flies and mosquitoes. (Basil is also rumored to attract lovers!)

There are 150 to 350 basil species (no one can agree) in a variety of fragrances, including ones that are lemon-scented and anise-scented.

You may as well plant basil from seed because it sprouts in only about one week. If you cut back the flower stalks, your plants stay compact and continue to produce more leaves throughout the summer for culinary delights like pesto, as well your aromatherapy projects.

Here's what you need to know about basil.

- ✔ Annual.
- ✔ Full sun.
- ✔ Dry, medium rich, and well-drained soil.
- ✔ Grows to 2 feet tall by 1 foot wide.
- ✔ Basil grows especially well in a container, even a small half-gallon-sized pot. It even thrives indoors if placed in a sunny window.

Bay

This attractive plant's main feature are its shiny, leathery leaves because its clustered yellow flowers, which bloom in June and July, are very small. The tradition of potting bay began in Europe, to make it easier to bring the plant indoors to winter and avoid the possibility of a hard winter (below 28°F) killing it. Potting bay also stunts its growth, so the scented leaves are easier to pick. Otherwise, bay grows into a huge tree. Add the leaves to your beans and soups, use them to keep the bugs out of your grains, and use them in your aromatherapy projects. The seeds seem to take forever to sprout, so start bay from a plant.

Here's what you need to know about bay.

- ✔ Perennial.
- ✔ Sun or partial shade.
- ✔ The best soil for bay is well-drained and sandy.
- ✔ If not planted in a pot, it can grow into a 25 to 60 foot tall tree. The milder the climate, the taller it grows. In a pot, it can grow several feet tall.
- ✔ If you plant bay in a pot, make sure that the pot is large enough. It can start off in a gallon-sized pot and grows very slowly, but will eventually graduate to at least a 5-gallon pot.

Chamomile, German and Roman

Both Roman and German chamomiles are spindly, feathery plants. They bloom in early summer with a profusion of small, daisylike flowers. Roman chamomile makes a fragrant ground cover. If you're planning on using chamomile for tea, grow the sweeter German chamomile. It prefers seeding directly where it will grow and will be up within a couple of weeks. Sow it early in the spring, or the plants become leggy in hot weather. Water the young seedlings gently so that they don't fall over into the mud.

Here's what you need to know about chamomile.

- ✔ Annual: German chamomile; Perennial: Roman chamomile.
- ✔ Full sun.
- ✔ Grows to 1 to 2 feet tall by 1 foot wide (German chamomile) or 6 inches tall by 6 inches wide (Roman chamomile).
- ✔ A rich soil produces lush growth, but fewer flowers. For more flowers, use a light, sandy, and well-drained soil.
- ✔ In a pot, Roman chamomile is a better choice than German, but either will work provided it has a fairly sunny location and you don't let it dry out too much.

Clary Sage

Clary sage's large, heart-shaped leaves grow from a central stalk that eventually bends with the weight of its showy, lilac or pale blue flowers in June and July. The resinous flowers are where you find this herb's fragrance. Clary sage is effective when planted in isolated groups, with other herbs in a mixed border, or by itself in a container. Start it from seeds — they sprout in less than two weeks — or from plants purchased at a nursery.

Here's what you need to know about clary sage.

- ✔ Biennial.
- ✔ Full sun.
- ✔ Clary sage likes a well-drained, fertile soil. It prefers soil that is always slightly moist but can tolerate dry spells in between waterings.
- ✔ Grows to 3 feet tall by 1 foot wide.
- ✔ A two-gallon pot is best for clary to reach full size and flower.

Lavender

Try to plant lavender where your garden visitors can sniff its fragrant buds and admire its soft, gray foliage. The very fragrant, vivid purple flowers cluster on tall spikes in the summer. They contrast well in your garden with pink-flowering herbs such as pink yarrow or roses. Collect the flower stalks when the buds are still tight, and they'll hold their scent for years. Lavender is difficult to grow from seed or cuttings, so buy plants. Once established, they live at least 12 years. Of the many subspecies and cultivars, English lavender is the most fragrant and the hardiest. French lavender is the best choice if the soil isn't well drained. If you live where the winter temperatures drop below freezing, then surround the base of the plants with straw or leaves and be sure that your plants are in a well-drained area.

Here's what you need to know about lavender.

- ✔ Perennial.
- ✔ Full sun.
- ✔ Sandy, very well-drained soil
- ✔ Grows to 2 to 3 feet tall by 2 to 3 feet wide.
- ✔ The dwarf Munstead lavender is best suited for a container. You can start off putting it in a half-gallon container, but will need a 5-gallon pot in a couple of years to keep it from becoming stunted.

Marjoram

Marjoram is a small, bushy herb that looks nice when placed near the edge of a bed or terrace. Plant it where it's easy to reach so that you can pinch its leaves and release its scent — unlike many culinary herbs, marjoram doesn't automatically perfume the air. The slightly hardier "pot" marjoram that hails from southeast Europe and Turkey is often grown as a substitute because it can make it through a winter if the ground doesn't freeze (although this type is less aromatic with a coarser flavor). Sowing marjoram from seed is tricky because, although the seeds sprout easily, the young plants are fragile and subject to damping-off disease or being knocked over by a forceful watering. It's easier to buy plants and then divide the roots once they're established. Tiny white flowers appear throughout the summer, but keep marjoram cut back to encourage leaf growth and to keep it from getting "leggy."

Here's what you need to know about marjoram.

- ✔ Perennial (although in cold climates, it's usually cultivated as an annual).
- ✔ Full sun.
- ✔ Well-drained, dry soil.
- ✔ Grows to 2 feet tall by 1 foot wide.
- ✔ Marjoram prefers at least a half-gallon container. In a hanging basket on your porch or patio, it gracefully hangs over the edge.

Melissa (Lemon Balm)

Lemon balm flowers are inconspicuous, but their yellow-green, lemon-scented foliage looks good in your garden growing next to deep greens. The cultivar golden lemon balm has especially attractive, variegated leaves. If you live in a climate where the ground can freeze, then plant lemon balm in a pro-tected location and put a straw or leaf mulch around its roots during the winter. You can start it from plants or seeds or divide the thick root clumps into individual plants. This is a prolific self-sower once it gets established. (In fact, if any of your neighbors have lemon balm, chances are that they have extra plants that they'd love you to take.)

Here's what you need to know about lemon balm.

- ✔ Perennial.
- ✔ The plants grow lusher in full sun, but tolerate partial shade.
- ✔ Grows to 3 feet tall by 2 feet wide.
- ✔ The soil should be fertile and moist, yet very well drained because soggy ground kills it.
- ✔ Use at least a 3-gallon pot for a full-sized bush.

Peppermint

Peppermint is common and grows so easily that you may want to curb its growth to keep it from taking over your garden by planting it in a container. The easiest way to grow peppermint is to separate the roots and replant them. There are a couple dozen species of mint. However, they've been hybridized so much that you now have quite a selection from which to choose. Very small, lilac-pink flowers bloom on short flower stalks throughout the summer.

Here's what you need to know about peppermint.

- Perennial.

- Sun. Partial shade is best because full shade or sun reduce peppermint's oil content.

- Moist plus soil is best. It can even handle excessive wetness.

- Grows to 3 feet tall by 1 foot wide.

- Peppermint will grow in just about anything, even a small, 4-inch container, but use something larger if you want lush growth.

Rosemary

Rosemary is a tall, graceful bush and an early bloomer, with its pale blue, flowers appearing in late winter in mild climates. It lends itself to pruning and being formed into interesting topiary shapes or trimmed into a hedge. To imitate the Tudor style, train it into patterns against a wall or fence. If you try this, be sure to get an upright or standard rosemary. The other, low-growing ground cover rosemary is nice to cascade over a hanging pot or terrace. The easiest way to start either one is to purchase the plants. Once it is established, you can propagate it by *layering*. For this technique, lay a few branches on the ground and cover them with a little mound of dirt. Keep this mound watered, and eventually roots will sprout. After a few months, cut the new plant off of the "mother" plant and replant. Mulch the roots in the winter with straw or leaves if your ground freezes and temperatures dip below 20°F.

Here's what you need to know about rosemary.

- Perennial.

- Full sun.

- Well-drained, fairly dry soil

- Grows up to 5 feet tall by 4 feet wide in a mild climate.

- Rosemary makes an attractive picture in a container due to its swooping branches. Grow it in a 5-gallon container if you want a larger plant.

Thyme

Thyme looks great when planted along a pathway, in a rock garden, or as a fragrant ground cover. It's particularly attractive cascading over a raised terrace or the side of a hanging pot. There are a couple hundred different species and numerous cultivars, including lemon, caraway, and creeping thyme. Planted together, different thyme plants play off each other's colors. Tiny, white to lilac flowers bloom profusely throughout the summer. Thyme's delicate root system makes it difficult to transplant except from a nursery pot. If you must transplant it, give thyme several months to re-establish its fine root system before a freeze. Even established plants can be damaged if the ground freezes solid, but a layer of sand on the soil helps prevent frost damage.

Here's what you need to know about thyme.

- ✔ Perennial.
- ✔ Full sun.
- ✔ Well-drained, light, rather dry, soil.
- ✔ Grows to 8 inches tall by about 8 inches wide. (The height varies with the different types.)
- ✔ Because thyme spreads, the container that you grow it in should be wide but can be shallow — say only 7 inches deep.

Two More Herbs to Consider

Two more wonderfully fragrant herb plants to consider growing are roses and jasmine. They're a little more ambitious to grow, but not very difficult. Obtain the plants and growing instructions from your local nursery. You can grow either one in a large, 10-gallon pot. I grow jasmine and many roses in my garden, but I also have them growing in pots on my deck. Choose a type of rose that is adaptable enough for container growing.

And, How about Another Hundred or So. . . ?

You may discover that you have a green thumb when you plant some of these herbs, or at least why so many people love to grow plants. If you find yourself interested in cultivating an even larger herb garden, then check out my book, *Herbs, An Illustrated Encyclopedia* (published by Freidman/Fairfax). It covers 150 herbs and even more varieties of my favorites that I've grown, with colored pictures so you can see what they'll look like in your garden.

Part IV
The Guides

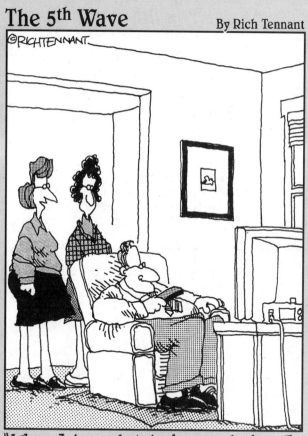

The 5th Wave   By Rich Tennant

"When I know he's had a rough day, I always put a few drops of lavender on the TV remote before he gets home."

In this part

In this part, I give you two handy guides. The Symptom Guide describes various conditions and tells you how you can use aromatherapy to improve or prevent them. In the Aroma Guide, I tell you all you need to know about the different essential oils that you'll encounter in aromatherapy.

Symptom Guide

• •

This *Symptom Guide* is a practical reference to using aromatherapy to treat 60 common conditions. These are my favorite aromatherapy remedies that I've seen work reliably during my last 30 years of experience working with holistic medicine. The problems that I describe typically are ones that you already self-diagnose and then treat yourself without seeing a doctor. Instead of using over-the-counter drugs, I suggest the aromatherapy products and treatments for you to use. In case you're feeling creative, I also give you recipes for making your own simple aromatherapy preparations.

Aromatherapy, like other forms of holistic healing, treats the individual. Most clinical aromatherapists prefer to custom-design a formula for an individual. Because that's not always practical, I am providing you with generic formulas. However, don't hesitate to be creative and change a suggested formula to better fit your personal needs. Refer to the Aroma Guide to find out more about oils that are appropriate substitutes. Many disorders that I don't describe can be helped with aromatherapy even though it doesn't offer a cure. For example, if you have diabetes, multiple sclerosis, a kidney or liver disorder, or some other serious problem, aromatherapy can still help relieve your symptoms. One of the many advantages of aromatherapy is that, unlike many herbs, it can often be used in conjunction with any pharmaceutical drugs you take.

It's an empowering thing to take your own health in your hands. It's your body and the more you learn about it and the various healing modalities, the better position you are in to make good choices. When you do so, be responsible. Make sure that you seek out more advice whenever you feel unsure of a treatment that you're pursuing. These suggestions are intended to complement your health but not replace the advice and care of a qualified health-care practitioner. If you suffer from serious disorders that would normally send you to a doctor, get professional help before you embark on your self-healing methods. A medical diagnosis is often valuable to make sure that you are treating the right thing. Sometimes a seemingly simple problem such as a lingering sore throat or headache is indicative of a far more serious, underlying problem.

I've organized the information on each condition into four categories to help you find a remedy easier:

Medical description: This defines the condition or symptom.

Aromatherapy remedies: In this category, I give you the specific aromatherapy solutions to treat your conditions and symptoms, and I suggest the type of aromatherapy products for you to buy.

Aromatherapy formula: In this section, I provide simple aromatherapy recipes that use essential oils in case you'd like to create your own formulas instead of buying them. In some cases, the remedy is so simple (say, an essential oil is added to water) you won't be able to buy it in a store so you do need to prepare it yourself.

Healthy habits: Aromatherapy is not always the only path to health and healing. It often works far better when used in conjunction with herbal medicine, and dietary and lifestyle changes. I heartily recommend that you further investigate holistic ideas for healing your condition and for staying healthy, and that you also refer to herb books for more information. You'll find the ones that I recommend in the Appendix. (And, of course, don't forget to check out *Herbal Remedies For Dummies* by Christopher Hobbs, L.Ac., IDG Books Worldwide, Inc. and my *Herbs for Health and Healing*, Rodale Press.)

Because so many disorders exist, you may not find the condition that you're looking for in this guide. If you don't, look up any of the symptoms that you experience. For example, if you have diabetes, no aromatherapy cure exists for the disease, but my suggestions on improving circulation can help you. (And you can also check out *Diabetes For Dummies,* by Dr. Alan Rubin, IDG Books Worldwide.) If you suffer from cancer or AIDS, look up what you can do to treat your immune system. Other conditions that I list here, such as insomnia and headaches, are symptoms of many different problems. Use my suggestions under these headings to at least ease your symptoms.

To translate the formulas in the guide (and throughout this book) into European measurements, 1 teaspoon (1/10 ounce) equals about 5 milliliters, 1 tablespoon (1/2 ounce) is about 15 milliliters, and 1 cup (8 ounces) is 250 milliliters.

Acne

Medical description: Acne is a skin inflammation that develops in the pores of your skin. It produces blemishes that can become infected, creating small sores. A hormonal imbalance is most often blamed as the cause, although holistic practitioners suspect that toxicity in the blood plays a role. If you have oily skin, you're more prone to acne because the excess oil easily traps dirt in your pores. (However, don't despair — oily skin also ages more slowly and gracefully than dry skin!)

Aromatherapy remedies: When shopping for aromatherapy products designed for acne, you'll encounter a large assortment that are sold in natural-food stores and some drugstores. Get something that you can apply directly to your acne. A general skin toner that will reduce future breakouts is also a good idea if you have an oily complexion. (Refer to my suggestions under Oily Skin or Dry Skin for other essential oils that aid your type of skin.) If you have a severe case of acne, use some type of herbal paste that you can dab directly on it. Look for acne products that contain lavender, chamomile, geranium, or sandalwood oils to reduce the swelling and irritation, help prevent infection, and heal your skin. Tea tree, cedarwood, lemon, eucalyptus or lavender or (Spanish) sage are good on oily skin that is prone to breaking out. (Any eucalyptus will do, although a slightly more expensive variety called dives or broad leaf eucalyptus, which is high in the compound cineole, is considered the very best type for acne.) Clary sage, fennel, frankincense, rosemary, and patchouli reduce inflammation, rejuvenate your skin, encourage oil production, and balance your hormones in case you have acne that is combined with dry or mature skin. Dermatologists say not to pop pimples, but if you do, use the following compress on the spot before and afterwards.

Aromatherapy formula: *To make an acne compress:* Pour ¼ cup boiling water over 1 teaspoon Epsom salts (also called magnesium sulfate — buy this muscle-relaxing salt in the grocery store). When the salts dissolve, add 4 drops each lavender and tea tree oils. Soak a small absorbent cloth in the solution, wring out, and press it directly on your pimples for a minute or two. Place the cloth back in the hot solution and then reapply it several times. *To make an acne paste:* Stir 12 drops tea tree oil into ½ teaspoon comfrey root powder and add enough distilled water to make a paste (about 1 tablespoon). Mix well, then dab the paste directly on your acne spots, and let it dry into a mask for 10 to 20 minutes before rinsing it off. Store any leftover paste in the refrigerator for the next treatment. Also read up on general skin care in Chapter 7.

Healthy habits: Avoid eating fried or sweet foods and drink plenty of water. Taking evening primrose oil capsules can help prevent recurring acne. If your acne is related to a hormonal imbalance, try taking vitex seeds in a tincture, tea, or pills. Herbs that improve liver function often help as well. One of my favorite combinations of liver herbs for the skin is burdock root, milk thistle seed, yellow dock root, and red clover blossom, but you'll find plenty of formulas from which to choose.

Appetite loss

Medical description: You can lose your appetite for many reasons; stress or depression are common culprits. Losing your desire to eat is also a side effect of some pharmaceutical drugs. Because loss of appetite can be a symptom of a far more serious physical or emotional disorder, be sure to check with a doctor if your appetite doesn't perk up after a couple of weeks. It's one of the most obvious signs of a eating disorder known as anorexia nervosa, which deals with psychological issues such as self-worth.

Aromatherapy remedies: Just smelling an aromatic herb or its essential oil stimulates your appetite and results in good digestion. Some of the best herbs to sniff are the culinary spices, such as anise, cardamom, cumin, coriander, and especially fennel and ginger. Conveniently, when you use herbs like these to flavor your food, both their direct action on the digestive tract and their scent help you digest your meal. They also aid anorexia nervosa, but only as a secondary treatment to psychological therapy. If your appetite decline is associated with stress or depression, then see my suggestions in those sections. Along with other aromatherapists, I find that the scents of bergamot and rose can help you deal with compulsive behavior and that geranium's fragrance encourages emotional stability. Also see the general information on digestion in Chapter 11.

Healthy habits: Exercise and eating a good, wholesome diet keeps your appetite on an even keel.

Arthritis and rheumatism

Medical description: Swollen, painful, and stiff joints are the uncomfortable symptoms of arthritis or rheumatism. What causes these disorders is not completely understood, so doctors and aromatherapists alike treat the symptoms: inflammation and the resulting pain.

Aromatherapy remedies: Essential oils such as rosemary and marjoram may not cure arthritis or rheumatism, but they penetrate deep into your joints to lessen inflammation, and thus pain, so they're used in many liniments. (See Chapter 9.) Clove oil, and to some degree ginger and peppermint oils,

directly numb arthritic and rheumatic discomfort. They also bring blood and heat to the area to further dull the pain. The scents alone of these oils also stimulate energy to encourage you to keep moving your stiff joints. Birch oil (usually sold as wintergreen because the two oils are almost identical) can be slightly toxic as an essential oil, but small amounts provide aspirinlike pain relief in a liniment. Other essential oils that you'll find in liniments for arthritis and rheumatism to reduce swelling are German chamomile, lavender, helichrysum, and lavender (or Spanish) sage. The scent alone of these oils helps to calm irritation you may feel from your discomfort. Frankincense helps athritis sufferers by improving blood circulation to the affected areas, repairing damaged blood vessels, and shrinking swollen tissue around painful and stiff joints. A liniment can have an alcohol or vegetable oil base, but I prefer aloe vera because it increases the pain relief. A liniment that contains St. John's wort or arnica flowering tops is especially effective to ease swollen joint areas. Besides using a liniment, take a warm bath that contains a few drops of these same essential oils now and then. Also see essential oils under Circulation, poor, to help relieve symptoms.

Aromatherapy formula: *To make a homemade liniment:* See the recipes and information in Chapter 10. *For a hot bath:* Use 3 drops each of rosemary and marjoram oil and 2 drops ginger oil in your tub. If your pain is localized in just your hands or feet, try soaking them in a pan or small basin of hot water that contains 1 drop of each of these oils.

Healthy habits: Work on arthritis and rheumatism from the inside as well as the outside with an herbal formula that contain devil's club root and the nutritional supplement glutamate to reduce inflammation and meadowsweet leaf or willow leaf to reduce pain. You'll find these available as pills. Also minimize the amount of meat, caffeine, and sugar in your diet, as well as vegetables in the nightshade family, such as tomatoes, potatoes, eggplant, and peppers. Do eat foods that are rich in benefical compounds called flavonoids, such as cherries and blueberries, and vitamins C and E, and make sure that you get plenty of minerals. Get moderate exercise, but don't strain your joints; bicycling and swimming are excellent.

Asthma

Medical description: This allergic condition is characterized by wheezing and shortness of breath, especially during an attack. The reaction intensifies if you're under emotional or physical stress. Likewise, having an asthmatic attack greatly ups your stress level. If you have asthma, chances are that you constantly battle a low-level lung congestion, which invites coughing and lung infection.

Aromatherapy remedies: Most aromatherapy books advise asthmatics to completely avoid essential oils, but you can rub your feet, do a foot bath, or hover over steam during the initial stages of an asthmatic attack to reduce its intensity. Frankincense, lavender, chamomile, helichrysum, rose, geranium, marjoram, mandarin, and neroli (orange blossom) are especially effective antihistamines that sedate the bronchial tubes in your lungs, yet are gentle enough to use with small children. And, the scent of these oils reduces stress. Eucalyptus, rosemary, and tea tree oils are sometimes used, but they're emotionally stimulating and are harsher, so you may react adversely to them if you have asthma. (If you do use them, the radiata species of eucalyptus or the verbenone type of rosemary are the best ones to use.) Between attacks, use them in a chest rub. Even though it's an excellent decongestant, avoid hyssop oil because it contains potent compounds called

ketones, which may bring on an asthmatic attack — that is, unless you use a special type of hyssop called *decumbens,* which treats allergic reactions and doesn't contain ketones. Also, see the other essential oils that I recommend under Lung Congestion.

Aromatherapy formula: *For a foot or chest rub:* Use 3 drops frankincense, lavender, or chamomile oils (or make a blend using 1 drop of each) diluted in a tablespoon of vegetable oil. Rub on your chest or feet. *For a foot bath:* Put the same oils and the same amounts in a basin of hot water and soak your feet. *To make an asthma steam:* Add 3 to 5 drops lavender oil to a 2 to 3-cup pot of water that is just hot enough to produce steam and inhale the steam. (If you have asthma, too hot a steam can be irritating. Also, pass on the typical technique of putting a towel over your head to capture the steam, which can make the steam too intense.) For a small child or baby, turn on the hot water in your bathtub and add about 10 drops lavender oil. Then hold her or him in the steam over the bathtub. The sooner this is done during an impending attack, the better it works to lessen the symptoms. *To make a chest rub:* Dilute 15 drops lavender oil (or 7 drops for a child) into a tablespoon of vegetable oil and rub this on your chest.

Healthy habits: Aromatherapy treatments help relieve the symptoms of asthma, but mullein leaf and elecampane root are examples of herbs that you'll find in products designed to strengthen and improve the general health of your lungs. If the herbal blend that you choose also contains immune enhancers such as echinacea root, shizandra berry, and vitamin C, it helps you to ward off further asthma attacks.

Athlete's foot/ringworm

Medical description: The most common fungal skin infection is ringworm. It's not a worm, but it does grow in a red, ringlike formation of itchy, peeling skin. Ringworm thrives in moist conditions, so it loves sweaty feet — your most likely spot to get the fungus. This is called athlete's foot, although everyone, even couch potatoes, can get it.

Aromatherapy remedies: Lavender, geranium, patchouli, lemongrass, cedarwood, and fennel oils, and especially tea tree, eucalyptus, myrrh, and clove oils do an excellent job of fighting fungal infections. Of these, lavender, geranium, tea tree, eucalyptus, and myrrh oils also heal injured skin. Sage oil decreases excessive perspiration, and small amounts of peppermint oil relieve itching. Look for an antifungal product that contains at least some of these essential oils and dab it directly on the infection at least twice a day. A powder or vinegar-based product dries out the area and discourages fungal growth unless the infected skin is cracked and dry. In that case, look for a salve or cream-based product. You can also wash with an aromatherapy soap that contains any of the antifungal oils that I just recommended. Also see the general information on fungal infection in Chapter 11.

Aromatherapy formula: *To make a foot powder:* Place ¼ cup cornstarch in a plastic sandwich bag. Drop in 25 drops (¼ teaspoon) tea tree oil or eucalyptus oil, 8 drops clove oil, 8 drops sage oil, and 3 drops peppermint oils. Close the bag and mix well with your fingers (through the outside of the bag). *For a liquid antifungal:* Add the same amounts of these essential oils to ¼ cup apple cider vinegar. Dab either preparation directly on the infected area 3 to 5 times a day.

Healthy habits: Completely dry the area after bathing or swimming. If the fungus persists, also take an immune and infection-fighting herbal combination, such as pau d'arco bark, echinacea root, and black walnut hull, in tincture or pills. When possible, wear cotton socks and open shoes to give your feet more air circulation and prevent sweating.

Baldness

Medical description: Hair falls out all the time, but then it grows back. Baldness occurs when empty hair follicles (the origins of hair in your scalp) take a rest and never get going again. Hair typically thins with advancing years. Often the scalp tightens and blood flow decreases, both of which cut off the supply of nutrients to hair follicles. The most common type of baldness is male-pattern baldness, which is hereditary and spurred on by the presence of the male hormone testosterone and enzymes that discourage hair growth. Once your hair is gone, there is little chance of it returning. Baldness can also be caused by hormonal disorders, drug treatments (especially including some types of antibiotic and cancer chemotherapy), radiation therapy, serious illness (especially nervous system disease), stress, malnutrition, and scalp disease. In these situations, your body doesn't consider hair one of your vital assets, so it's one of the first things to go, but it often grows back in when the disorder or treatment is over.

Aromatherapy remedies: Aromatherapy helps re-establish hair growth. In the case of male-pattern baldness, it usually can only slow further hair loss. Stimulate circulation with a scalp formula that contains vitamin E and essential oils that improve circulation to your scalp. Rosemary oil is the age-old favorite. Other circulation stimulants are basil, eucalyptus, ginger, lemongrass, juniper, cypress, fennel, peppermint, and geranium oils. To some degree, so are some of the citrus oils, but watch out about using them if your balding head is exposed to the sun because they are all, to varying degrees, photosensitizing agents that can cause skin reactions. (See my suggestions under Circulation for more ideas.) Cedarwood and ylang ylang are also sometimes recommended. Aloe vera is another good ingredient because it may promote hair growth, and apple cider vinegar enhances the health of your scalp (and has a folklore reputation for improving hair growth). Look for something that you can leave on your hair. Massaging this formula on your head further enhances your circulation and stimulates hair follicles. Also, find a hair conditioner that also contains these same essential oils and try to leave it on your head for longer than the typical few seconds before you rinse it off. Hair conditioners that contain balsams may not make your hair grow fuller, but they do make it seem thicker.

Aromatherapy formula: *To make a hair-loss conditioner:* Combine ½ cup aloe vera gel, 2 tablespoons apple cider vinegar, 1 tablespoon wheat germ or jojoba oil, and ½ teaspoon (25 drops) rosemary essential oil. Shake well and massage into scalp for 10 minutes nightly.

Healthy habits: Take vitamin E supplements and herbs, such as ginkgo leaves, to increase the blood flow to your scalp and nettles for scalp health. Eat a healthy diet and watch that cholesterol. Studies show that a high blood cholesterol limits blood flow to the scalp and also chokes out hair growth. (See Cholesterol for my tips on keeping it low.)

Bladder infection/cystitis

Medical description: Cystitis, or an inflammation of your bladder, is often caused by an infection, which is most often due to *E. coli* bacteria. If you don't already know the extent of your bladder

infection, head straight for your doctor to make sure that you don't have a kidney infection.

Aromatherapy remedies: Many essential oils both promote urination and kill germs, a perfect combination to counter a simple bladder infection. These include sandalwood, pine, chamomile, cedarwood, juniper, tea tree, bergamot, and fennel oils. Studies show that bay laurel, thyme, clove, and cinnamon are some of the strongest essential oils to fight *E. coli*. See the general information on infection-fighting essential oils in Chapter 11. Find a massage or body oil that contains several of these oils (or make one yourself) and rub it directly over your bladder area, which is located in your lower abdomen, above your pubic bone.

Aromatherapy formula: *To make a cystitis massage oil:* Add 14 drops tea tree oil, 5 drops fennel oil, and 5 drops bergamot oil in 2 ounces vegetable oil or a lotion. Rub this on twice a day. To help prevent the infection's return, put a tablespoon of this same oil in your bath once a week.

Healthy habits: To properly treat a bladder infection, you need to take antiseptic and anti-inflammatory herbs, such as uva ursi, pipsissewa, and marshmallow, along with your aromatherapy treatment. Or, you can drink cranberry juice to destroy the infection and make your urine more acidic and less hospitable to bacteria. At the same time, stay away from caffeine, sugar, and hot, irritating foods, except for garlic, which contains a strong, infection-fighting essential oil. Avoid perfumed soaps, vaginal sprays, and toilet tissue, wear loose underwear and clothing that allow for good air circulation, and keep the genital area very clean. You can use the witch hazel wipes sold in drugstores and natural-food stores.

Blood pressure, high

Medical description: Medical researchers aren't exactly sure what causes your blood pressure to go up, but living a high-paced life that involves eating a high cholesterol and fatty diet, drinking, smoking, and lots of stress are likely contributors. Because high blood pressure may be a life-threatening situation, be sure to consult your doctor.

Aromatherapy remedies: Simply smelling the citrusy scents of neroli (orange blossom), orange, melissa (lemon balm), and tangerine oils, as well as rose, ylang ylang, and geranium oils, can relax you enough to drop your blood pressure a couple of points. Marjoram, and clary sage oils also slightly lower your blood pressure. You can sniff either the essential oils or the herbs themselves. Fortunately, this doesn't interfere with any blood pressure medication you take. Purchase a massage or bath oil that contains these oils or carry around smelling salts that contain them to inhale throughout the day.

Aromatherapy formula: *For a blood pressure-reducing massage oil:* Combine 8 drops geranium oil, 3 drops orange oil, and 1 drop cinnamon oil in 2 ounces of any vegetable oil or in a lotion. *To make a bath oil:* Place 4 drops geranium oil and 1 drop orange oil in the water. (Go easy on orange oil because it can burn the skin if you use too much.)

Healthy habits: Aromatherapy alone isn't enough to treat high blood pressure, so add garlic or onion to your meals, every day if possible, to lower both blood cholesterol and pressure. Herbs to regulate your blood pressure include hawthorn, ginseng, and Siberian ginseng. Take them as tea, tincture, or pills. Eat a lowfat, low cholesterol diet, avoid smoking cigarettes, and limit how much alcohol you drink. Also, relax and see my suggestions in the section on Stress.

Blood pressure, low

Medical description: When your blood pressure falls too low, you can feel dizzy, weak, and disoriented. Even worse, that means that not enough blood and oxygen reach your cells. Also known as hypotension, low blood pressure can be due to many things. Because it can signal a serious problem like internal bleeding or a heart condition — and it can be serious in itself — make sure that you to see your doctor.

Aromatherapy remedies: The scents of cypress and rosemary oils increase blood pressure, while geranium is used to regulate both high and low blood pressure up or down, depending upon what you need. For even more of an effect, use massage or body oils that contain them. German pharmacies sell a rosemary ointment designed to rub over your heart to increase blood pressure, improve poor circulation, and ease the headaches and dizziness that often accompany low blood pressure. The ointment is based on an old European formula that infused rosemary leaves in white wine for the same purpose.

Aromatherapy formula: *To make a chest rub:* Add 12 drops rosemary oil, 5 drops geranium oil, and 4 drops cypress oil to ¼ cup white wine. Rub this solution on your chest every day. (You can also make the same remedy by chopping ⅛ cup rosemary leaves and covering them with ½ cup white wine. Keep this in a clean glass jar at room temperature for two weeks and then strain out the leaves. Add 10 drops geranium oil and shake well before using it.)

Healthy habits: Herbs that you can take in a tea, tincture, or pills to help raise your blood pressure and keep it regulated are hawthorn, ginger, ginseng, and Siberian ginseng.

Bowel disorders

Medical description: Bowel problems represent any of a number of conditions that are caused by infection or irritation in your intestines. They all result in problems with ingestion and diarrhea or constipation. Examples are *colitis,* which is an ulceration of your large intestine, and *irritable bowel syndrome,* which is related to nerves and unknown causes. In fact, many bowel disorders are tied in to emotional or nervous system problems.

Aromatherapy remedies: When used in abdominal massage, Roman chamomile and peppermint oils ease all sorts of stress-related bowel problems in two ways. They directly relax your intestine muscles, and at the same time, their fragrances ease your mind and your worries. To relieve intestinal gas, try a tea of peppermint, or anise, cardamom, cinnamon, coriander, cumin, ginger, and caraway. (The tea's hot water draws out the herb's essential oil.) European doctors treat irritable bowel syndrome with capsules of peppermint oil that are specially coated to not release their contents until they reach the large intestine. The safest and most enjoyable way to eat herbs like these is in food. You can also take the herb itself as a tea, tincture, or in pills. If it relates to you, also see my suggestions under Stress, Depression, and associated conditions.

Aromatherapy formula: *To make tea:* Pour 2 cups boiling water over a teaspoon each chamomile flowers and peppermint leaves. Steep about 5 minutes, strain, and drink at least 1 cup a couple hours after each meal. *To make a massage oil:* Add 7 drops fennel, 4 drops teaspoon Roman chamomile, and 3 drops ginger oils to 1 ounce vegetable oil or a lotion and massage over your abdomen.

Healthy habits: Eat small, leisurely meals of easy-to-digest foods. Herbal teas, tinctures, or pills that help your bowels include chamomile flowers, wild yam root, licorice root, marshmallow root, and fenugreek seed. Include fermented foods, such as yogurt or miso, in your diet or take the acidopholus supplements that are sold in natural-food stores to support the growth of beneficial flora in your intestine and to reduce populations of destructive organisms. (Acidopholus is a natural bacteria that causes milk to ferment into yogurt.) For constipation, massage the abdomen is a clockwise direction with the massage oil and add natural bulk, such as eating vegetables and fruits, to your diet, or take psyllium seed husk with lots of water if you're constipated.

Burns and sunburn

Medical description: Burns from heat, fire, the sun, or radiation redden your skin and cause it to swell and blister. You can treat a minor burn at home, but have a doctor tend to any serious or extensive burns.

Aromatherapy remedies: The first step after you are burned is to quickly immerse the area in a cold water bath that contains skin-healing essential oils. (If that's not possible, at least hold the burned area under cold water.) Follow this with any of the numerous natural burn remedies that contain aloe vera and the essential oils of lavender, chamomile, geranium, or neroli (orange blossom) to reduce inflammation, pain, and the possibility of infection. These essential oils also speed new cell growth and healing. Convenient if you have a sunburn, these same oils cool down your body if you feel overheated. You probably won't find a burn remedy containing helichrysum or rose oils because they're quite expensive, but both of these essential oils have similar properties. Tiny amounts of peppermint also relieve the pain. A burn remedy in a spray bottle is handy so that you don't have to touch the painful area. For an extra tip, keep the bottle or tube in refrigerator to provide extra cold relief on a burn.

Aromatherapy formula: *For a cold water burn bath:* Plunge the burn into a basin that contains 5 drops chamomile oil or 8 drops lavender oil for every cup of very cold water. (If ice cubes are available, use them to chill the water.) *To make a homemade burn remedy:* Add ¼ teaspoon (25 drops) lavender oil, 2 drops peppermint oil, and 1 teaspoon vitamin E oil to 2 ounces aloe vera juice. Shake well before using and apply as often as needed.

Healthy habits: To keep from getting sunburned in the first place, apply a good sunscreen. Try to find one that contains less of the chemical cocktail found in the average drugstore brands. For two weeks before your next tropical vacation or summer outing, you can take a daily dose of 500 units of vitamins C and 200 units of vitamin E. Evidence suggests that these vitamins reduce the likelihood of a burn.

Candida

Medical description: Candida is a yeastlike fungus that occurs naturally in most people's digestive tract. However, it can multiply so much that you end up with gas, indigestion, fatigue, and feelings of fuzzy-headedness. It's the same fungus that is responsible for thrush, a patchy white infection inside your mouth, and for the vaginal yeast infections many women experience. Candida can also grows under your nails, making them cracked and discolored. It's especially prevalent after taking antibiotics, which encourage it to multiply. If the problem isn't clearing up within a week, consult a health practitioner.

Aromatherapy remedies: The essential oils of chamomile, lavender, bergamot, tea tree, and thyme inhibit about 70 percent of candida growth in lab experiments. Studies also show clove, cinnamon, lavender, eucalyptus, lemongrass, lemon verbena, and garlic oils likewise slow its growth. So does thyme oil, although the gentle variety called geraniol is more effective than regular thyme oil, which easily burns sensitive skin. Look for a mouthwash, nail soak, or douche formula that includes some of these oils. For a vaginal yeast infection, douching is very effective, but has met with recent criticism because some gynecologists fear it upsets the normal vaginal balance and may spread infection into the uterus. If you douche, suspend the bag no higher than shoulder level so that the flow of water isn't too strong. As an alternative, you can buy tea tree suppositories at natural-food stores.

Aromatherapy formula: *To make a candida remedy:* To 1 ounce black walnut husk tincture, add 5 drops lavender oil and 8 drops tea tree oil. Shake very well before using and take 30 drops internally twice a day. (Studies show that black walnut husk destroys candida better than a commonly prescribed antifungal drug.) You can also swab this formula directly on thrush a couple times a day. *To treat nail fungus:* Add 12 drops tea tree oil to 2 tablespoons castor oil. Soak your nails in this solution for 5 to 15 minutes a day. *To prepare an aromatherapy douche:* Add 3 drops each of lavender and tea tree oils to 3 cups warm water. (You can also add 2 tablespoons yogurt to restore the vagina's natural flora and 1 tablespoon vinegar to restore acidic enironment.) Mix well, put in a douche bag, and use once a day.

Healthy habits: Avoid sweets in your diet because they feed candida and lower your resistance to prevent it extensive growth. Build up your resistance to candida with immune herbs such as pau d'arco and echinacea. If you keep getting vaginal infections, avoid sweets and clothes that prevent air circulation, such as tight pants and leg tights.

Canker sores

Medical description: Canker sores are tiny, but painful, ulcerations with white patches that occur in your mouth. They make the inside of your mouth red and swollen. You can get them when your defenses are down from emotional or physical stress, or if you have a poor diet, an infection, or a chronic disease. Sometimes the use of antibiotics brings them on. These sores generally take a couple weeks to heal. If they remain longer than that, see your doctor as they may be something more serious.

Aromatherapy remedies: Use one of the natural mouth washes that contains tea tree oil, or the more tasty fennel, chamomile, sage, or peppermint oils, to promote healing and discourage further infection.

Aromatherapy formula: *For a home-made mouth wash:* Combine 3 drops tea tree, 2 drops fennel, and 1 drop peppermint oils in ½ cup warm water. Stir well and slosh around the mouth for a few minutes before spitting out. (If there's any left over, it will keep in the refrigerator for a couple days.) Once a day, you can also put a drop of tea tree oil on your toothbrush before adding the toothpaste.

Healthy habits: Try to avoid stress and eat a good diet that includes plenty of foods that are high in B vitamins and vitamin C or take these supplements. Avoid drinking coffee and alcohol and eating foods that are high in acid, such as tomatoes and oranges, because all of these irritate the sores. If you keep getting canker sores, build up your immune system with herbs.

Carpal tunnel syndrome and repetitive strain injury

Medical description: You can get a repetitive strain injury from doing lots of the same work that repeatedly uses the same movement. Carpal tunnel is an example. In this case, the meridian nerve in your wrist (which runs through a narrow opening called the carpal tunnel) can become compressed from an activity such as typing, massage, or hammering. This makes your wrist feel numb with sharp, shooting pain so that it's difficult or impossible to use it.

Aromatherapy remedies: Look for a product that contains lavender, rosemary, and/or marjoram oils that you can rub over the injured area to ease the inflammation and pain. Although not proven, I've observed that these oils also seem to help to heal damaged nerves. I also think that these same essential oils help to prevent you from developing the strain in the first place.

Aromatherapy formula: *To make your own remedy:* Combine 15 drops lavender oil, 5 drops marjoram oil, and 4 drops rosemary oil with 1 ounce St. John's wort tincture. (It counters inflammation and nerve damage and is sold in natural-food stores.) If you prefer a remedy with an oily base, use St. John's wort oil instead of the tincture.

Healthy habits: Massage, chiropractic treatments, and stretching exercises all help to ease a repetitive stain injury and to discourage its return. Also take herbal nerve tonics such as St. John's wort flower/leaf and scullcap leaf tinctures or pills internally. To treat or to prevent the problem, take a break once in awhile from any repetitive work to stretch out and exercise the strained area.

Cholesterol, high

Medical description: Cholesterol is a type of fat that is measured in your blood. When excessive amounts build up inside your arteries, it can cause you to have heart and circulation problems. Eating a high fat diet is only part of the cause because there are cultures that eat plenty of cholesterol, yet the people don't develop this condition. Stress may be one of the culprits.

Aromatherapy remedies: The essential oils in onion, garlic, cayenne, rosemary leaf, fenugreek seed, and ginger root reduce high cholesterol, but it's best to eat all of these as foods rather than using them as pure essential oils. You only need to eat three onions or five cloves of garlic a week for results. If you find garlic good for your heart, but not your social life, try garlic capsules. Lavender helps normalize cholesterol and can be used in a massage oil. Although the amount that any massage oil directly lowers cholesterol is questionable, it certainly will decrease stress. Cayenne and ginger essential oils help your body break down cholesterol into bile acids, which is an important step in eliminating cholesterol. (The best way to utilize these oils is to season your food with the spices cayenne and ginger rather than using the pure essential oil.)

Aromatherapy formula: *To make a cholesterol-lowering massage oil:* Add 8 drops lavender oil, 3 drops ginger oil, and 2 drops rosemary oil in 2 ounces vegetable oil.

Healthy habits: Eat a balanced diet of vegetables and grains that includes onion, garlic, cayenne, rosemary, fenugreek seed, and ginger root. Also get plenty of exercise and, just in case stress does contribute to cholesterol, take the advice of the section in this chapter on stress.

Circulation, poor

Medical description: If you tend to have cold hands and feet, you may have poor blood circulation. Because poor circulation is a symptom of some other disorder — often low blood pressure (which I also cover in this guide) — look for the source of your problem and treat it as well. It can signal a serious condition, so get a doctor's evaluation. If you have the circulation disorder called Raynaud's disease, the small blood vessels, particularly those in your hands and feet, are so sensitive that they go into spasm. This decreases the flow of blood to these areas and can eventually lead to the damage of your cells, including nerves. Also look at the suggestions that I give for nerve damage caused by repetitive strain injury.

Aromatherapy remedies: Plenty of essential oils can get your blood moving. These include eucalyptus, ginger, lemongrass, juniper, cypress, rosemary, fennel, and geranium oils. Chamomile, frankincense, bergamot, grapefruit, lemon, and cedarwood oils are also fairly effective and also help the integrity of the blood vessels themselves, and frankincense also improves blood circulation. All these oils decrease swelling and bloating. One of the best ways to encourage circulation is to combine aromatherapy with *hydrotherapy,* which is the therapeutic use of water (*hydro* means water). Alternating between hot and cold water is a way to increase circulation. (If you have Raynaud's syndrome, you may need to stick to only hot water because cold water can lead to spasms.) Essential oils that increase circulation can be incorporated into a massage oil. You can also drink a tea made from ginger, lemongrass, rosemary, fennel, or geranium. (The hot water pulls the essential oils from the plants).

Aromatherapy formula: *To do a hand or foot bath:* Stir 2 drops each ginger, rosemary, cypress, and juniper oils into a basin or pan of hot water and soak your hands or feet for at least five minutes. To increase circulation and water elimination even more, also have a pan or basin of cold water and go back and forth several times between the hot and cold. *To make a circulation oil:* Combine 8 drops lemon, 3 drops rosemary, 3 drops geranium, and 2 drops cypress oils in 1 ounce vegetable oil or a skin lotion and rub on your hands, feet, back of neck, or legs. *To make a tea:* Take 2 teaspoons total of your choice of these herbs and cover them with 2 cups boiling water to steep 5 to 10 minutes. Then strain the herbs and drink.

Healthy habits: Exercise to improve your circulation and eat a good diet that includes lots of vitamin E and vitamin C with bioflavonoids. Take supplements to improve the integrity of your blood vessel walls, such as the anthrocyanidins found in bilberry, blueberry or proanthrocyanidins from pine bark and grape seeds.

Cellulite and fat

Medical description: Cellulite is just fat, but what gives it a distinction from just any fat is the lumpy, orange peel texture of the skin that covers it. Really a fancy word for puckered fat, it occurs in women more that men and most often in the thighs and buttocks. The likelihood of having it depends on the number of fat cells you have (although thin people do develop it), how good your circulation is, and if it runs in your family. Hormones may also play a role.

Aromatherapy remedies: You can find cellulite massage and body oils. Essential oils to look for in them are geranium and fennel, which both help balance your hormones. Along with grapefruit, these oils have traditionally been used to facilitate weight loss, and I suspect that they increase metabolism to help with weight loss. Even their scent conveniently encourages you to eat less. (Believe it or not, another fragrance that isn't available as an aromatherapy oil but that research found helps along these lines is chocolate. So, you can sniff a chocolate bar, but you'll need iron willpower to keep from putting *it* in your mouth!) Use the scent of bergamot if you have trouble with compulsive eating. Cypress and juniper are good adjuncts because they stimulate your circulation and ease fluid retention, problems that are often associated with cellulite. There are quite a few aromatherapy products to treat cellulite available.

Aromatherapy formula: *To make a massage or bath oil:* Add 5 drops each cypress, geranium, grapefruit, bergamot oils and 2 drops each juniper and fennel oils in 2 ounces vegetable oil. You can add the same proportion of essential oils to 2 ounces body lotion. The concentration of the resulting oil or lotion is too strong to use as a total massage, but you can rub it directly on cellulite areas once a day, if possible. (I'd also better warn you ahead of time that this is one of the few formulas in this book that doesn't smell too good. I find that people who want to work on their cellulite usually don't care a bit.) *In your bath:* Add 2 tablespoons of this blend to the water.

Healthy habits: A deep, rolling massage on the cellulite area (with an aromatherapy oil, of course!) seems to stimulate fat reduction. If you're trying to lose fat, aromatherapy is much more effective when you combine it with a total weight-loss plan. Restrict your dietary fat and, most important, get plenty of exercise that focuses on that area. For hips and legs, that means fast walking, bicycling, swimming, tennis, or any activity that works your legs.

Colds/sinus infection

Medical description: Colds and sinus congestion go hand in hand because a cold virus is the most common type of sinus infection. The symptoms include inflamed and congested sinuses and a runny nose, which makes it uncomfortable for you to breath. Smoking cigarettes, irritation from environmental sources, and some medications can also make your nose stuffy.

Aromatherapy remedies: Eucalyptus, lavender, tea tree, lemon, thyme, marjoram, rosemary, basil, and peppermint oils inhibit a cold virus. These same oils also clear your sinuses by relieving inflammation and congestion. In addition, they fight the bacterial infection that often follow a cold (as well as staph, strep, and pneumonia infections). Plus, if your cold makes you feel down in the dumps, the scents of lavender, lemon, and marjoram lift your spirits. Peppermint, ginger, anise, and chamomile stop inflammation by slowing the release of the body's *histamine* (which causes allergic-related inflammation). Use an aromatherapy steam to carry the therapeutic oils into your sinuses where it can counter the infection and inflammation. (The steam alone makes it easier for you to breath when you're congested.) When steaming is impractical, get a nasal inhaler that contains some of these same essential oils. Eating hot herbs that contain essential oils, such as cayenne, horseradish, garlic, and onions, drains your sinuses and can even stop a cold in its tracks if you catch it soon enough.

Aromatherapy formula: *To prepare a steam:* Put 5 drops eucalyptus oil (or another of the oils listed) in 3 cups simmering water. Turn off the heat, place your face over the steam, and drape a towel over the back of your head to collect the steam in a mini-sauna. Take deep breaths through your nose, coming out for fresh air as needed at about 2 minute intervals. Repeat this for at least three rounds. If possible, do this routine a few times a day. *As an alternative method:* You can steep 2 tablespoons of these same herbs (fresh or dried) in 3 cups simmering water for a few minutes so that the heat releases their essential oils and the steam carries it up into the air. You can also take a hot, steamy bath that has 3 drops each eucalyptus and lavender oils and 2 drops ginger oil. *For a nasal inhaler:* Combine 5 drops eucalyptus (or other) oil and ¼ teaspoon coarse salt in a small glass vial that has a tight lid. (Salt absorbs the oil and is convenient to carry without danger of spilling it.) Throughout the day, open the vial and inhale the scent.

Healthy habits: Treat sinus infection with goldenseal root (buy only cultivated roots, please, because the wild plant is endangered), the Chinese herb coptis, yarrow flowers, and/or elder flowers. A hot tea or elder flower, peppermint leaf, and yarrow flower help clear your sinuses (and also lower a fever). Get extra rest because sleep, along with herbs like echinacea root and baptisia root, amp up your immune system so that you get well sooner. Take extra of the anti-infection vitamins A and C and zinc supplements.

Coughs, sore throat, and laryngitis

Medical description: You typically get a sore throat — an inflammation of your throat — if you have a cold, have a cough, smoke, strain your voice, or are exposed to air pollution or some other type of irritation. If you have a persistent cough and can't figure out why, have your doctor check it.

Aromatherapy remedies: Anise, eucalyptus, tea tree, fennel, myrrh, ginger, peppermint, and thyme oils are ingredients in all sorts of cough drops, syrups, gargles, and sprays for sore throats. They make these products tasty, but more importantly, they stop coughing, possibly by suppressing the brain's cough reflex. Along with sage, hyssop (use the variety called decumbens), thyme, and marjoram oils all relieve laryngitis and tonsillitis. You can follow the example of European singers who traditionally preserve their voices by drinking marjoram or sage tea sweetened with a little honey! (The tea pulls the essential oils from the herb into the water.) I give a lot of weekend seminars, and I find that a steam of lavender, tea tree, or eucalyptus particularly good to keep my throat from being strained and to fend off laryngitis. (See the directions for making steams under Sinus congestion.) Other germ-fighting and soothing essential oils to treat a sore throat are cardamom, clary sage, benzoin, rose, rosemary, sandalwood, and bergamot.

Aromatherapy formula: *To make a gargle:* Add 3 drops tea tree oil (or your choice of another of the above oils) to ¼ cup cold water or apple cider vinegar with ¼ teaspoon salt dissolved in it. Several times a day, gargle with this solution and then spit it out. Or, make a strong tea by pouring a cup of boiling water over a teaspoon each of marjoram and sage herbs, let this steep about 5 minutes in a covered pan, and then strain out the herbs. Add ½ teaspoon salt. When the salt is dissolved, gargle with this solution. If your neck is stiff or the lymph that run along it are swollen, make a neck wrap: Add 8 drops ginger oil to about 1 cup hot water. Soak a soft cloth, preferably soft, absorbent flannel, in the water. Then wring it out and wrap it completely around your neck. To keep in the warmth, wrap a thin towel or a flaxseed neck pillow (available in stores) that has been warmed in the microwave oven around this. Remove the wrap before it cools. Repeat this treatment as many times as needed to ease the discomfort.

Healthy habits: Herbal cough syrups that contain herbs such as marshmallow root and horehound leaf are excellent. Commercial versions usually also contain some essential oils. Eat garlic to obtain the essential oils that counter infection. Don't overdo talking until your throat fully recovers. Meanwhile, to regenerate your immune system, get extra sleep, take it easy, and take immune stimulating herbs like goldenseal (buy cultivated only because the wild roots are quite rare).

Cuts

Medical description: Broken skin is usually the result of injuring your skin or having a skin disorder in which the skin breaks open. Get medical treatment if you get a serious wound.

Aromatherapy remedies: Treat superficial cuts and scrapes with a spray or salve that contains antiseptic and wound-healing essential oils, such as eucalyptus, lavender, lemon, thyme, marjoram, rosemary, tea tree and/or basil. Numerous salves that contain antiseptic and skin-healing essential oils to use on cuts are available along with a few liquid preparations. A spray container is a convenient way to spritz antiseptic essential oils on a cut. In fact, spraying eucalyptus or lemon oils through the air increases their antiseptic properties as the oils combine with oxygen. The germ-fighting abilities of tea tree oil also improves when it's in the presence of blood or the pus from an infection. Use the same highly antiseptic essential oils to treat an infected wound. Surround the infected wound with a diluted antiseptic oil, applying it directly to the reddened area around the wound. When dealing with a deep or dirty cut, first thoroughly clean the wound with hydrogen peroxide to counter any initial infection before applying the aromatherapy antiseptic.

Aromatherapy formula: *To make an antiseptic spray:* Add 12 drops tea tree oil and 6 drops lemon oil to ½ ounce distilled water and ½ ounce vinegar (which is also antiseptic) and put in a spray bottle. (For extra action, use an herb vinegar such as oregano, garlic, or calendula.) Shake well to disperse the oils before spraying it on minor cuts, burns, and abrasions to prevent infection. *For a direct application:* Dilute 15 drops of tea tree for every 1 tablespoon vegetable oil or vodka (which is simply a combination of alcohol and water) and rub it all around the outside perimeter of the wound, but not directly in an open wound.

Healthy habits: Keeping in good general health reduces your risk of developing a serious infection.

Dandruff

Medical description: This scalp condition is characterized by flaking skin on your scalp that often causes itching. If you have dry skin in general, you're more likely to also have dandruff. Like dry skin, your dandruff may be associated with a food allergy.

Aromatherapy remedies: Look for a hair conditioner that contains geranium, lavender, clary sage, and bergamot oil and especially rosemary, sandalwood and/or tea tree oils. Cedar, juniper, and patchouli oils are good additions if your dandruff is a result of an overly oily scalp. If your flakes are due to a dry scalp, chamomile, myrrh, and sandalwood are good. Also see the essential oils that are suggested for Dry Skin and Oily Skin in this guide for more ideas and general hair information in Chapter 7. Once a day, you can dab a couple drops of rosemary or sandalwood oil on your fingertips and massage your head or put a couple drops on your comb before combing your hair.

Aromatherapy formula: *For a quick, homemade hair rinse:* Combine 4 drops rosemary oil, 4 drops lavender oil, 2 drops tea tree oil, ⅓ cup vinegar, and ⅔ cup water. Shake this mixture well before using it to rinse your hair. Vinegar in itself is an excellent hair rinse. You can rinse it out in a few minutes, but it's even better to leave it on. (Don't worry; I promise that the smell of vinegar will dissipate within a few minutes after applying this rinse.) *For another hair rinse technique:* Use superstrong rosemary tea. (The hot water draws out the rosemary's essential oils.) Prepare the tea by pouring 2 cups boiling water over 3 teaspoons rosemary leaves (dried or fresh). Steep for 10 minutes and then strain. Add ⅓ cup vinegar and use to rinse your hair. Keep any leftover rinse in the refrigerator.

Healthy habits: Drink plenty of water, make sure that you're getting an adequate amount of vitamin C, and include flaxseed in your diet and/or take evening primrose oil capsules. Also avoid fried foods — and that includes fried health food corn and potato chips. If food allergies or digestive problems plague you, then also see my suggestions for those problems.

Depression/anxiety

Medical description: Depression is a mental state in which you feel emotions that can range from chronic sadness to despair. It often makes you unable to feel joy. Anxiety is another emotional condition that is closely related to depression. Unjustified fear, insomnia, and difficulty concentrating can accompany either problem. Physical imbalances in brain chemistry is most often the cause, so you may need professional advice to help you deal with it.

Aromatherapy remedies: The citrus scents of orange, bergamot, lemon, lemon verbena, melissa (lemon balm), petitgrain, and neroli (orange blossom) oils act as antidepressants. So does the fragrance of chamomile, and to some degree, that of rose, lavender, and angelica oils. The scent of orange, according to research, and of fir and juniper reduces anxiety. In India, basil's fragrance is used to prevent agitation and nightmares. In addition, aromatherapists find that the scents of cedarwood, cypress, clary sage, marjoram, and geranium oils ease emotional upset caused by feelings of apprehension, loneliness, or rejection. I find that any of these oils also help anyone undergoing a major life transition. If you get heart palpitations and chest pains or dizziness along with your anxiety attack, also use a relaxing scent. Ylang ylang, sandalwood, frankincense, and marjoram are particularly effective. Look at the fragrances that I mention under Stress for more ideas. Choose any aromatherapy method described in Chapter 5, such as a light bulb ring, potpourri, or an aromatherapy diffuser, to dispense these scents into the air. If you're on the go a lot, carry them with you in an aromatherapy inhaler (easy to purchase) or as smelling salts that you make yourself. If you are already taking antidepressive or anti-anxiety drugs, it's safe to use aromatherapy with them.

Aromatherapy formula: *To make antidepressive or anti-anxiety smelling salts:* Add 3 drops bergamot oil, 2 drops geranium oil, and 1 drop neroli oil (orange blossom), or 3 drops petitgrain oil, to 1 tablespoon rock or other coarse salt. Carry in a closed container and sniff as needed. *To make massage oil:* Add the same essential oils (in the same amount) to 4 ounces vegetable oil. If you can't get a massage, then add a couple teaspoons of this massage oil to your bath water and enjoy!

Healthy habits: Aromatherapy helps you deal with depression and anxiety, but for a permanent solution, seek a more complete and holistic approach. Relaxation techniques, counseling, a wholesome diet, and exercise are all good ideas. Herbal antidepressants, such as a tincture or pills of St. John's wort leaf/flower, help ease some kinds of depression. (Have a knowledgeable health professional help you select antidepressive herbs if you're already on medication to treat depression.)

Dermatitis, psoriasis, and eczema

Medical description: If you suffer from any of these skin conditions, your skin may be inflamed, red, itchy, and flaky, develop unsightly skin lesions that ooze, and then crust over. Secondary skin infections can occur if your skin is rough or broken. The cause is not completely understood, but if you're under stress, allergies and exposure to environmental toxins worsen and can even cause the problem.

Aromatherapy remedies: Turn to products containing skin-healing and anti-inflammatory essential oils that also kill any bacterial or fungal infections to treat a wide range of skin problems. Lavender, chamomile, tea tree, melissa (lemon balm), neroli (orange blossom), and spikenard oils all fit the bill. If you can't find a herbal salve that contains these essential oils, then add essential oils to a store-bought salve following the recipe in the next paragraph. Use your salve directly on your skin condition a few times a day. If you also have dry skin, which is often associated with these skin conditions, look at my suggestions under that heading. For healthy skin care, also see Chapter 7.

Aromatherapy formula: *To custommake a dermatitis salve:* Using a toothpick, stir 10 drops tea tree oil, 8 drops lavender oil, and 5 drops chamomile oils into a ready-made 2-ounce jar of skin salve. (A salve containing calendula and comfrey is a good choice.) *For a more intensive skin treatment:* Stir in

¼ teaspoon each tinctures of pau d'arco bark and goldenseal root (or barberry bark). This makes the salve semi-liquid but still easy to apply.

Healthy habits: Follow the advice of herbalists and some progressive dermatologists and clear up your skin condition by improving the functioning of your liver — the primary organ of detoxification. Your liver also helps keep your hormones in balance. Other herbs that aid your liver and that are especially good for skin conditions are burdock root, Oregon grape root, red clover flower, milk thistle seed, and yellow dock root. Take them as a tea or in pills. You can cook burdock as a vegetable. (It's sold fresh in Oriental markets and some natural-food stores; treat it like a carrot.) Or you can grind up milk thistle seeds and sprinkle them on your food. Taking supplements of evening primrose oil often helps. Eat wholesome meals that do not include fried food and refer to the section on using aromatherapy for Stress control. If you have psoriasis, exposure to the sun and to heat in general are two nontoxic ways to treat it.

Diaper rash

Medical description: Skin irritation from diapers chafing baby's delicate skin causes a rash, reddening, and inflammation. Moisture from wet diapers makes it worse.

Aromatherapy remedies: Using a baby powder and an herbal salve with every diaper change protects your baby from diaper rash by absorbing moisture and preventing chafing. Better yet, select a baby powder that contains essential oils that reduce inflammation, soothe irritated skin, and promote skin healing. Two gentle essential oils that do this are lavender and chamomile. Baby powder that is made with white (or China) clay, cornstarch, or arrowroot powder is much better than talc, which is

sometimes contaminated with harmful substances like asbestos. Be sure to choose a diaper salve that is made with vegetable oil rather than mineral (petroleum) oil.

Aromatherapy formula: *To make your own baby powder:* Put ½ pound cornstarch (sold in grocery stores) in a plastic bag and add 25 drops lavender oil, drop by drop. Distribute the drops throughout the starch. (It clumps if you pour it all in one spot). Seal the bag, breaking up any clumps with your fingers on the outside of the sealed bag. Let it stand for four days to evenly distribute the scent. Spice or salt shakers with large perforation holes in their lid make handy containers for your powder.

Healthy habits: Keep wet diapers changed and try to give your baby some diaperfree time. An herbal salve designed for babies — available at any natural-food store — further protects baby's skin from moisture and chafing.

Dry skin

Medical description: Dry skin is obviously dry, containing very little water. It doesn't have any luster and chafes and peels easily.

Aromatherapy remedies: Increase your skin's oil production and rejuvenate it by encouraging the growth of new cells with a cream that contains essential oils such as lavender, geranium, neroli (orange blossom), rosemary, sandalwood, chamomile, jasmine, and rose. Less common essential oils that you may encounter in dry skin creams are spikenard, carrot seed, and vetivert. Lavender, chamomile, geranium, jasmine, rose, and carrot seed are especially good on skin that is mature or very sensitive or cracked. Tea tree or the variety of thyme called geraniol (which is much less harsh on skin than regular thyme) make good additions to dry skin products if you're prone to any type of skin infection. A small amount of peppermint activates your skin's glands to produce more oil. Avoid the use of bar or liquid soaps, which are very drying and can irritate dry skin, except when you're really dirty. Otherwise, wash with a soap substitute such as powdered oatmeal tied in a loose-weave cotton bag. Also read about dry skin care in Chapter 7.

Aromatherapy formula: *To make a skin moisturizer:* Put 6 drops geranium, 4 drops sandalwood, 1 drop chamomile, and 1 drop jasmine or rose oil (expensive so these are optional), 2 ounces aloe vera gel, 2 ounces orange blossom water, and 800 IUs vitamin E oil (use liquid E oil or pop open a couple of 400 IU vitamin E capsules) in a blender and mix. If you don't object to its smell, 1 teaspoon vinegar helps retain skin health by maintaining natural acidity. Shake before each use and apply as a daily dry-skin conditioner. *To make a soap substitute:* Add the same amount of essential oils to ¼ cup powdered oatmeal. (Powdered oatmeal can be achieved by putting oatmeal in your blender or coffee grinder.) Place in a piece of loose-weave cotton fabric that is about 8 inches square and tie the ends to make a bag. Use this in place of bar soap at the sink or in the tub or shower. It usually lasts for a couple washings. Then empty the bag and replace it with a new mixture.

Healthy habits: Drink water and be sure to get plenty of vitamin C in your diet or to take supplements. Also, eat vegetable oils like olive oil that are rich in essential fatty acids and avoid fried foods, which interfere with your body's oil metabolism. For excessively dry skin, try taking supplements of evening primrose capsules.

Ear infection

Medical description: A bacterial or fungal infection in the ear causes inflammation that can be very painful. Simple ear infections of the external ear canal can be self-treated, but infections in the middle ear need a doctor's care. Don't hesitate to see your doctor if you're unsure of the source of your infection because it can eventually damage your eardrum and lead to other, more serious consequences.

Aromatherapy remedies: To treat an infection in your ears, massage antiseptic oils that relieve inflammation and pain, such as lavender, tee tree, garlic and chamomile oils around the outside of your ear. You can find a selection of herbal ear oils available in natural-food stores, some of which contain essential oils. A few drops of garlic-mullein flower oil several times a day often takes care of an ear problem. Never drop an essential oil directly into your ear, although you can put one drop on a piece of cotton and place this in your ear. If your eardrum is injured, see your doctor. Always treat both of your ears, even if only one hurts, because when one ear is infected, it's likely the other is on it's way. Continue the treatment several days after your pain disappears to make sure that the condition doesn't return. If your ear problem began with a throat infection, also use the antiseptic gargle that I describe under Sore throat.

Aromatherapy formula: *For an ear oil:* Add 8 drops each lavender and tea tree oils to ½ ounce olive oil. Rub a little of this oil around the outside of your ear and down the side of your neck. If your child comes down with an ear infection, use the same formula, but half the amount of essential oils (4 drops each) and remember to use this around, not in her ear. For baby and toddlers, use an even milder blend of 2 drops of each oil in ½ ounce olive oil.

Healthy habits: If you get ear problems often, you may have a food allergy. Many foods cause allergies, and dairy and wheat seem to be the predominate culprits in ear infections. Immune herbs help fend off allergic reactions, so see the section on Immunity for more suggestions.

Eyes inflammation/strain

Medical description: If your eyes are red, swollen, and sore from eye strain or lack of sleep, aromatherapy remedies can help. See a doctor if your eye problem continues for more than a few days, your eyes start oozing, your vision is affected, or they're very painful. Also get checked if you have an eye infection.

Aromatherapy remedies: Sties, eye inflammations, and strained eyes respond well to placing a compress over your eyes. Lavender or chamomile are good choices because both ease inflammation and sore muscles, and they smell great! Don't ever put essential oils in your eyes, even when they're diluted. However, hydrosols of rose and other gentle herbs are okay if they're pure and are not contaminated with bacteria — unfortunately, these are two things that you can't always be sure about.

Aromatherapy formula: *To make an eye compress:* Put 4 drops lavender oil in about a cup of water and slosh a soft cloth around in it. (Use cool or hot water depending upon which feels best to you. Swollen eyes usually respond better to cold because it reduces inflammation. Hot often feels better if you have eye strain.) Wring out the cloth and place it over your closed eyes and leave on this compress at least three minutes. *Another compress method:* Use herbs instead of essential oils by first preparing a strong tea of chamomile or lavender. Pour boiling water over 2 heaping teaspoons of the herbs and steep for five minutes. Strain out the herbs and soak the cloth in the tea. *For a quick compress:* While you're traveling or at work, steep two tea bags of chamomile or regular black tea for a few minutes in hot water. Then squeeze the excess water from the bag and place a tea bag over both of your closed eyes. If convenient, also put a small, folded cloth over the tea bags to hold them in place and block out any light. Keep the mini-compress on for at least three minutes.

Healthy habits: Your eyes use many different muscles. Just like other muscles in your body, they benefit from slow, relaxing exercises. Close your eyes and move them up and down several times, then side to side, and draw a box, a circle, and diagonals with your eyes moving them one way and then the next. If you do much close work with your eyes — say, you stare at a computer screen all day — be sure to look away now and then at an object in the distance. If you're stuck in a cubicle, at least pretend to look out to the horizon. Supplements that increase blood circulation and increase the oxygen flow to your eyes include vitamin E and anthrocyanidins and proanthrocyanidins, which are derived from herbs like bilberries, grape seed, and pine bark. Also, eat carrots and other foods that are rich in betacarotene or take supplements of this precursor to vitamin A.

Fatigue

Medical description: Whatever causes your chronic tiredness, remember that it's just a symptom of another disorder. Try to determine its source and treat that. A few of the many causes of fatigue are chronic illness, depression, chronic fatigue syndrome, infection, allergies, immune system impairment, or simply burning the candle at both ends. Adrenal insufficiency can develop if you're subjected to long-term stress. After a while, you become fatigued and find that you no longer respond quickly to crisis or joy.

Aromatherapy remedies: The sharp scents of eucalyptus, cypress, pine, and rosemary oils and the spicy scents of clove, basil, black pepper, cinnamon, and ginger oils all pep you up and reduce drowsiness, irritability, and headaches. To a lesser degree, the aromas of orange, bergamot, patchouli, and sage are also stimulating. Sniffing any of these scents helps counter fatigue that involves muscle weakness, such as chronic fatigue syndrome, but specific oils for this condition are ginger, and a cultivar of rosemary oil called cineole. Sniff these oils or, better yet, incorporate them into a muscle massage oil. Other oils for chronic fatigue are those that have a combination of both stimulating and focusing effects, such as lavender, petitgrain, and lemon eucalyptus. A nice thing about aromatherapy stimulants is that they don't over-amp your adrenal glands and then leave them flat the way coffee, cola, and black tea can. In fact, these oils counter an adrenaline rush and prevent the sharp drop in attention that typically occurs after working about 30 minutes. Some even offer specific treatments for adrenal problems. Along with other aromatherapists, I suggest that you use the scents of clary sage, spruce, and pine (particularly the species of pine called *sylvestris*) to help counter adrenal insufficiency in massage and body oils. When you're trying to stay awake, sniff your choice of these aromas every five minutes or so. Use your choice of the methods that I describe in Chapter 4 to fill your room with scent, such as a few drops of essential oil in a diffuser, on a light bulb ring, or in steaming water. Or, use a commercial aromatherapy inhaler or smelling salts or carry a sprig of the herb itself when you're on the run.

Aromatherapy formula: *A good anti-fatigue combination:* Combine 6 drops bergamot oil, 4 drops lemon oil, 2 drops eucalyptus oil, 1 drop cinnamon oil, and 2 drops peppermint oil (and 1 drop cardamom oil, if you have it). Use this in one of the many methods I mention in Chapter 4 or add it to 2 ounces vegetable oil to create a massage or body oil. You can also add the same blend of essential oils to a hand or body lotion.

Healthy habits: For sustained energy throughout the day, eat well, get at least 20 minutes of aerobic exercise, and take Siberian ginseng root or ginseng root. Then get a good night's sleep. (If sleeping's a problem, then look at my suggestions under Insomnia.)

Fever

Medical description: A fever increases your body temperature so that it can burn off a viral or bacterial infection. Until a fever gets near a dangerous level of 104°F, do yourself a favor and let it cook (unless you're generally in poor health, very weak, or treating a baby or small child). Because a fever is only a symptom of something else, be sure to treat the problem directly. Many essential oils have antibacterial and antiviral properties. Lower a fever with a cold water wash that contains the essential oil of lavender.

Aromatherapy formula: *To make the fever wash:* Add 5 drops lavender oil to every cup of cold water and use this to wash off or sponge down the hands and feet or the entire body.

Healthy habits: Aromatherapy is only an adjunct treatment to lowering a fever. In addition to the wash, drink a hot cup of fever-lowering herbs. My favorite fever tea is an old standby: Equal parts of yarrow flower, peppermint leaf, and elder flower. Pour boiling water over the herbs, steep them for about five minutes, and then strain and drink. Also drink plenty of fluids, such as lemon water, natural ginger ale, or plain water to replace water lost when you sweat.

Fever blisters (cold sores)

Medical description: Cold sores are an infection that is caused by the herpes virus. It manifests as small, painful blisters around your mouth that inflame nerve endings. The virus stays dormant in your nervous system until it's triggered by stress, low immunity, or sunlight. These same suggestions work to treat genital herpes and another herpes infection, shingles.

Aromatherapy remedies: Several commercial herpes ointments, including a capsaicin cream, are sold in natural-food stores and drugstores. They generally contain the essential oils of tea tree, eucalyptus, or myrrh. These oils, along with geranium and lavender oils, are effective treatments (lemon eucalyptus is preferred over other types.) Studies on melissa (lemon balm) oil show that it's a deterrent to herpes, although it's also quite expensive and these other oils work fine. (Any tea tree will do, although the type called niaouli is especially effective.) Small amounts of peppermint oil or capsaicin, the hot essential oil compound in cayenne, may be included to deaden the nerve-tingling pain. Also see the general information on viral infections in Chapter 11.

Aromatherapy formula: *To make a cold sore remedy:* Add 20 drops (¼ teaspoon) tea tree oil, 10 drops myrrh oil, 10 drops geranium oil, and 4 drops peppermint oil to 1 teaspoon echinacea tincture. (If the tincture stings too much, then use an infused calendula oil instead.) Apply directly on blisters several times a day. This recipe contains a high percentage of essential oils, so apply it only to the blistering area. (If the alcohol stings too much, use ½ teaspoon vegetable oil of St. John's oil instead.)

Healthy habits: Increase your immunity with echinacea root and heal your nerves with St. John's wort leaf/flower. Both come in tinctures or pills. Also, take supplements of the amino acid lysine. Avoid nuts, especially peanuts, and other foods that are high in another amino acid called arginine, and citrus and other acidic foods that irritate the blisters. In addition, seek out ways, including aromatherapy, to reduce your emotional and physical stress levels.

Fibrocystic breasts

Medical description: Breast lumps or cysts that are nonmalignant lumps are common in women. They're associated with hormones, especially an overabundance of estrogen and associated hormonal compounds, but why they form in the first place is not completely understood. Make sure that you have the lump checked out by a doctor before self-diagnosing.

Aromatherapy remedies: To ease inflamed and painful breasts, use a compress made from chamomile, ginger, or lavender oils. Go easy on your use of cypress, angelica, and coriander oils, and especially anise, clary sage, fennel, sage, and anise oils because they have estrogenic properties. Actually, no one knows yet if any of these essential oils help or hinder the situation. (Estrogenic herbs, due to the complex way that plants work on your physiology, often are beneficial in conditions that are associated with too much estrogen.)

Aromatherapy formula: *To make the compress:* Add 4 drops lavender oil, 2 drops ginger oil, and 1 drop chamomile oil to 1 cup strong calendula tea. (Make the tea by pouring 1¼ cups boiling water over 2 teaspoons calendula flowers, steep about 10 minutes, and then strain.) Or, instead of using tea, add a teaspoon of calendula flower tincture (you can purchase this at a natural-food store) to the water. Soak a small, soft cloth in the solution. Wring the cloth out, fold it into several layers, and place it over your swollen breast. Run another cloth under cold water and wring out.

After 5 to 10 minutes, exchange the hot compress for the cold cloth, and leave it on about 2 minutes. Repeat this procedure several times a day if possible.

Healthy habits: Research shows that breast cysts disappear within three months in about 80 percent of the women who discontinue caffeine. Herbal formulas that contain vitex berry, which helps balance women's hormones, reduce the size of breast cysts. For more detailed herbal information on fibrocystic breasts, see my book *Women's Herbs, Women's Health* (Interweave Press).

Fluid retention

Medical description: Swelling from fluid buildup can occur just about anywhere in your body, but the most common location is your extremities — in your hands, feet, ankles, and legs. The problem is often twofold: The body isn't moving water out of your cells fast enough, and your kidneys are not eliminating enough of it. Retaining fluid is a symptom of some other disorder, such as high blood pressure, varicose veins, constipation, PMS, arthritis, kidney and heart disorders, and general *edema* (a fancy name for fluid retention). Seek your doctor's evaluation to make sure that you don't have a serious heart or kidney condition. Find the source of your problem so that you can treat it as well. (Then look it up in this guide for more of my treatment suggestions.) Many women also experience fluid retention in the last trimester of their pregnancy, although if you're pregnant, be sure that you read the safety precautions for pregnancy in Chapter 3.

Aromatherapy remedies: Quite a few essential oils reduce fluid retention, including grapefruit, lemon, lemongrass, juniper, cypress, rosemary, eucalyptus, fennel, sandalwood, and geranium oils. Chamomile, frankincense, and cedar wood oils are also fairly effective. All these essential oils encourage general circulation and the elimination of excess water through sweating and via your kidneys. They also decrease swelling and bloating. Carrot seed oil (although it smells rather strongly of carrot) also aids water elimination. Use these essential oils in a compress or massage oil that is used directly over the bloated area or in a full or foot bath. You can also ingest one or a combination of the herbs as a tea. (The hot water pulls the essential oils from the plants.)

Aromatherapy formula: *To make a massage oil:* Combine 5 drops grapefruit oil, 3 drops rosemary oil, 3 drops cypress oil, and 1 drop fennel oil in 1 ounce vegetable oil or a lotion. (Be forewarned that this is one of the few blends in this book that doesn't smell great.) *For a compress:* Use these same oils in about ½ cup hot water. Soak a soft cloth in the solution, wring it out, then fold it, and apply it over the area that you want to treat. To increase circulation and water elimination even more, alternate this cloth with one soaked in cold water and go back and forth several times. *Prepare a hand or foot bath:* If your hands, ankles, or feet swell, stir 2 drops each grapefruit, rosemary, cypress, and fennel oils into a basin or pan of hot water and soak your hands or feet in the water for at least five minutes. You can get immediate results if every couple minutes, you place your hands or feet in a cold water soak for about 30 seconds and then return them to the hot, scented water. *Make a tea:* Cover 1 teaspoon each fennel and chamomile with 2 cups boiling water and steep for 5 to 10 minutes. Then strain the herbs and drink.

Healthy habits: Limit the amount of salty foods that you eat so that you don't retain as much water. Eat foods that are high in potassium, such as bananas, to balance the sodium in salt and fresh vegetables that are natural diuretics, like asparagus. Also, exercise as much as you can and sit and stand as little as possible.

Forgetfulness

Medical description: If you have trouble with a poor memory, chances are that you have too little blood and therefore not enough oxygen reaching your brain. A common reason is hardening of the arteries due to aging, but other things can be responsible, such as continual stress, which affects brain chemistry so that you can't think properly.

Aromatherapy remedies: Sniffing spicy scents such as cinnamon, bay leaf, basil, pimento bay, clove, rosemary, and sage perk your memory. These same essential oils also stimulate blood circulation when used in a massage oil. Sniff the essential oil or the plant throughout the day whenever you need to remember something or use any of the aromatherapy techniques I describe in Chapter 5.

Aromatherapy formula: *For a nice-smelling blend:* Combine 10 drops lemon oil, 5 drops rosemary oil, 3 drops sage oil, and 1 drop cinnamon oil. If stress affects your memory, use these essential oils with the calming oils that I recommend under Stress.

Healthy habits: The herbs ginkgo leaf, gotu kola leaf, ginseng root, and Siberian ginseng root as a tincture or in pills improve your memory, especially if you're experiencing definite memory problems (rather than simply wanting to be smarter). Other things that help improve your thinking ability are to reduce stress, get enough sleep, and breathe deeply to assure that enough oxygen reaches your brain. As you get older, research shows that if you keep your mind active by learning new things, your brain capacity is less likely to decline. This is especially true if you learn a new language, or study music or math.

Gum problems

Medical description: The gum problem that you're most likely to face is an infection, which can lead to inflammation and bleeding, a problem known as gingivitis. Plaque buildup, smoking or chewing tobacco, a severe nutritional deficiency, and even overzealous tooth brushing can also cause this condition.

Aromatherapy remedies: Many of the toothpastes and mouthwashes sold in both natural-food stores and drugstores rely on essential oils such as myrrh, eucalyptus, peppermint, and thyme, which studies show fight bacteria and reduce the buildup of plaque on your teeth. Other oils that effectively reduce bleeding gums are sage and rosemary. Toothpicks and dental floss that are soaked in antiseptic tea tree oil are also available. Many of the sticks from various bushes and trees that are traditionally used throughout the world to clean the teeth contain essential oils that help to prevent gum disease.

Aromatherapy formula: If you'd rather make your own *herbal gum treatment:* Add 20 drops tea tree oil and 8 drops myrrh oil to 1 ounce tincture of echinacea root (sold in natural-food stores.) Shake very well and then put ¼ teaspoon of the solution in ⅛ cup water and swish in your mouth for at least one minute. Spit it out or swallow it. You can add a couple drops of this same mixture to your toothbrush before adding toothpaste and then brush your teeth as usual.

Healthy habits: Be diligent with your dental hygiene. Floss at least one a day and brush your gums for several minutes after every meal. Also, eat a wholesome diet, avoiding sweets.

Headache

Medical description: Your headache may be related to allergies, stress, and immune system imbalances. Vascular headaches such as migraines are caused by constrictive blood vessels in the head. If you get chronic headaches, get an examination by a medical doctor because they sometimes result from an injury, a tumor, or other serious disorders. Stress or a tight neck or shoulders increase the intensity of a headache.

Aromatherapy remedies: Inhale lavender or melissa (lemon balm) or a combination of peppermint and eucalyptus to reduce your headache. Studies show that it can also be effective to rub a balm made with these essential oils on your temples. Take a hot bath if it eases your headache pain. (Some people, especially if they have a migraine, find that heat only make it worse.) One way to stop a migraine is to place your hands in a basin of 110°F water with 5 drops of lavender oil. Relieve the pain of a cluster headache with capsaicin cream. It blocks a neurotransmitter called substance P (the P stands for pain) to stop the brain from registering pain impulses. However, it does need to be used four to five times a day for about a month to work. Other essential oils to sniff when you develop a headache are basil, chamomile, lemongrass, and marjoram. Bay, jasmine, and spikenard are examples of essential oils that heal a headache in small doses, but may cause one if you smell too much. Coriander and cumin are good if your headache is associated with indigestion. If problems such as insomnia, indigestion, or sinus congestion prompt your headache, then see the suggestions that I give under those headings.

Aromatherapy formula: *To make a headache compress:* Add 5 drops lavender oil to 1 cup cold water and swish a soft cloth in the solution. Wring out the cloth and place it over your forehead and eyes as often as you like. If it feels better, use hot water instead of the cold or alternate cold and hot water. If your headache is prompted by muscle or emotional stress, it often helps to place a second hot compress under your neck. (If you have a migraine headache, you probably prefer a cold compress, although it may be that the smell of any essential oil and the slight pressure of the compress is bothersome.) If you don't have time for a compress or it feels too uncomfortable, dab a small dot of lavender oil, eucalyptus oil, or peppermint oil on each temple instead.

Healthy habits: A tincture, tea, or pills of fresh feverfew leaves help migraine headaches, especially if taken on a regular basis rather than just when you feel the first pangs of a headache approaching. Ginkgo leaves, also as a tincture or pills, and ginger root in any form increase circulation to relieve migraine and other types of headaches. Valerian root or scullcap soothe muscle tension and pain in general. Be patient; some people need to take herbs regularly for several months before the intensity and frequency of their headaches diminish. If you suffer from migraines, stay away from cultured cheese, wine, sausage, pickles, nuts, chocolate, and caffeinated drinks like coffee and sodas. (A cocktail party sounds like a real bad idea.) If you're like most people with a headache, you can benefit from having your neck and shoulder, as well as your head, massaged.

Heartburn

Medical description: The heat and pain produced by heartburn may make you feel like you're experiencing a heart problem, but this complaint is actually caused by a spasm in the stomach or esophagus as gas and acid from your stomach move up the throat. Severe heartburn may be the result of a hiatal hernia, a condition in which the top of the stomach bulges into the diaphragm.

See your doctor to get a correct diagnosis of any chronic stomach pain before you embark on self-treatment.

Aromatherapy remedies: Chamomile, lemon, melissa (lemon balm), and fennel oils reduce stomach acid, inflammation, and infection and even help protect your stomach lining from its own acid. The best way to take them is as a tea made with your choice of these herbs. (The hot water draws the essential oils out of the herbs.) Fortunately, they're all quite tasty. Drink a cup with each meal. Rubbing a massage oil that contains these essential oils over the chest area also helps relieve this condition.

Aromatherapy formula: *To make a heartburn massage oil:* Combine 4 drops each chamomile, fennel seed, and lemon oils in 1 ounce vegetable oil and use daily. This oil will ease your symptoms, although not necessarily cure the problem.

Healthy habits: At mealtime, choose grains and steamed vegetables instead of fried, spicy, or high protein foods. Eat slowly, chew your food well, and try to stay relaxed while you eat. An herb tea that soothes heartburn discomfort include marshmallow root, licorice root, and wild yam root.

Hives

Medical description: Hives are rashlike skin bumps that itch like crazy. They often result from a food allergy.

Aromatherapy remedies: Use a skin wash, compress, or poultice to stop the itching, decrease inflammation and sensitivity, and to slow the allergic reaction. Good essential oils to choose are lavender and especially chamomile (it helps counter allergic reactions). A cool bath with essential oils and oats also helps relieve your itching.

Aromatherapy formula: *To make either remedy:* Start off by adding 10 drops chamomile oil, 3 drops peppermint oil, and 3 tablespoons baking soda to ½ cup cool water (or better yet, to cooled elder flower tea). *To make a compress:* Soak a soft cloth in this solution and wring out the excess water. Apply to irritated skin. Reapply every 10 minutes or so until itching is alleviated. *To make a poultice (paste):* Stir 3 to 4 tablespoons ground oats into the solution. Allow it to thicken for a few minutes and then apply the paste with your fingers or the back of a spoon directly on the hives. Leave the paste on the skin for at least 20 minutes before washing it off. This poultice is the most effective treatment, but if you want to avoid the mess, you can use the same liquid solution without the oats to rinse your skin. *For a bath:* Add 5 drops lavender oil and 2 drops peppermint oil and a cup of ground oatmeal to a cool bath water and soak in it. (Be sure to place a strainer over the tub drain to prevent the oatmeal from clogging the drain.)

Healthy habits: Look into why you get hives in the first place and try to resolve this to prevent them from reoccurring.

Immune system problems

Medical description: If you have allergies or come down with frequent infections, even colds or sinus trouble, it signals that you have a weakness in your immune system. Lymph nodes located in the throat, groin, breasts, under the arms, and in other areas of the body, act as filtering centers for cleansing the blood of waste residues that are produced by the body's metabolic functions or infection.

Aromatherapy remedies: Many antiseptic essential oils, such as lemon, myrrh, lavender, thyme, eucalyptus, and tea tree, also support your immune system. These same oils promote faster healing by encouraging new cell growth.

Some of the best essential oils to use are those that are also strong antivirals, such as tea tree, bay, and melissa (lemon balm). Low immune cell counts are corrected with eucalyptus, thyme, spike lavender. (The species of eucalyptus called dives, polybractea, and radiata are especially potent for the immune system. So are the linalol, thuyamol, and satureioides types of thyme.) Other good immune essential oils are myrtle, and peppermint. One way to increase immunity is to use at least one of these essential oils in a castor oil pack treatment. Lemon, rosemary, grapefruit, and bay oils stimulate the drainage of your lymph system, which runs throughout your body gathering toxins.

Aromatherapy formula: *To make a lymphatic massage oil:* Put 12 drops each lemon, rosemary, and grapefruit oils in 4 ounces vegetable oil (preferably castor oil). If available, also add 6 drops true bay oil. *To make a castor oil pack:* Soak a cotton flannel cloth in 2 to 4 cups warm castor oil that contains 3 drops lavender oil per cup. (The size of the area treated determines the size of the cloth and the amount of oil needed to thoroughly soak it.) Fold the cloth and place it over the afflicted area. Cover the oily cloth with a towel (protected by a sheet of plastic wrap if you want to avoid getting the towel oily). Then place a heating pad, hot water bottle, or heated flaxseed pillow on the towel to retain the warmth. Remove everything when it cools in about half an hour. If this sounds a little messy, you're right, but at least one study found that these packs increase immunity (although *how* they work is not known).

Healthy habits: Try treating yourself to a lymphatic massage, which uses long, deep strokes that move from the extremities toward your heart. The massage practitioner moves up your legs and arms towards the lymph nodes located in your groin and armpits. You can do this massage yourself, but I'm sure you'll agree it is so much nicer if someone else gives it to you. Eat a wholesome diet that includes plenty of foods rich in vitamin A and C, plus supplements of these if necessary. Get lots of sleep and use relaxation methods such as yoga and meditation to build your immune system reserves. Herbs that improve your immunity include echinacea root, pau d'arco root bark, and the Chinese herbs astragalus and shizandra berry. Mullein leaf, red root, cleavers leaf, and prickly ash bark are some of the herbs that facilitate lymph drainage.

Indigestion

Medical description: Indigestion encompasses many disorders, including gas pains, stomachache, nausea, and stomach ulcers. Frayed nerves, anxiety, and overexcitability restrict your digestive juices and digestive tract muscles. If you don't have enough hydrochloric acid in your stomach to properly break down protein, you can develop a food allergy.

Aromatherapy remedies: The same aromatic herbs that make food tasty — rosemary, sage, fennel, cumin, anise, basil, caraway, cardamom, cumin, dill, thyme, and coriander — also improve digestion. You can sniff them directly from the spice rack or use them in cooking. They stimulate the release of digestive juices to relieve belching, stomach pains, and intestinal gas. Some essential oils have specialty jobs for digestion. These oils are best taken in food or as teas. (The essential oils are extracted into the hot water.) You can also put them into massage oils to rub directly over the area. Rosemary improves poor food absorption, lemongrass, chamomile, fennel, and melissa (lemon balm) oils relieve nervous indigestion and inflammation, and black pepper and juniper berry increase

stomach acid. All these oils, but especially peppermint, ginger, fennel, coriander, and dill oils relieve gas pains. One
clinical study showed that irritable
bowel syndrom or general stomach
upsets, such as belching, nausea, heartburn, spasms, and loss of appetite, one
herbal combination that contains
mostly peppermint, caraway, and some
fennel works better than the indigestion
drug metoclopramide. If you have a
problem digesting fatty foods, then
rosemary, peppermint, lavender, and
black pepper stimulate bile production.
Use them as herbs in your meals and as
essential oils for abdominal massage.
Also read the general digestive information Chapter 11.

Aromatherapy formula: *To make a
massage oil:* Add 12 drops peppermint
oil, 12 drops orange oil, 8 drops ginger
rhizome oil, and 5 drops fennel oil in 4
ounces vegetable oil or a lotion. *To
make tea:* Select one of the herbs mentioned and pour boiling water over 1
teaspoon of the herb. Let steep 5 to 10
minutes and then strain and drink.

Healthy habits: Indigestion is simply a
symptom of an underlying problem. It
may be that you're not digesting your
food properly, and you need to take an
herbal bitter formula that includes
herbs such as gentian and bitter orange
before each meal to promote your
digestive juices. Instead of gulping it
down, take time to fully chew and
digest your food in a peaceful setting. A
couple drops of grapefruit seed extract
(not an essential oil) in a glass of water
or the capsules reduce diarrhea, constipation, intestinal gas, bloating, and
abdominal discomfort. It effectively discourages *E. coli,* candida, and geot-
richum, a fungus responsible for
intestinal problems. Studies show that
bay laurel, thyme, clove, and cinnamon
are some of the strongest essential oils
to fight *E. coli.*

Insect bites and stings

Medical description: A bite or sting
from an insect. If you get bit by a poisonous insect or experience any allergic
reaction, be sure to see a doctor.

Aromatherapy remedies: Chamomile,
cedarwood, eucalyptus, tea tree, and
lavender oils reduce the swelling, itching, and inflammation and help stop
allergic responses when you're bitten or
stung by an insect. For mosquito or
other tiny insect bites that don't
demand much attention, a simple dab
of one of these essential oils provides
relief. If you're bitten by spiders or
stung by a bee, use a clay paste that
contains essential oils. As the clay
dries, it pulls toxins from the bite or
sting to the skin's surface to keep them
from spreading. This method is also
good to draw out pus or splinters that
are imbedded in your skin. Lots of natural bug repellents are available in all
sorts of stores. The most effective ones
contain citronella or some other lemon-
scented essential oil.

Aromatherapy formula: *To make a bite
oil:* Put 5 drops lavender oil and 3 drops
German chamomile oil into a teaspoon
of vegetable oil or alcohol (either vodka
or rubbing alcohol). Dab this directly on
insect bites. For a bite and sting poultice
recipe and bug repellent, see Chapter 6.

Healthy habits: During bug season,
wear long sleeves and natural insect
repellent. Eat garlic and brewers yeast
so that bugs don't bother you as much.
(This combo also keeps fleas from biting your pets.)

Insomnia

Medical description: Lack of sleep
leaves you feeling tired the next day. If
you don't get adequate sleep for weeks
or months, you easily develop symptoms
of sleep deprivation, such as dizziness,
confusion, agitation, and depression.

Aromatherapy remedies: For insomnia due to mental agitation or overwork, you can try sniffing several scents: bergamot, chamomile, lavender, clary sage, frankincense, sandalwood, or rose. Other relaxing scents come from the essential oils of neroli (orange blossom), melissa (lemon balm), bergamot, tangerine or mandarin, and geranium. Even better, get a massage with a massage oil that contains these essential oils. One of the most relaxing treatments before bedtime — or anytime — is a warm aromatherapy bath. An old-fashioned, but effective, treatment is to stuff a small pillow with dried hops. Its scent has sedative effects.

Aromatherapy formula: *For a general insomnia massage:* Put 6 drops bergamot oil, 5 drops lavender oil, 5 drops sandalwood oil, 2 drops chamomile oil, 1 drop frankincense oil, and 1 drop rose oil (expensive, so optional) in 2 ounces vegetable oil or a lotion. *For a bath oil:* Add 1 teaspoon of this massage oil to your bath. You can also add 5 drops total of any combination of the oils listed in the massage directly to the water. If you don't have time for a bath, rub a little of the blend under your nose and on your wrists to sniff. To make a sleep pillow and for even more ideas: See Chapter 9.

Healthy habits: Exercise and eat well during the day. Make sure that you get enough calcium and magnesium in your diet or take them as supplements. Eat mostly carbohydrates for dinner and go light on the protein. Before bed, relax with massage, yoga, meditation, visualization, or in a bath and avoid mentally stimulating activities. Take teas, tinctures, or pills of sedative herbs like valerian root, kava root, catnip leaf, hops strobiles, scullcap leaf, and passion flower leaf. If you suspect that your insomnia is related to stress, depression, or other problems, see those sections in this directory.

Lung congestion/bronchitis

Medical description: General congestion or inflammation of your *bronchioles* (the small air tubes in your lungs) can make it difficult for you to take a deep breath. If you have almost constant lung congestion, it may be due to an allergy such as asthma or food allergies.

Aromatherapy remedies: Decongestant essential oils that clear lung congestion include eucalyptus, peppermint, lavender, and frankincense. Use any of these essential oils as a steam or in a vaporizer to bring these antibiotic oils directly into your lungs. The steam also opens your bronchial passages and makes it easier for you to breathe. You can also use these same essential oils in a massage oil. Rosemary, tea tree, thyme, or ginger oils are recommended when congestion is due to an infection in your lungs. A good way to use them is to rub a salve that is loaded with essential oils (called a *vapor balm*) over your chest and throat to increase circulation and warmth in these areas to help fight infection. This way, the essential oils are both absorbed through your skin and inhaled into your lungs. A piece of flannel fabric on your chest after rubbing in the balm holds in the heat to increase absorption of the essential oils. Vapor balm made with a vegetable oil and beeswax base (a healthier solution to petroleum oil) are available in natural-food stores. Other useful oils (although they are more difficult to find) are helichrysum and the variety of hyssop called decumbens.

Aromatherapy formula: *For a homemade vapor balm:* Add 12 drops eucalyptus oil, 5 drops peppermint oil, and 5 drops thyme oil to 1 ounce vegetable oil (such as olive oil). Shake well before using. Gently massage onto your chest and throat several times a day.

Healthy habits: Aerobic exercise expands your lung capacity and helps your overall breathing. Build up your immune system and lungs with herbal tonics. For your lungs, turn to herbs such as mullein leaf, elecampane root, hyssop leaf, and horehound leaf as a tea, tincture, or pills. Echinacea root and the Chinese herb shizandra berry treat both your immune and lung problems.

Menstrual cramps

Medical description: Painful uterine muscle cramping during menstruation. Either emotional or physical stress can worsen your cramping.

Aromatherapy remedies: Muscle relaxants that reduce menstrual (and other muscle) cramps are chamomile, ginger, lavender, marjoram, and melissa (lemon balm) oils. These same essential oils also ease cramps resulting from disorders such as endometriosis and uterine fibroids. For general information on pain-relieving essential oils, turn to Chapter 11. If you have a uterine problem, also see my advice in this section.

Aromatherapy formula: *To make a muscle-relaxing massage oil:* Combine 12 drops lavender, 8 drops ginger, 4 drops marjoram, 4 drops chamomile in 1 ounce vegetable oil. Rub over the cramping area as needed to relieve the pain. Use St. John's wort infused oil instead of plain oil for an even more effective remedy. For severe cramping, after you rub on the oil, cover the area with a thin cloth and then with a hot water bottle, heating pad, or a flax-filled pillow that has been heated in a microwave oven to provide long-lasting heat. *For your bath:* Add a total of 6 drops essential oil to a hot bath. (Choose one oil or a combination of those suggested.)

Healthy habits: Herbs that ease your uterine cramping are cramp bark and wild yam root in a tea, pill, or extract. General herbal muscle relaxants such as valerian root and relaxation techniques also help. Some women report relief from their cramps by taking evening primrose capsules throughout their cycle to help adjust the hormone-like substances that cause the cramping. For the same reason, use olive oil and unheated flaxseed in your diet and avoid hydrogenated oils like margarine and fried and processed food, including fried corn chips sold in natural-food stores. Ease off of eating heavy protein, especially meat (unless this makes you weak or anemic), just before menstruation and during menstruation. For more detailed herbal and nutritional information on relieving menstrual cramps, see my book *Women's Herbs, Women's Health* (Interweave Press). Regular exercise, especially aerobic exercise where you keep a steady pace for at least 20 minutes, is good throughout your menstrual cycle — belly dancing classes are a great way to tone uterine muscles. Last, but not least, try to plan ahead to take some time for yourself during the worst cramping.

Menopause

Medical description: Menopause is the slow down and cessation of the menstrual cycle and, along with it, fertility. This happens as your ovaries slow down their release of eggs. The average age is 52, but menopause can occur earlier or later. The many symptoms, which include hot flashes, bone fragility, confusion, depression, and a dry, less elastic vagina due to a thinner lining, are apparently caused by the reduced and erratic hormonal activity.

Aromatherapy remedies: Several essential oils that have hormonelike activity can help you through menopause. Use estrogenic oils, which include clary sage, sage, anise, fennel, and to some degree, cypress, angelica, and coriander, in your bath and as body lotion or cream. Geranium, neroli (orange blossom), rose, and lavender help balance hormones and are useful not only in facial creams to reduce aging and wrinkles, but to counter vaginal dryness. Hot flashes are partially relieved by peppermint, sage, and lemon oils.

Aromatherapy formula: *To enhance a body lotion or cream:* Purchase your favorite cream or lotion or buy a basic, unscented lotion at a natural-food store or body shop. Stir in 6 drops geranium oil, 6 drops lavender oil, 2 drops neroli oil (orange blossom), 1 drop rose oil, and 1,500 units vitamin E oil to a 2-ounce jar (or into 2 ounces pure vegetable oil). Use daily. (Vitamin E oil improves the strength and flexibility of the vaginal lining and heals abrasions. Buy the liquid or pop several vitamin E capsules and squeeze out the oil.) *To cool hot flashes:* Add 10 drops lemon oil, 5 drops peppermint oil, and 2 drops clary sage oil to 1 ounce aloe vera gel. Shake, stir, or blend to mix it all together. Dab or spray on your wrists, face, or neck whenever a hot flash threatens to hit. *To make a hot flashes tea:* Cover a teaspoon of sage leaves with a cup of boiling water and steep about 5 minutes. Then strain and drink a cup or two every day or at the first sign of a hot flash. (The water pulls out sage's essential oil.)

Healthy habits: Natural treatments can make your menopause smooth. Read my *Women's Herbs, Women's Health* (Interweave Press, 1998) for detailed information about herbs such as black cohosh root, dong quai root, and vitex berry and foods like soy to balance hormones.

Muscle cramps and back pain

Medical description: Persistent pain in your muscles. If you don't know why you're in pain, get it checked out by your doctor to make sure that you don't have a kidney, lung, heart, or bowel problem or that your discomfort is not the result of some injury of which you weren't aware.

Aromatherapy remedies: Rub a massage oil that contains muscle-relaxing essential oils like lavender, Roman chamomile, and marjoram on sore muscles and they relax twice as fast than with just rubbing alone. (And, the scent of these same oils also help to de-stress you in case that is part of the source of your aches.) Juniper, rosemary, and peppermint oils are pain-relievers that penetrate into your muscles. (For the ultimate relaxation, have a friend or a professional do the massage.) If you can, take a hot bath before your massage using the same essential oils, or if you must, in place of a massage. To help alleviate pain, alternate hot and cold compresses on the area. If the area around your backbone is inflamed and/or you have pinched nerves, apply only cold compresses for the first 12 hours after the injury to help reduce the inflammation. If you plan to exercise enough to strain your muscles, limber up beforehand not only with warmups, but also rub a liniment into muscles you'll use. (See Arthritis in this section and Chapter 11 for information on buying or making a liniment.)

Aromatherapy formula: *To make a muscle cramp massage oil:* Combine 8 drops lavender oil, 4 drops marjoram oil, 6 drops German chamomile oil, and 4 drops peppermint oil in 2 ounces vegetable oil. For an even more effective massage oil, use a vegetable oil that is infused with St. John's wort oil or arnica oil instead of plain vegetable oil. (You'll find these sold in natural-food stores.) *In your bath:* Add 2 drops each of these same essential oils to the hot water, along with ¼ cup Epsom salts to further relax tight muscles. *For a compress:* Add 3 drops ginger oil and 2 drops lavender oil to ½ cup hot water.

Soak a soft cloth in the solution and wring out the excess. Fold the cloth and lay it on the painful area. To hold in the heat, cover the cloth with a towel, a hot water bottle, or a flaxseed pillow that has been heated in the microwave. Before it cools, replace the hot cloth with another one that has been soaked in plain cold water. Leave the compress on 5 to 10 minutes, or until it starts to cool, and then replace it with another hot one. Repeat this procedure several times.

Healthy habits: Muscle relaxant herbs include chamomile, valerian, scullcap, and kava. Many formulas contain these herbs. Exercise, especially gentle stretches like yoga and tai chi, help your body and back stay flexible. You can take classes or get an instructive video. A chiropractor or an osteopath can spot problems and point out any harmful habits that contribute to your muscle or back pain by looking at the way that yoy walk or hold your weight. If it isn't uncomfortable, aerobic exercise like running, swimming, skiing, and bicycling can help ease your back pain. Also, wear shoes that have proper support, watch how you stand, and bend your legs when you lift anything.

Nausea and motion sickness

Medical description: Feeling sick to your stomach and nauseous can be due to an illness, eating spoiled food, drinking bad water, the flu, emotional distress, hormonal imbalance (as in pregnancy), or motion sickness. Chronic bouts of nausea can also signal something even more serious, so be sure to see your doctor about it.

Aromatherapy remedies: Basil, ginger, chamomile, and peppermint oils relieve nausea. The best way to take these oils is in a breath freshener, mint, natural ginger ale, or as tea. (The hot water pulls essential oils out of the plant into the water.) You can also rub a massage

oil that contains any of these oils over your stomach. This approach is good for children who refuse to drink the tea or take other medications. In a pinch, you can put some water in your mouth and put a half drop of peppermint or ginger on your finger and then lightly lick it — but be prepared, they're both very hot and produce a burning sensation on your tongue. Sometimes, just inhaling a little of peppermint's aroma is all you need. See the general discussion on oils for digestion in Chapter 11.

Aromatherapy formula: *To make an antinausea tea:* Pour 2 cups boiling water over 2 teaspoons of the herb or herbs of your choice listed in the preceding bullet. Cover and steep for 5 to 10 minutes and then strain and drink. *For a massage belly oil:* Mix 8 drops chamomile and 4 drops ginger into 1 ounce vegetable oil and rub as needed over the stomach area. This blend is also good for general digestive tract upset, and the massage that goes along with rubbing on the oil also helps to ease digestive distress.

Healthy habits: Nausea can be due to poor eating habits and poor choices of foods. If so, you know what to do. If you're subject to motion sickness, try watching a stationary object outside the vehicle to explain to your confused mind what is really happening.

Nerve pain

Medical description: Pain that is caused by injured or pinched nerves.

Aromatherapy remedies: The essential oils of lavender, chamomile, marjoram, and helichrysum relieve nerve pain. To some degree, so do sandalwood, caraway, and lemongrass oils. Use these oils to reduce the pain of any condition related to nerves, such as a pinched nerve, sciatica, carpal tunnel syndrome, and shingles (a painful skin eruption related to herpes). These essential oils can even give you some relief if you suffer from nervous system conditions like multiple sclerosis and chronic fatigue syndrome. General information on essential oils and pain is in Chapter 11.

Aromatherapy formula: *To make a massage oil for your nerves:* Combine 8 drops lavender oil, 4 drops chamomile oil, 4 drops helichrysum oil (if available), and 3 drops marjoram oil in 2 ounces of an infused oil of St. John's wort. Apply as needed for relief.

Healthy habits: Nerve conditions are difficult to heal, so talk to someone skilled in natural medicine for more ideas on how to treat your particular problem.

Oily skin

Medical description: Oily skin has a lot of luster and may even be slightly shiny from all the oil. It also tends to have a coarser texture, with large pores, and is prone to acne because the excess oil attracts dirt and clogs your pores with dead cells, which can breed bacteria and infection. The oil also protects it from drying out, so skin looks plump and takes longer to develop wrinkles.

Aromatherapy remedies: Basil, eucalyptus, tea tree, cedarwood, cypress, lemongrass, spike lavender, and ylang ylang oils help to normalize skin that has overactive oil glands. Sage and lemongrass actually slow down oil production. (They also reduce sweating.) Use these essential oils in aromatherapy steams and facial masks, which help unclog your pores and encourage the release of excess oil. Any citrus, such as lemon or orange, is appropriate for use on oily skin. (Keep in mind that these oils can have a photosensitizing effect if you're one of the people who is sensitive to this reaction and you're in the sun after using them. Except for

bergamot, you typically need to have a lot of essential oil in a product for your skin to react.) A skin lotion is better for your oily skin than a cream. A little oil is fine, but look for products that are based more on aloe vera or aromatherapy hydrosols. (See the explanation of hydrosols in Chapter 1.) Vinegar is also good to use on oily skin, although most products don't contain it due to its strong smell, even though the smell does dissipate in a few minutes once you apply it to your skin. Some witch hazel and grain alcohol help to dry your skin, but don't overdo it because putting too much drying substances on your skin only encourages more oil production. Find more on oily skin in Chapter 7.

Aromatherapy formula: *To make a skin toner:* Combine 5 drops cedarwood oil, 3 drops lemongrass oil, 1 drop ylang ylang oil, ¼ cup aloe vera, and 1 ounce witch hazel distillate. Shake well before applying to your skin.

Healthy habits: Cleanse your oily skin a couple times a day with an aromatherapy soap to remove excess oil.

PMS (Premenstrual Syndrome)

Medical description: Irritability, mood swings, depression, headaches, bloating, and swollen breasts are a few of the symptoms that can occur during the few days just before menstruation. Known as premenstrual syndrome, or PMS, it's thought to be caused by the rise and fall of hormones just before menstruation. What classifies these symptoms as PMS is that your symptoms disappear after menstruation begins. PMS is mildly unpleasant for some women and temporarily debilitating for others.

Aromatherapy remedies: Try to begin your PMS treatment a couple of days before you expect the symptoms to hit. Essential oils that help in general are angelica, chamomile, lavender, marjoram, and especially geranium and clary sage, both of which help to balance hormones. For problems with water retention, use a massage oil that contains grapefruit, carrot seed, and/or juniper. For depression associated with PMS, use clary sage, neroli (orange blossom), jasmine, or ylang ylang. If you experience fatigue, acne, fluid retention, headaches, or other symptoms, refer to these specific sections in this guide for more advice on how to deal with them.

Aromatherapy formula: *For a PMS massage/body oil:* Add 10 drops geranium oil, 6 drops chamomile oil, 3 drops clary sage oil, and 3 drops angelica oil, and 2 drops marjoram oil to 2 ounces of vegetable oil. Use as a body oil — or better yet, have someone give you a massage with it.

Healthy habits: Vitex berries in any form balance hormones, but you may need to take them two to three months for results. Dandelion root tea or tincture treats water retention and evening primrose capsules help relieve most symptoms. For more detailed herbal and nutritional information on PMS, see my book *Women's Herbs, Women's Health* (Interweave Press). Go easy on salt and sugar at least a week before menstruation and if you have breast cysts, try to eliminate caffeine and chocolate. Relaxation methods and taking time for yourself are good ideas.

Poison oak/ivy/sumac rash

Medical description: An allergic reaction from contact with one of three plants causes a rash with extreme itching.

Aromatherapy remedies: Look for a remedy that combines herbs with essential oils. Chamomile and helichrysum are examples of essential oils that help ease the painful rash and heal the skin, while cypress dries it up. The menthol in peppermint relieves the painful burning and itching. You can wash with a liquid peppermint soap. (Purchase this at a natural-food store.) Stay away from oil-based products during the first stages. Later, you can use a lotion during the subsequent dry stage of a poison oak, ivy, or sumac rash.

Aromatherapy formula: *For a homemade poison oak, ivy, or sumac remedy:* Add 3 drops lavender oil, 3 drops cypress oil, and 2 drops peppermint oil to a solution of 1 tablespoon apple cider vinegar or distilled witch hazel (from the drugstore) and 2 tablespoons water. Dissolve ½ teaspoon Epsom salt into this and use it as a skin wash. *For a paste to dry up an oozing rash:* Stir 1 teaspoon ground oatmeal into this solution to make a paste. Dab the paste on your rash as often as needed. *For a bath to relieve itching:* Pour 1 tablespoon of the solution, ½ cup Epsom salts, and 4 cups quick-cooking oats (they dissolve best) into a tepid bath and bathe in it. (When you let out the water, be sure to put a catcher designed to catch hair over your drain so that the oats don't go down your drain and clog it.

Healthy habits: Take supplements of vitamin C and pantothenic acid. Echinacea root and chamomile flower tincture, tea, or pills help reduce the inflammation. Good external washes include mugwort leaf, manzanita leaf, and jewelweed leaf. And, try not to itch.

Sprains and bruises

Medical description: When you injure a *ligament,* the springy tissue that holds your muscles to your bones, it's called a sprain. You get bruised when soft tissue is damaged. In either case, the result is pain and often discoloration as the area swells. If this happens to you often without apparent reason, get a check up to make sure that your bruising isn't the result of an underlying disorder, such as a kidney disorder.

Aromatherapy remedies: Both sprains and bruises are treated similarly with essential oils like lavender, chamomile, or helichrysum in an oil or alcohol base. They reduce swelling and bruising and also help relieve the pain. General information on essential oils to reduce swelling is in Chapter 11.

Aromatherapy formula: *To make a sprain and bruise oil:* Add 12 drops lavender oil to ½ ounce St. John's wort tincture or arnica flower tincture. This oil is a great item to carry in your aromatherapy first-aid kit.

Healthy habits: If you do warmups, such as slow stretching exercises, you're not as likely to develop a sprain. If you bruise or get sprains easily, be sure that you get an adequate amount of vitamin C that includes bioflavonoids in your diet. If not, take supplements. Anthrocyanidins or proanthrocyanidins supplements improve the integrity of your ligaments and blood vessels.

Stress

Medical description: Emotional stress occurs when you feel overly pressured, nervous, or anxious. It takes a toll on your adrenals and the rest of your hormonal system, your nervous system, and your brain. Continuous stress can permanently damage these areas.

Aromatherapy remedies: Fragrance alone can make you less tense. Lavender, bergamot, marjoram, sandalwood, lemon, and chamomile (in that order) have a relaxing effect on brain waves. The citrusy scents of neroli (orange blossom), petitgrain, and tangerine or mandarin oils, and also ylang ylang, chamomile, valerian, and opopanax (with a fragrance that is similar to myrrh) oils are sedating. Anise's aroma is for stress that develops from working too hard. You can find more on stress in Chapter 9.

Aromatherapy formula: *For an anti-stress scent:* Combine 10 drops lavender oil, 4 drops sandalwood oil, 4 drops bergamot oil, 4 drops chamomile oil, 4 drops ylang ylang oil in 4 ounces vegetable oil. Use as a body oil or, better yet, as a massage oil. Add 1 to 2 teaspoons massage oil to your bath. You can use 5 drops of any of the suggested oils individually in a bath or hot tub.

Healthy habits: Sure, I know that it's easier said than done, but do try to relax! You can take many herbs, such as valerian root, kava root, catnip leaf, scullcap leaf, and passion flower leaf, on a regular basis to relax your mind. If you seem to be under continual stress, also take adaptagenic herbs like Siberian ginseng, ginseng, licorice, fresh oat berry, and the Ayurvedic herb ashwaganda in tincture or pills. Antistress nutrients to have in your diet are vitamin C and the B vitamin complex, especially pantothenic acid. Eat well and stay healthy to reduce your stress level. Go on a mini-retreat from your work and personal problems by emptying your mind and getting physical with your choice of yoga, meditation, tai chi, workout at the gym, aerobic exercise, swimming, sailing, skiing, bicycling, and so on. Take a class, join a club, read novels, or buy a hammock *and* use it. Also refer to the sections on depression and nervous system problems if that's appropriate for you.

Toothache and teething

Medical description: Painful teeth due to disease or, in babies and young children, from new teeth emerging.

Aromatherapy remedies: Dull your tooth pain with a diluted essential oil such as clove bud. Clove works great to numb tooth pain, but it's hot stuff so dilute it before sticking it in your mouth. It's also one of the potentially toxic essential oils so use it with care. Although it's an old teething remedy for babies, it's probably too strong. Instead, use chamomile oil.

Aromatherapy formula: *To make a toothache oil:* Dilute 4 drops clove bud oil in 1 teaspoon vegetable oil and rub this on your gums just in the area where the tooth hurts. Repeat this as needed. If it is too hot, dilute it with more vegetable oil. *To make a teething oil:* Mix 1 drops chamomile oil in 1 teaspoon vegetable oil and rub about a half drop on your baby's sore gum. Apply a half drop up to six times a day. This can also be rubbed on cheeks externally.

Healthy habits: Practice good oral hygiene by brushing your teeth and flossing them after every meal. To ease teething pains, give your baby an arrowroot teething biscuit.

Uterine problems

Medical description: Uterine problems include endometriosis, uterine fibroids, and cervical dysplasia. What causes these disorders is varied, complicated, and not well understood. It's likely that hormones are involved, especially estrogen. These disorders are difficult to treat either naturally or with drugs, so aromatherapy is only an adjunct therapy to use along with other treatments.

Aromatherapy remedies: A sitz bath with rosemary, lavender, and chamomile oils promotes circulation and ease inflammation.

Aromatherapy formula: *To make a sitz bath:* Fill your bath tub with just enough hot water to reach your navel when you're sitting in the tub. Add 2 drops each of rosemary, lavender, and chamomile oils. Fill a plastic washing basin (like the kind sold in hardware stores to wash your dog) half full of cold water. Switch back and forth, staying in the hot bath about 5 minutes and the cold one for a minute or so. If you have the time, do this four times. Also see Immune problems for instructions on how to do a castor oil pack.

Healthy habits: Turn to health professional to help you deal with uterine problems and refer to my book, *Women's Herbs, Women's Health,* cowritten with Christopher Hobbs (Interweave Press), which devotes individual chapters to these conditions. What you can do on your own is to take herbs such as red raspberry leaf to tone your uterus. Eat as healthy as possible, especially avoiding caffeine and tobacco, and get exercise.

Varicose veins and hemorrhoids

Medical description: Believe it or not, these two conditions are closely related. In fact, hemorrhoids are a type of varicose vein. Because your circulation relies on leg and pelvic muscles to push the blood back up to the heart, varicose veins and hemorrhoids occur when the flow bogs down. The extra load stretches out your veins. If you sit or stand for long periods of time, are overweight, pregnant, constipated, or wear skintight pants or a girdle, blood flow through your pelvic area is especially restricted and encourages their development. Surgery is the only medical solution.

Aromatherapy remedies: Chamomile, lavender, myrtle, and juniper oils, and especially neroli (orange blossom), frankincense, and cypress oils diminish the inflammation, pain, and size of your varicose veins or hemorrhoids. Look for a products that contains at least some of these essential oils. Use myrrh and carrot seed oils if the problem is so bad that the veins are breaking.

Aromatherapy formula: *To make a varicose vein compress:* Add 3 drops each of chamomile, lavender, and helichrysum oil and 1 drop neroli (orange blossom) oils to 1 ounce distilled witch hazel (from the drugstore). Soak a soft cloth in the solution, wring out, fold the cloth, and apply externally. *For seriously extended or broken varicose veins:* Add 3 drops each of myrrh and carrot seed oils to this solution. For hemorrhoids, pour 2 tablespoon of this solution into a jar of the witch hazel or aloe vera cotton wipes that are available in drug and natural-food stores. Apply as a compress directly to your hemorrhoids.

Healthy habits: Improve your circulation with increased exercise that involves moving your legs, eat a good diet that includes lots of vitamin C with bioflavonoids, or take supplements to improve the integrity of your blood vessel walls and help prevent them from extending. The anthrocyanidins found in bilberry, blueberry, and other herbs and proanthrocyanidins from pine bark and grape seed have similar properties and are available as supplements. If you have hemorrhoids, try to get up and move around and increase the roughage in your diet to avoid constipation.

Warts

Medical description: Warts are small, hard growths on the skin caused by a viral infection. If genital warts don't begin to disappear after a couple weeks, have a doctor remove them because this virus (the human papilloma virus, or HPV) is passed to sexual partners and can lead to cervical dysplasia in women.

Aromatherapy remedies: Tea tree and especially thuja oils fight wart viruses. Thuja oil is very strong so should be used only in small amounts.

Aromatherapy formula: *To make a wart oil:* Add 12 drops tea tree oil and 12 drops thuja oil to 1 ounce castor oil, along with 800 IU vitamin E oil (pop open a vitamin E capsule and squeeze it in). Apply two to four times a day with a glass rod applicator, rounded toothpick, or dropper directly — and only — to the warts. Avoid getting the oil anywhere else because this is a very concentrated brew and thuja can burn sensitive skin. You may want to protect surrounding skin around the warts with a coating of herbal salve. If possible, cover the wart with a bandage to keep it moist after applying the oil.

Healthy habits: Build up your immune system so that you're better able to fight the virus by taking immune herbs, especially pau d'arco bark. For the same reason, make sure that you have plenty of vitamin C and A in your diet.

Aroma Guide

. . . .

*I*n this Aromatherapy Guide, I offer a quick reference to more than 40 fragrant plants that produce the most popular essential oils. I list each plant by its common name, followed by the Latin name. (This two-part name has the genus first, which is capitalized, followed by the species.) Latin names are better to positively identify a plant than common names, which can refer to several different plants. Knowing the Latin name is interesting for other reasons. Plants that occur in the same genus quite often share similar characteristics and scents. Examples are the citrus: Orange, lemon, and lime.

I also give you a description of the plant and its scent — an important factor when discussing *aroma*-therapy. I explain the healing properties that the essential oils have on the body and the mind. I tell you the most common method of producing each oil. I also provide cautions when necessary, but always keep in mind that any essential oil is very concentrated and can be toxic if used improperly. Always dilute an essential oil before applying it to the skin (except in a few cases) and do not ingest them.

Fragrant plants and the essential oils they contain offer tremendous health and healing benefits. I hope that this guide provides you with a ready-reference to an exciting and healthful exploration of aromatherapy.

Angelica

Latin name: *Angelica archangelica*

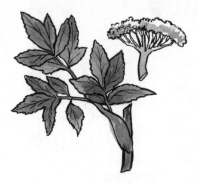

Description: Thought to have originated in Syria, this tall, stately herb now grows throughout much of Europe and in many herb gardens throughout the world. Two similar essential oils are either distilled or solvent-extracted into absolutes. One is made from the seed and the other from the root.

Scent: The angelica plant offers little fragrance until you bite into the seed or break the root. Then the aromatic scent is spicy, almost peppery. The root oil also has a spicy aroma, but smells even stronger and more "rooty."

Uses: Angelica is related to a Chinese herb called dong quai *(Angelica chinensis)* that is a popular women's tonic. Similarly, angelica's essential oil helps regulate the menstrual cycle and relieve menopausal symptoms. It also aids digestion and breathing and relieves coughing. Angelica is typically used for these conditions in a massage oil. The scent alone counters depression and calms nervousness. Summed up, this is an ideal essential oil for women who experience nervousness that is associated with hormonally related problems or an upset stomach.

Caution: Use both the seed and root essential oils carefully because they can overstimulate the nervous system. The root's essential oil also contains a compound called *bergaptene,* which makes skin photosensitive in a few individuals.

Basil

Latin name: *Ocimum basilicum*

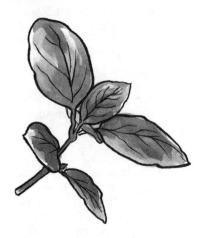

Description: Basil seasons culinary delights like pizza and pesto. Originally from India, Mediterranean peoples have cultivated the fragrant, compact bush for thousands of years. In fact, the name *Ocimum* is probably derived from the Greek word "to smell." The essential oil is distilled from the leaves and flowering tops as an inexpensive substitute for *mignonette* (lily-of-the-valley) in perfume and soap.

Scent: The scent is sweet and spicy and smells just like basil from the spice rack.

Uses: Sixteenth-century herbalist John Gerard said that basil's scent "taketh away sorrowfulness." Modern aromatherapists agree, using it to overcome emotional negativity and mental fatigue. I recommend sniffing basil whenever you need a lift. Basil also aids in memory recall and stimulates blood circulation. Its scent can help make you alert and keep you attentive. It can also relieve a headache, sinus congestion, or a head cold. Basil is an excellent choice to treat indigestion and nausea — even when due to chemotherapy — and it eases the pain of sore muscles and menstruation. All this makes basil an obvious choice during a cold or flu. Plus, it will help to knock out the virus and can even fight off fungal infections A salve containing basil treats herpes blisters and shingles. It is sometimes used in cosmetics for oily skin and hair. In addition, basil promotes childbirth and breast milk, although more often as a tea rather than as an essential oil.

Caution: Use basil in recommended doses because it is a very potent oil and large amounts are overstimulating to your nervous system. It may relieve nausea, but it's way too strong to use it if you're pregnant.

Bay

Latin name: *Laurus nobilis*

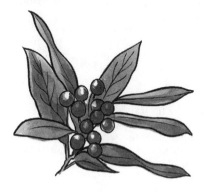

Description: The ancient Greeks loved the bay laurel tree and placed its leaves on the heads of scholars. (Today, Americans still honor graduates with a degree called a Baccalaureate — which means "noble berry tree" in French.)

Greek soothsayers at Delphi sniffed the smoke from burning bay leaves to increase their prophetic visions. The essential oil is distilled from the leaf and occasionally the berry. However, the source of most present-day bay, including the oil used in the men's cologne Bay Rum and "bay" soap, is really from berries of the bay rum tree *(Pimenta racemosa),* which grows in the Virgin Islands. To differentiate between the two, I always refer to bay laurel when discussing the true bay in this book. I call the Virgin Island tree bay rum (pimento).

Scent: The strong, spicy, and pungent aroma may remind you of cooking because this is the same bay that is used to flavor food.

Uses: Bay's most popular aromatherapy use is in a liniment or massage oil to stimulant lymph and blood circulation. The oil also produces a heat sensation, which alleviates muscle tension when rubbed on the body. Studies prove what the Greeks already knew, that bay's aroma improves the memory. Inhaling it also relieves headaches, as well as sinus and lung congestion. A massage oil made with bay is perfect when your lymph glands (tonsils, for example) swell and your head feels foggy due to any type of infection. It boosts the immune system and helps ward off viral and bacterial infections. Bay also helps indigestion and relieves gas, making the leaves a popular addition to bean dishes. The smell alone deters insects like grain weevils and moths, so many cooks also place a few bay leaves in their stored grains to keep insects "at bay."

Caution: Sniff this essential oil lightly because too much produces the reverse effect; you end up with a headache instead of curing one! Overdoses seem to have a slightly narcotic effect, thus the use at Delphi. Also, be careful to dilute the oil when applying to your skin; it could cause irritation.

Benzoin

Latin name: *Styrax benzoin*

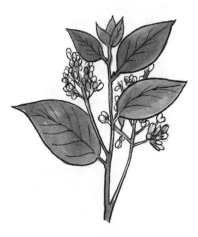

Description: The trunk of this tall Southeast Asian tree, when cut, exudes a gum resin. The Arabic name for benzoin, *luban jawi* means "incense of Java." Tongue-tied European traders shortened this to banjawi, then changed it to "Benjamin," and eventually to benzoin. An absolute is made, but is so thick, it is usually thinned for use with the chemical ethyl glycol. I prefer buying the pure absolute and then thinning it myself with less toxic alcohol.

Scent: With its sweet, warm, vanillalike odor, benzoin is the closest essential oil to real vanilla, although it carries a slight bitterness. It is sometimes used in place of the much more expensive true vanilla.

Uses: The essential oil of benzoin is most popular in a cream or salve to protect chapped skin, improve skin elasticity, and to heal redness, irritation, and itching. As an added benefit, benzoin is a natural preservative that delays spoiling in creams and lotions. It also is a "fixative" that retains the scent in potpourri, perfume, and other fragrant products. A balm or massage oil for chest rub is sometimes used to treat lung and sinus infection. When inhaled, benzoin can also reduce drowsiness and irritability and has been known to improve mental energy.

Bergamot

Latin name: *Citrus bergamia*

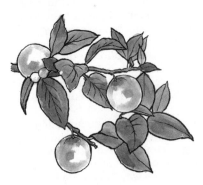

Description: The small citrus tree produces an attractive round, green fruit, but one that tastes too bitter to eat. The green-tinted bergamot oil is pressed from the rinds before the fruit is ripe. Originally from tropical Asia, it now is grown commercially in Italy, mostly as a flavoring for many beverages and candies, including Earl Gray tea. It also scents men's colognes and aftershaves.

Scent: The fragrance is fresh, citrus, and refreshing, but slightly spicy and balsamic compared with other citruses. It mixes well with other scents, making the overall fragrance rich, but mellow.

Uses: Bergamot destroys bacteria, viruses, and fungi, so it's used to treat urinary tract, mouth, and throat infections and for the flu. It also increases the production of white blood cells, which helps the body rid itself of the aforementioned offenders even faster. Diluted in a salve or massage oil, bergamot is applied externally on a variety of skin problems, including eczema, herpes blisters, shingles, and chicken pox. It also makes a pleasantly scented, natural deodorant that kills odor-causing bacteria. The aroma is second only to lavender in its ability to relax brain waves when sniffed, and thus is very calming. But don't inhale too much, bergamot also has sedative properties and can relax you right to sleep! You can also use the oil as an antidepressant.

Caution: Bergaptene, a compound in the essential oil, can be photosensitizing. A bergaptenefree essential oil is available and is a safer choice.

Birch

Latin name: *Betula lenta*

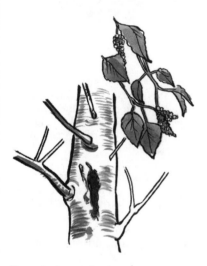

Description: North American birch is a large tree with a fragrant inner bark. It is the real source of the "wintergreen" essential oil used for chewing gum, breath mints, and many medicines because true wintergreen is much more expensive. The two oils share a similar chemistry and so have the same properties, fragrance, and flavor. Birch essential oil is the main ingredient in the men's fragrance "Russian Leather" (so named because the Russians used birch oil to keep their leather book bindings soft and free of insects).

Scent: The aroma is of wintergreen chewing gum or candy: Clean, sweet, sharp, invigorating, and minty. Many people say that birch smells medicinal, probably because it flavors so many over-the-counter drugs.

Uses: A birch salve or lotion softens roughness caused by skin problems, such as eczema. Muscular and arthritic pain and stiffness are relieved when a birch massage oil or liniment is rubbed over painful areas. The essential oil can also be added to your bath to ease pain. Birch is known to help dull pain by delaying the "pain" messages from reaching your central nervous system. What your brain doesn't know won't hurt! The oil also increases blood circulation and menstruation that has been delayed by physical or emotional stress. I like to use birch in tingling, pain-relieving, circulation-promoting foot baths and foot massage oils, which soften calluses and soothe tired feet. It helps prevent dandruff when incorporated in hair conditioners.

Caution: Birch may smell like candy, but it's a potent essential oil. Do not use more than the quantities suggested in recipes in this book because high doses can be toxic. And, store it away from the reach of children so that they won't taste it.

Cardamom

Latin name: *Ellettaria cardamomum*

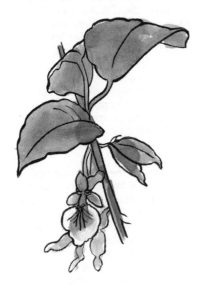

Description: Cardamom is a relative of the common ginger root. It's native to the Middle and Far East where it's used as a condiment in sweet dishes. It gives Turkish coffee and East Indian chai tea a warm, spicy flavor. The essential oil is distilled from the seed.

Scent: The best quality essential oil has a warm, sweet, and spicy scent, while the inferior oil is harsher, with a slight hint of eucalyptus. A little of this potent fragrance goes a long way, so it's mainly used in a blend to accent other essential oils.

Uses: Cardamom essential oil is pricy, but almost everyone who inhales the aroma falls in love with it. I always think of it as a warm and happy aroma. East Indians have long considered the aroma invigorating, warmly romantic, and an aphrodisiac — an obviously good combination! This is its most popular use, but in case illness threatens to destroy your love life, the essential oil also treats digestive problems, such as poor appetite and upset stomach, and it eases coughs and muscle spasms. It is a bacteria and virus fighter and relieves the swelling and irritation that result from inflammation — headaches, menstrual cramps, bruises, insect bites, and so on. This multipurpose oil can also improve your concentration by reducing drowsiness and irritability.

Carrot Seed

Latin name: *Daucus carota*

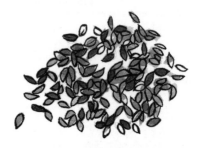

Description: Carrot essential oil is distilled from the seeds of wild Queen Anne's lace, the ancestor of the common vegetable carrot. Indeed, the lacey plant closely resembles the carrots in my vegetable garden.

Scent: Not surprisingly, this essential oil has a carrotlike fragrance, which makes it pungent enough to require that it be used in small quantities. Despite its strong aroma, it is in expensive perfumes as a contrasting note to sweeter fragrances.

Uses: Carrot seed's best claim to fame is the care of dry or damaged skin and hair, dermatitis, eczema, rashes, and even precancerous skin conditions. Despite its carrot smell, it is used in some complexion creams to improve skin tone, elasticity, and general skin health. It may even slow the progression of wrinkles. I find that carrot seed makes a good essential oil for anyone who spends a lot of time outside because it seems to reduce the frequency of skin problems produced by the sun. The essential oil in a massage oil also increases blood circulation, improves liver function, and helps treat various reproductive, urinary, and digestive complaints. You may have difficulty finding this oil in stores and need to order it through the mail. (I list mail-order companies in the Appendix.)

Cedarwood

Latin name: *Cedrus deodora* and *Cedrus atlantica*

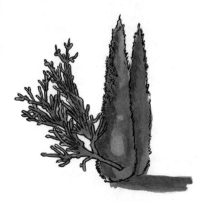

Description: The majestic cedar tree grows to 100 feet tall and lives more than 1,000 years. It was the lumber used to build ancient temples, such as that of King Solomon, because the fragrance of its wood was believed to lead worshipers closer to God. It also resists insect damage. The modern source of most "cedarwood" essential oil is really juniper *(Juniperus virginiana)*, a coniferous evergreen known as "red cedar."

Scent: The scent is similar to camphor, but with a richer, woodsy, balsamic undertone.

Uses: An aromatherapy steam with cedar essential oil treats respiratory infections and clears sinus and lung congestion. In a sitz bath, it reduces the pain and irritation of a bladder infection. The essential oil is also an astringent that dries oily or blemished skin when used in a facial wash or spritzer. Added to a salve or hair conditioner, it relieves eczema, psoriasis, skin inflammation, and dandruff, especially when these conditions are related to excessively oily skin. Cedarwood is also good for dry hair because it increases the ability of your skin and scalp to hold in water. You can also put it on itchy bug bites. Although I have no proof, it is reported to slow hair loss.

Caution: Cedar, and also juniper, are best avoided during pregnancy. Inhaling the fragrance is stimulating and possibly counteracts the sedative effects of drugs like pentobarbitol.

Chamomile, German

Latin name: *Matricaria recutita,* formerly *M. chamomilla*

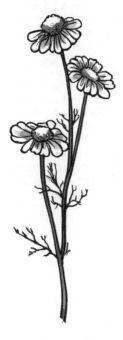

Description: Chamomile resembles tiny daisies with its miniature white-petaled flowers and yellow centers. A chemical reaction during distillation, which creates the compound chamazulene, makes the essential oil a blue-green (azulene means "blue"). This increases its already potent anti-inflammatory properties. Several other chamomiles produce pale yellow essential oils that have similar properties. These include Roman chamomile *(Chamaemelum nobile)* and mixta *(Anthemis mixta),* which is sold as "gold" chamomile.

Scent: Sweet and herbaceous, the chamomile scent is so applelike that the Spanish call it manzanilla, or "little apple," and the Greeks know it as "earth-apples."

Uses: Research show that both the aroma and essential oil when used externally relax the mind and body, soothing those who feel stressed, anxious, depressed, or can't sleep. As a result, a massage oil, aromatherapy bath, or compress are popular treatments for insomnia, depression, PMS, menopause, headaches, hyperactivity, and nervous indigestion. I often use the essential oil when the skin, as well as the emotions, are oversensitive, inflamed, or bruised. Chamomile also reduces the inflammation of burns, eczema, skin rashes, allergic reactions, and numbs the pain of stiff joints and cramping muscles. It also helps the body fight off infection by increasing the production of white blood cells. A cream, compress, or salve is suitable for all complexion types, enlarged capillaries, and varicose veins. It is an ideal treatment for acne. Added to shampoos, the essential oil brightens the hair and brings out highlights.

Cinnamon

Latin name: *Cinnamomum zeylanicum*

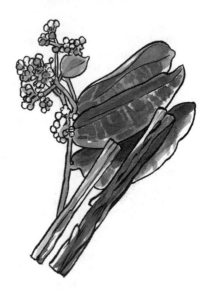

Description: Cinnamon is a large, sub-tropical tree with fragrant bark that can be harvested twice a year for 30 years. A reddish-brown essential oil is distilled from both leaf and bark. Yardley's famous Brown Windsor soaps are based on cinnamon.

Scent: Cinnamon has a sweet, spicy-hot fragrance that is so potent, only small amounts are needed to perk up an aromatherapy blend. The scent is well known for its use in cinnamon rolls, candies, and many other foods.

Uses: The essential oil of cinnamon is best described as a mover and shaker. It is a physical and emotional stimulant that gets the blood and mind moving. It also affects the libido and is known as an aphrodisiac, as well as an antidepressant. Researchers found that just having the aroma in the room reduces drowsiness, irritability, and the pain and frequency of headaches. In one study, it helped the participants concentrate and perform better on mental work. The essential oil provides the heat in a warming liniment to relax tight muscles, ease painful joints, relieve menstrual cramps, and increase circulation. It also increases the action of enzymes that break down food in the body, aiding the metabolic process. The essential oil fights viral, fungal, and bacterial illnesses and boosts the immune system.

Caution: Both the leaf and bark essential oils can irritate, redden, and even burn sensitive skin so use them carefully — no more than ½ drop in a bath. Avoid their use altogether in cosmetics.

Citronella
Latin name: *Citronella nardus*

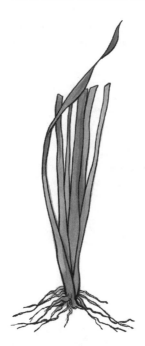

Description: This tropical grass releases an intense odor when broken. A story from 332 B.C. says that Alexander the Great, while riding an elephant near the Egyptian border, became intoxicated when he smelled "nard" (the old nickname for citronella) as it was crushed underfoot. The deep yellow essential oil is distilled from the grassy leaves.

Scent: Distinctly lemony, the scent is sharp and camphorlike.

Uses: Citronella essential oil treats colds, infections, and oily complexions, but its main use is in insect repellents — flea collars, bug sprays, and candles — to keep away mosquitoes, ticks, fleas, and other pesky insects. The scent is very relaxing and can help relieve insomnia. It often is used to adulterate the far more expensive and more mellow-scented oils, lemon verbena, and melissa (lemon balm).

Caution: The essential oil is safe to use, but it can irritate skin, so it is rarely used in cosmetics.

Clary Sage

Latin name: *Salvia sclarea*

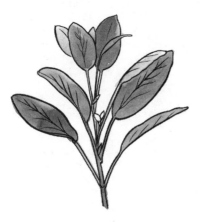

Description: Distilled from the flowering tops and leaves of a three-foot tall perennial, clary sage is produced mostly for flavoring foods. It is related to common garden sage, but it has different fragrance.

Scent: The scent of culinary sage is obvious, but there is also a nutty, wine-like aroma that I can only describe as heady.

Uses: Added to a massage oil or used in a compress, clary sage essential oil eases muscle and nervous tension, pain, and indigestion. It slightly promotes the action of the female hormone estrogen, so it is especially good for woman's ailments, easing menstrual cramps, PMS, and menopausal hot flashes. The fragrance alone helps relieve depression and insomnia and slightly lowers blood pressure. It rejuvenates tired adrenal

glands, which are responsible for controlling anxiety levels in the body. It is an obvious favorite of menopausal women. It is also useful for blemished, mature, wrinkled, or inflamed skin in a complexion cream and can help regulate oily hair. It is sometimes is used in natural deodorants for its fragrance and its ability to reduce perspiration and destroy odor-causing bacteria.

Caution: Watch out! Clary sage can cause giddiness, headaches, and nightmares. Large amounts raise the blood pressure. It increases the effects of drinking alcohol, so do not sniff and drink. It also causes problems in conjunction with some antipsychotic pharmaceutical drugs. Because it has an estrogenlike component, it may be ill-advised in disorders that involve too much estrogen (but there is no research on this).

Clove Bud

Latin name: *Syzygium aromaticum,* formerly *Eugenia caryophyllata*

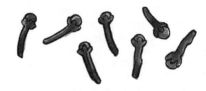

Description: Clove buds — the same as used in cooking — are the unripe flower buds of a short, slender evergreen tree that bears cloves for at least a century. Most of the trees are grown in Indonesia and the African island Zanzibar, and the pale yellow essential oil that is distilled from them is used to flavor food and in dental products.

Scent: If you're already familiar with cloves, you will readily recognize their sweet-spicy, but also strong and hot aroma, with their slight fruitiness.

Uses: One of the most potent antiseptics, Europeans doctors once breathed through clove-filled leather beaks to ward off the plague. Modern dental preparations contain clove essential oil, or its main constituent, eugenol, to numb toothache and teething pain and to stop infection. It is also a potent germ-fighter and antifungal for other conditions, such as flu, colds, bronchitis, and athlete's foot. The essential oil gives heat to a liniment, helping relieve muscle and arthritic pain. Researchers found that sniffing the spicy aroma reduces drowsiness, irritability, and headaches, assists memory recall, and increases blood circulation. This powerful essential oil also has the ability to abate depression, relieve indigestion, and contribute to sexual stimulation.

Caution: The essential oil is irritating to skin and especially to mucous membranes. Although clove bud smells stronger, the leaf contains almost pure eugenol — a very irritating compound — and is rarely used. Don't put either oil undiluted on a baby's gums for teething as is often suggested, or you will soon have a baby who is screaming from the heat.

Cypress

Latin name: *Cupressus sempervirens*

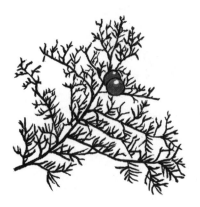

Description: The essential oil is distilled from the needles or twigs and sometimes the cones of this statuesque evergreen. Most of the oil is used in men's colognes and aftershaves.

Scent: The scent is fresh, woody, and pinelike, but more pungent and almost smoky compared to the fragrance of a pine tree.

Uses: A massage oil or compress of cypress essential oil treats circulation problems, such as low blood pressure, poor circulation, varicose veins, and hemorrhoids. The same technique works well to diminish excessive menstruation, urinary infection, or water retention. A drop of the essential oil on your pillow or a steam will lessen laryngitis, spasmodic coughing, and sinus congestion. In cosmetics, it reduces excessive sweating and an overly oily complexion as well as controls oily hair. Smoke from the burning resin was inhaled in southern Europe to relieve sinus congestion, and the Chinese chewed its small cones to reduce gum infection and inflammation. Long associated with death, French and Northern Americans plant the tall, narrow cypress in their graveyards, and aromatherapists use the scent to comfort those who are grieving. Perhaps then, it is not surprising that the oil is also used as an antidepressant. Cypress can increase mental energy and attentiveness by reducing drowsiness and irritability.

Eucalyptus

Latin name: *Eucalyptus globulus*

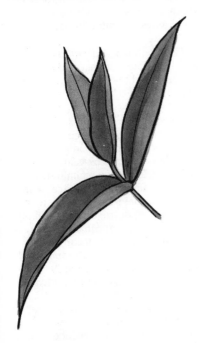

Description: Eucalyptus trees hail from Australia and Tasmania, but are now found in subtropical regions all over the globe. They are one of the tallest and fastest growing trees. Out of the more than 600 species, the blue gum is the most widely cultivated variety and provides most of the essential oil. Aromatherapists also use several others, including lemon eucalyptus (*Eucalyptus citriodora*) with its relaxing qualities and pleasant, lemony scent.

Scent: Pungent and camphorlike, the scent of eucalyptus is so sharp, it seems to hit the top of your nose when inhaled.

Uses: Eucalyptus essential oil is highly antiseptic but also very inexpensive, so it's used liberally in aftershaves, colognes, mouthwashes, and household cleansers. Researchers found that the scent provides a real wake-up call, so using these products should help you get through the day. The essential oil of eucalyptus, or its main component eucalyptol, is used in many drugstore products as a liniment for sore muscles, in vapor rubs for lung and sinus congestion, in skin blemishes/oily complexions lotions and creams, and in shampoo for oily hair. Many people use either eucalyptus leaves or the essential oil in steam baths and saunas by placing a few drops on the hot rocks so that the scent fills the room. Eucalyptus is also one of the strongest essential oils to fight viral infections like flu, herpes blisters, and chicken pox and helps boost the body's immune system.

Caution: Do not use eucalyptus during an asthma attack. Some people are sensitive to the smell and their eyes water just from inhaling the aroma, so be cautious using it in a public sauna.

Fennel

Latin name: *Foeniculum vulgare*

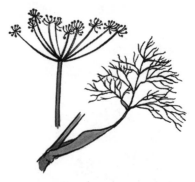

Description: This tall, featherlike Mediterranean herb is often referred to as "licorice" plant or anise because it tastes and smells so much like licorice. A clear essential oil is distilled from the seed.

Scent: The scent is herbaceous, sweet, and very licoricelike.

Uses: The most popular uses of the essential oil are to reduce water retention and urinary tract problems and to soothe an upset stomach. Historically, both the aroma and the essential oil in a massage oil are said to be good for weight loss. I suspect that it does promote the body's metabolism and slightly stimulates the adrenal glands. Modern aromatherapists use fennel's scent to improve self-motivation, including the ability to diet, although it can both reduce and stimulate the appetite. The essential oil heals bruises and is especially useful for rejuvenating mature skin, as well as dry skin prone to acne. In previous centuries, a fennel cream was said to remove complexion wrinkles, perhaps due to the essential oil's estrogenlike properties. It increases mother's milk, but a nursing mom should drink the tea instead because the dose is much safer.

Caution: Because it can overexcite the nervous system, use fennel oil carefully. Individuals with nervous system problems, epilepsy should completely avoid it. It has estrogenlike properties, so use cautiously if you have estrogen-associated problems.

Fir

Latin name: *Abies alba* and other species

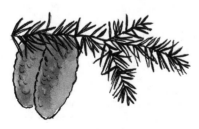

Description: A native of northern Europe, the fir is well known as the Christmas tree. It produces a clear essential oil that is distilled from the needles. Sometimes the essential oil from pine (*Pinus* species) needles is sold as fir. Pine has the same properties, but its aroma is sharper and harsher.

Scent: Fresh, softly balsamic, invigorating, and forestlike, the essential oil is the fragrance of walks through the woods and of Christmas time.

Uses: The essential oil of fir soothes muscle and rheumatic pain and increases poor circulation when used in a massage oil, liniment, or bath. It also helps prevent bladder and kidney infections and reduces coughing from lung congestion, bronchitis, or asthma when used in an aromatherapy steam or a chest rub. According to research, the scent of fir is stimulating and increases energy. All this makes it a good winter remedy. Aromatherapists say the Christmaslike, woodsy smell makes most people happy and may be one reason the traditional European Yule log and Christmas tree were brought into the home at the time of year when the daylight hours are so short and people tend to get depressed. The essential oil is occasionally added to a salve or other skin preparation as an antiseptic for skin infections.

Caution: Fir is good to treat asthma, but only use it in between attacks as a preventative rather than while an attack is happening.

Frankincense

Latin name: *Boswellia carteri*

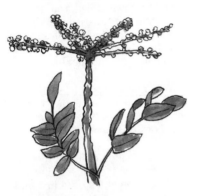

Description: This small tree is planted on rocky, dry ground in Yemen, Oman, North Africa, Somalia, China, and India. The clear to pale yellow oil is distilled from hard "tears" of gum resin that ooze from the tree when the trunk is cut. It is one of the three priceless gifts that the Magi brought to the Christ child, and its fragrance still fills Greek Orthodox churches and churches during high Mass.

Scent: Soft and balsamic, the heady fragrance can seem slightly lemony or camphorlike.

Uses: Frankincense is an expensive essential oil, but also an important healer. It rejuvenates skin, so it's used on mature and aging complexions and to fade old scars, reduce inflammation, moisturize dry hair, and cure acne. Its antiseptic properties fight bacterial and fungal skin infections in a salve, lotion, or as a compress. It also treats infection of the lungs, the reproductive organs, and the urinary tract, and it increases the menstrual flow. The oil works in two ways to help the body fight infection and pain. It first numbs nerve endings to reduce the amount of pain sensations that reach the brain. And then it boosts the body's immune system to accelerate the healing process. As an added bonus, the oil's aroma relaxes the brain, which helps bring on sleep. However, due to its expense, it's primarily used in cosmetics — expensive ones. The fragrance has been valued for thousands of years to inspire one to prayer and meditation.

Geranium

Latin name: *Pelargonium graveoloens*

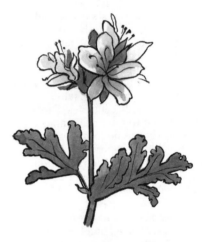

Description: Known as rose geranium to herbalists, this small, South African perennial is one of 600 varieties of scented geraniums that have been hybridized. The deep green essential oil produced from it is a relative newcomer because it was not distilled until the 19th century. The pharmaceutical industry uses the main chemical compound, geraniol, to make synthetic rose oil and to adulterate true rose oil.

Scent: The fragrance is an herblike combination of rose, with some citrus and a suggestion of wood.

Uses: Aromatherapists sum up the reaction to rose geranium as physically and emotionally "balancing." The scent is good for those who feel overly emotional and need more stability. Experimental clinics in Azbajian found it successful for this and also to stabilize blood pressure, increasing or lowering it a few points depending upon the individual needs. It also acts as a sedative to induce sleep. In cosmetics, it's suitable for all complexion types and is said to slow the skin's aging process. As a salve, cream, lotion, or massage oil, geranium essential oil treats a long list of skin problems and fights bacteria, viruses, and fungi. As a result, it is known to relieve inflammation, eczema, acne, burns, infected wounds, ringworm, lice, shingles, and herpes blisters. It also helps remove, or at least prevent, scarring and stretch marks. It's excellent for treating hormonally-related problems, such as PMS, menopause, and fluid retention. In its native Africa, the herb tea is used to stop diarrhea and internal bleeding.

Ginger

Latin name: *Zingiber officinale*

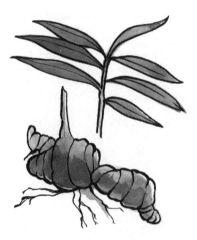

Description: Ginger grows in the tropics with tall, narrow leaves and a knotty root (botanically speaking, a *rhizome*). The root is used in cooking around the world and also distilled into a pale yellow essential oil that is used extensively in the food industry.

Scent: The scent is best described as peppery, sharp, pungent, aromatic, and warm, sometimes with a hint of camphor or lemon. You already know the aroma well if you have had ginger ale or ginger snap cookies or dined on Oriental food containing it.

Uses: Ginger is a multipurpose essential oil with a special knack for reducing inflammation. In a massage oil or liniment, its heating action relieves pain from arthritis or sore muscles, menstrual cramps, and headache. It also combats pain by delaying pain sensations from registering in the brain. Ginger stimulates both appetite and poor blood circulation and relieves nausea and motion sickness. It also acts as a sexual stimulant. For a sore throat, laryngitis, or lung and sinus congestion, try wrapping a warm ginger compress around the neck. Ginger also reduces drowsiness and irritability and jump starts the brain to keep concentration and mental energy high.

Helichrysum

Latin name: *Helichrysum angustifolium,* sometimes *Helichrysum orientale*

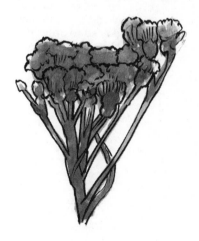

Description: This everlasting flower, also called everlast and immortelle, is a Mediterranean and North African native. Distilled from the flowers, the French oil is green while the less refined and less expensive Yugoslavian oil has an orange hue. A related species (*Helichrysum stoechas*) is extracted into an absolute.

Scent: The pleasant fragrance is spicy, sweet, almost fruity, and a little reminiscent of curry powder. (In fact, the common name is curry plant.)

Uses: Helichrysum stimulates production of new cells, so it's used in skin products to treat acne, scar tissue, bruising, mature skin, and burns. It also helps to prevent sunburn. It treats bacterial infection and inflammation and helps to boost the body's immune system. Its healing properties can quell a chronic cough, bronchitis, or fever, and it can alleviate pain by numbing nerve endings. It also lessens muscle pain, arthritis, enlarged veins, liver problems and counters allergic reactions like asthma. Its scent helps relieve depression, nervous exhaustion, and stress. With all this going for it, I am surprised that commercial products seldom use it. You may even have difficulty finding this oil in stores and need to order it through the mail. (I list mail-order companies in the Appendix.)

Jasmine

Latin name: *Jasminum officinalis* and *J. grandiflorum*

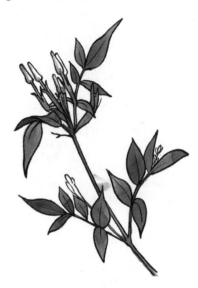

Description: Jasmine has captured the imagination of poets and been the mainstay of expensive perfumers for centuries. The flowers of the twining shrubs are responsible for its exquisite fragrance, which is solvent-extracted into an absolute from two of the dozens of different species. Probably an Iranian native, the most prized oil today comes from France and Italy, although about 80 percent is Egyptian. Synthetic jasmine is much cheaper but is also harsh, so it needs the addition of true jasmine oil to soften it.

Scent: The aroma is distinctively rich, warm, floral, and sweetly exotic. Jasmine's fragrance varies, and it sometimes has a fruity-tea undertone.

Uses: The scent sedates the nervous system, so it's good for jangled nerves, headaches, insomnia, and depression and for taking the emotional edge off PMS and menopause. Seventeenth-century herbalist Nicholas Culpeper recommended rubbing the oil into "hard, contracted limbs," and indeed, it eases muscle cramping, including menstrual cramps, when used in a massage oil. The essential oil is used in cosmetics for sensitive or mature, aging skin. In India, jasmine flowers are applied to difficult-to-heal sores. The scent stimulates brain waves and sharpens mental awareness. In one study, it allowed computer operators to reduce the number of mistakes they made by one-third. However, its age-old reputation is as an aphrodisiac.

Juniper Berry

Latin name: *Juniperus communis*

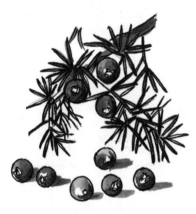

Description: The needles and berries from the prickly, large, evergreen bush offer the highest quality essential oil, although sometimes an inferior oil is made from the branches or from the "exhausted" berries that have already been distilled into gin. The wood also produces a thick, black juniper tar that was previously used in skin ointments.

Scent: Pungent, herbaceous, peppery, pinelike, and camphorlike, the lively scent of juniper is familiar to anyone who has ever sharpened a pencil, because pencils are made from this wood.

Uses: Juniper oil is used in massage oils, liniments, and baths because of its ability to treat the pain and inflammation of arthritis and rheumatism, varicose veins, and hemorrhoids by warming and thereby relaxing the muscles. It increases circulation and can also help release fluid retention during PMS and bladder infection. The essential oil helps the body eliminate metabolic waste by aiding the digestion process and easing nausea. Inhale it as a steam to relieve bronchial congestion, infection, and spasms. Sniffing the oil serves as a pick-me-up to counter tiredness and reduce anxiety. It is suitable in cosmetics for acne and eczema and in shampoos for greasy hair or dandruff. It repels wool moths.

Caution: It's not known for certain, but many herbalists say that juniper can overstimulate the kidneys, so do not use it if your kidneys are inflamed or infected.

Lavender

Latin name: *Lavandula angustifolia*

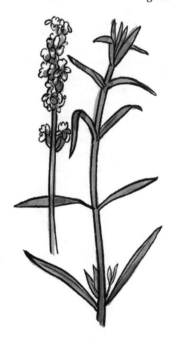

Description: The name of this well-loved Mediterranean herb comes from the Latin lavandus, meaning to wash, because the Romans added it to their bathing water. Lavender still remains the most popular scent for soap. A less expensive spike *(Lavendula latifolia)* and lavandin *(Lavendula intermedia)* are produced in greater quantities, but they have a more camphorlike and harsher scent, with inferior healing properties.

Scent: Lavender has a sweet, floral, but very herbal fragrance with balsamic undertones.

Uses: Among the safest of all essential oils, lavender is also one of the most antiseptic. This antiviral and antifungal oil treats lung, sinus, vaginal, and skin infections and reduces inflammation and relieves muscle pain and headaches. It is suitable for all complexion types and hastens the healing of skin cells, so it's used on burns, sun-damaged skin, wounds, and rashes. It also relieves the pain of injuries by numbing nerve endings. Lavender can be used to treat oily skin and acne and prevents scarring and stretch marks and reputedly slows the development of wrinkles. A lavender massage oil or bath improves digestion and boosts immunity. Of several fragrances tested by aromatherapy researchers, lavender was most effective at relaxing brain waves and reducing stress. It also eliminated almost one-quarter of computer errors made by office workers. Lavender acts as a sedative and an anti-depressant and can reduce the stress that causes asthma flare-ups. No wonder it is the most widely used aromatherapy oil!

Lemon

Latin name: *Citrus limonum*

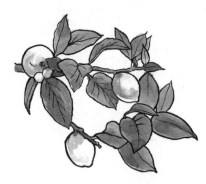

Description: The lemon tree hails from Asia, but has been cultivated in Italy since at least the 4th century. The essential oil is produced by cold-pressing the peel. (For descriptions of this and other forms of extracting essential oils, see Chapter 1.) Like other citruses, the oil keeps for only about a year unless you prolong its life by storing it in a cool place or even in the refrigerator.

Scent: Lemon carries a well-known citrus scent that is clean and sharp. The better the quality, the smoother the aroma.

Uses: Lemon is best known medicinally throughout the world as a remedy that relieves fevers, sore throat, coughs, and indigestion. Studies show that the essential oil counters a wide range of viral and bacterial infections and increases immune system activity by stimulating the production of the white corpuscles that fight infection. It is most often used in massage oil or as an aromatherapy steam. The massage oil also relieves lymph glands congested from infection and reduces bloating, and some say that it promotes weight loss. It also reduces inflammation and works particularly well at relaxing stiff muscles. Incorporated into cosmetics, lemon is best used on oily complexions and skin blemishes. It also regulates oily hair. After being researched, the scent is diffused through the air systems of some Japanese offices and factories to increase worker's concentration, ability to memorize, and cut the number of mistakes they make by half. One way it does so is to relax brain waves. Inhaling the scent also slightly lowers blood pressure and can be used as an antidepressant.

Caution: The essential oil of lemon is photosensitizing to the skin of a few people.

Lemongrass

Latin name: *Cymbopogon citratus*

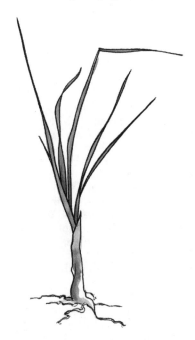

Description: This tall perennial grass is originally from India and Sri Lanka, but has found its way into the traditional cuisines throughout Southeast Asia. An

inexpensive essential oil, it is the source of most of the lemon scent found in cosmetics and hair preparations, soaps, perfumes, and deodorants. It also flavors processed foods. In fact, lemongrass is one of the bestselling essential oils in the world. The distilled oil is an amber-yellow color.

Scent: Rose and lemony, but herbal and slightly bitter. It gives Ivory soap its familiar scent.

Uses: Lemongrass essential oil is found most often in cosmetics such as hair conditioner, facial water, lotion, and vinegar for oily hair and skin. Added to water or vinegar and sprayed in the air, on a countertop, or along walls and floors (or on your pet!), it is an insect repellent and attacks fungi by discouraging mold growth. An antiseptic wash or compress is used on skin infections, especially ringworm and infected sores. According to researchers, it is more effective against staph infection than either penicillin or streptomycin. Other uses are to reduce headaches, indigestion pain, rheumatism, and nervousness. One of the ways in which lemongrass decreases the pain of the preceding ailments is by reducing the amount of pain sensations that reach the brain. It also numbs nerve endings, which dulls the intensity of the pain. The scent alone is used to decrease irritability and drowsiness.

Caution: The oil is nontoxic, but causes skin sensitivity in some people.

Marjoram

Latin name: *Origanum majorana,* formerly *Majorana hortensis*

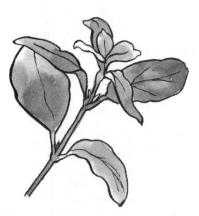

Description: The low, bushy perennial is native to Asia, but was naturalized in Europe where it was a favorite of the ancient Greeks, who named it "joy of the mountain." The greenish-yellow oil is distilled from the plant's flowering tops. The scent and properties are milder than the closely related and potentially toxic oregano *(Origanum vulgare).*

Scent: The sweet, herblike, pungent, sharp, and spicy scent has just a hint of camphor. It smells a lot like pizza, which contains marjoram as a seasoning.

Uses: Marjoram is a good sedative. Testing shows that it's one of the most effective fragrances to relax brain waves. A calming massage oil, the essential oil eases stiff joints and muscle spasms, including tics, excessive coughing, indigestion, menstrual cramps, and headaches, especially migraines. It slightly lowers high blood pressure and is known to penetrate pain. In a steam, compress, or vapor rub, it fights the viruses and bacteria responsible for colds, flu, and laryngitis. It's used in salves and creams to soothe burns, bruises, and inflammation.

I think of marjoram as a comfort oil, good for people who have been through a lot physically or emotionally, or both.

Melissa (Lemon balm)

Latin name: *Melissa officinalis*

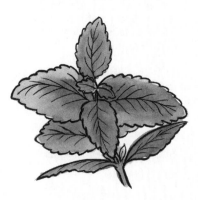

Description: Melissa, known to herbalists as lemon balm, is a southern European native. The essential oil is distilled from the leaves, but it's expensive because so little is produced. As a result, oil sold as melissa is often adulterated or replaced altogether with the far less costly lemon or citronella. A medieval favorite, it was the main ingredient in the famous "Carmelite Water," a combination of alcohol and essential oil that women splashed on their faces to ease nervous headaches and nerve pain, to improve their complexion, and also to sip when no one was looking.

Scent: The sweet smell is soft and distinctly lemon.

Uses: The 17th-century herbalist Gerard said that melissa "maketh the heart merry, joyful, strengtheneth the vital spirits." The scent is a sedative that helps reduce shock, distress, depression, nervousness, and insomnia. It also helps relax stiff, sore muscles, as well as calms the mind. The essential oil of melissa treats indigestion, lung congestion, and menstrual irregularities and slightly lowers high blood pressure. It reduces inflammation and fights viral infection such as strep throat, herpes blisters, and chicken pox, as well as fungal diseases.

Caution: Melissa can increase the effects of the sedative pentobarbital.

Myrrh

Latin name: *Commiphora myrrha*

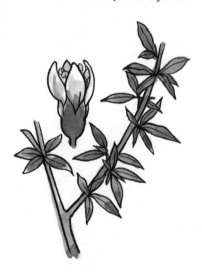

Description: Myrrh is a small, scrubby, spiny tree that is found in arid regions of the Middle East and North East Africa. For several thousand years, the valuable gum it exudes was an important trade item for use in cosmetics and incense and to inspire prayer and meditation. Despite its bitter taste, this deep, amber-colored oil distilled from the gum is used in toothpastes and gum preparations as an antiseptic to heal mouth ulcers, gum inflammation, and infection.

Scent: The aroma is warm, spicy, and bitter, with smoky and musky undertones.

Uses: Myrrh's essential oil is a strong antiseptic and fights viral and fungal infections. A salve containing it effectively treats eczema, bruises, infection, athlete's foot, and difficult-to-heal wounds. Myrrh also reduces the swelling of infection and can even hasten the healing of infections by increasing the production of white blood cells. It is used on varicose veins, chapped, cracked, aged skin, candida (thrush), and herpes blisters. Its moisturizing properties work well to treat dry hair. A remedy for mouth and gum diseases, it's found in gargles, mouthwash, and toothpaste. It activates the immune system, so lozenges or a syrup containing myrrh is good for coughs, colds, and flu. There is some evidence that it helps to regulate an overactive thyroid and that it increases menstrual flow. To top it all off, myrrh's essential oil works as an aphrodisiac.

Caution: Due to it possibly increasing thyroid activity, do not use myrrh on a continuous basis if you have an overactive thyroid.

Myrtle

Latin name: *Myrtus communis*

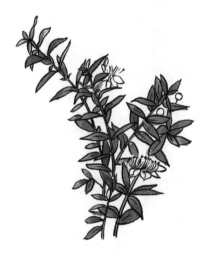

Description: This small, attractive North African tree now grows throughout the Mediterranean. It was a favorite in the ancient gardens of Baghdad, Grananda, and Damascus. The Greeks and Romans honored poets with myrtle leaves to symbolize that their fame would never die. It was the main ingredient in a 16th-century complexion water called "Angel Water." The essential oil is distilled from the leaves and twigs, and sometimes the flowers are included.

Scent: The scent is spicy and slightly camphorlike.

Uses: The essential oil of myrtle is an antiseptic that is particularly useful in treating lung and respiratory infections. It also relaxes muscle spasms and takes the inflammation out of hemorrhoids and enlarged surface veins. The oil also has the ability to calm and relax the mind, as well as increase the libido. It is useful in cosmetics for oily complexions and acne.

Neroli or Orange blossom

Latin name: *Citrus aurantium*

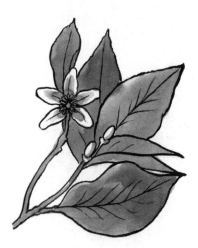

Description: The tree that produce flowers for this essential oil, the bitter orange, is a different species from the sweet orange. The name *neroli* is used for the blossoms of the bitter by perfumers and aromatherapists. It is said to have been named after a 16th-century princess from Nerola, Italy, who loved the scent of orange blossom. Petitgrain *(Citrus aurantium),* which means "little fruit," is a less expensive essential oil that is made from the twigs, leaves and small immature fruit of the same tree. Its scent is less elegant and more herb-like, but it also costs much less than neroli.

Scent: The scent is bittersweet, floral, spicy, and quite strong until it is diluted.

Uses: Neroli's favored use is to regenerate skin cells and to tone mature, dry, and sensitive skin, although its healing properties are appropriate for all skin types. It helps circulation problems, especially hemorrhoids, and reduces high blood pressure. I find it one of the best of the aromatherapy antidepressants, although it is also one of the most expensive. It may seem contradictory, but this oil both stimulates brain waves and has sedative properties to relax the body. The cost of products that contain reflect the oil's value. A by-product of distilling orange blossoms, "orange flower water" is the main ingredient of the original eau de cologne, which was used both as a body fragrance and as a skin toner. Not surprisingly, this sweet-smelling aroma also doubles as an aphrodisiac.

Orange

Latin name: *Citrus sinensis*

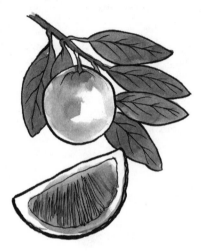

Description: The orange tree was brought to the Mediterranean from Asia by the Saracens during the Crusades. It now grows in Sicily, Israel, Spain, and the United States, with the essential oil having different characteristics depending upon the country of origin. The essential oil is cold-pressed from the orange fruit peel from the sweet orange tree.

Scent: The perky, lively scent is distinctively scent of the orange that is eaten as fruit — which this is.

Uses: Although not as antiseptic as lemon, orange essential oil still combats flu and colds. A massage oil eases indigestion and overcomes a light case of insomnia or depression. The scent of orange reduces anxiety and slightly lowers high blood pressure.

Caution: The essential oil is only slightly photosensitizing, but go easy in baths or any skin preparations because it can burn the skin — just 4 drops in a bath tub can irritate and redden sensitive skin. Related essential oils from tangerine or mandarin *(Citrus reticulata)* make a milder and safer choice for pregnant women and very young children.

Patchouli

Latin name: *Pogostemon cablin*

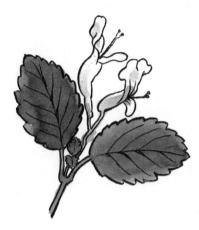

Description: The succulent leaves of this pretty, East Indian bush carry little indication of their potential, because the scent is developed by exposure to air while the leaves are drying and aged. Even after being distilled, the harsh, translucent yellow oil must age to a syrupy brown before it develops a rich patchouli scent.

Scent: Patchouli's scent is quite heavy, earthy, musty, and penetrating. It is the fragrance in many famous perfumes, including Tabu and Shocking.

Uses: The oil rejuvenates skin cell, so it's used on mature, aging skin and also treats dry skin prone to acne problems. It is also antiseptic and antifungal on skin problems, such as eczema, inflamed or cracked skin, and athlete's foot. In India, it is even a traditional treatment for snakebite and poisonous insect stings. The aroma reduces appetite and relieves headaches. As a hair conditioner, it helps eliminate dandruff. It repels wool moths and other insects.

As a "fixative," it retains the scent in pot-pourri, perfume, and other fragrant products. It's also an aphrodisiac.

Pepper, Black
Latin name: *Piper nigrum*

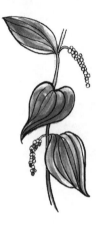

Description: This climbing shrub from India supplies the black (or white) pepper in your peppercorn shaker used for seasoning. The essential oil is distilled from the unripe fruits for extensive use in prepared foods and a pinch in perfumery.

Scent: Pepper's pungent and spicy scent, along with its hot taste, is so well-known that we pepper our conversation with comparisons. It also has a warm, herbaceous aroma that is often not detected because sniffing pepper is more likely to make you sneeze before you detect this.

Uses: Use pepper in a chest rub during a cold or flu to counter congestion and infection. It improves poor circulation and helps to heat up tight muscles and sore joints when used in a liniment. It improves digestion and appetite and eating the peppercorn itself aids digestion by increasing production of stomach acid. Sniffing it is definitely a stimulating experience and the scent has a

reputation as an aphrodisiac. Inhaling steam containing black pepper essential oil can help relieve physical and anxiety symptoms of withdrawal from smoking tobacco.

Caution: Although nontoxic, pepper can redden and irritate your skin if you use too much.

Peppermint
Latin name: *Mentha piperita*

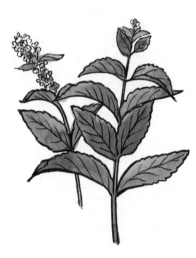

Description: Peppermint is a creeping herb with fragrant leaves that make a popular tea. It's used in beverages, ice cream, sauces and jellies, liqueurs, medicines, dental preparations, cleaners, cosmetics, tobacco, desserts, and chewing gums.

Scent: The minty-fresh and slightly camphorlike scent of peppermint is familiar to many because it's used in gum and candy and is one of the most popular herbal teas.

Uses: Peppermint essential oil as a massage oil over the abdomen relaxes the muscles to help in the digestion of heavy meals and relieves flatulence, cramping, nausea, and specific disorders such as irritable bowel syndrome. It is a warming oil, so it's found in most liniments to relieve painful muscle spasms and arthritic conditions. Peppermint oil relieves the itching of ringworm, herpes blisters, scabies, and poison oak and ivy and stimulates oil production in dry skin and hair. Many bacterial, fungal, and viral infections are destroyed by it and when inhaled or when a vapor balm is rubbed on the chest, it clears sinus and lung congestion. The scent is energizing, and historically, it was said to be an aphrodisiac.

Caution: At first, peppermint feels cooling, but watch out — too much can burn. Although peppermint is good for nausea, use a mint tea instead of the essential oil if you're pregnant.

Pine

Latin name: *Pinus* species

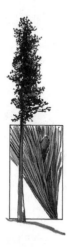

Description: The Pine is a stately tree that graces many North American forests and is found throughout most of the world. Several of the many different species are distilled. Common species used to produce the oil are *palustris, abies,* and the Scotch pine, *sylvestris.*

Scent: Pine's fresh, pungent smell is easy to imagine if you've ever been in a pine forest. Perhaps unfortunately, most people's associate pine with cleaning solution or paint (because it's also used to make turpentine).

Uses: Pine is popular in cleaning solutions. It's also in European bath preparations to increase circulation and for its fresh, invigorating scent. The scent is stimulating to the senses and the species of pine called sylvestris is used in massage and body oils to help counter adrenal gland insufficiency. Because it's sharper and less sweet than the fir tree of Christmas tree fame, fir is usually preferred in an aromatherapy blend that needs a forestlike scent. However, as a disinfectant and an infection fighter, pine can't be beat. It's also very good in a penetrating liniment for sore muscles or joints.

Rose

Latin name: *Rosa damascena, R. gallica,* and other species

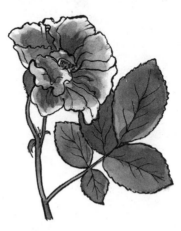

Description: Originally from Asia Minor, Turkish merchants brought rose bushes to Bulgaria where the most valued essential oil is now produced. Due to the small yield from distillation and the

care required to cultivate the bushes, the essential oil is expensive, so it's used in costly perfumes. Not all of the oil separates during distillation, so a highly scented rose water is a by-product of the process. The oil congeals to a waxy thickness when the temperature is cool.

Scent: Intense, sweet, and floral. The fragrance inspires poets such as the Greek poetess Sappho, who christened it "queen of flowers."

Uses: Suitable for all complexion types, rose essential oil is a cell rejuvenator, an antiseptic, and an anti-inflammatory that is used in skin creams and lotions to soothe and heal various skin conditions and cuts and burns and to reduce swelling. Due to these properties and its wonderful scent, rose is used in many facial-care products. In addition, it can be inhaled by asthmatics, and it relieves a variety of female problems, including menstrual cramps and PMS symptoms. Sniffing the oil or using a rose massage oil has been suggested to reverse impotency, but it's more likely to be used by women to lessen moodiness during menopause. The scent is also used as an aphrodisiac, an antidepressant, a sedative, and a stress reliever. And if that weren't enough, it also stimulates brain waves to keep the mind focused and alert.

Rosemary
Latin name: *Rosmarinus officinalis*

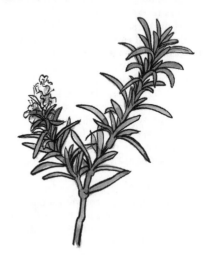

Description: Rosemary's name is derived from *rosmarinus,* which means "dew of the sea." It is cultivated worldwide, but France, Spain, and Tunisia are the main essential oil producers.

Scent: The scent is herbaceous, woody, sharp, and camphorlike.

Uses: Japanese researchers have preliminary evidence that rosemary improves memory, as Shakespeare's character says, "There's rosemary for remembrance." It is also a stimulant to the nervous system that increases energy. Rosemary aids in the assimilation of enzymes that break down food in the stomach and helps the lymphatic system eliminate waste from the body. It also reduces the discomfort of nausea. In a massage oil, liniment, compress, or bath, the essential oil improves poor circulation and eases and penetrates muscle and rheumatic pain. Rubbing a rosemary vapor balm on the chest relieves lung and sinus congestion. Cosmetically, it encourages dry, mature skin to produce its own oil and also treats acne for those with dry skin. It also helps get rid of canker sores and other viruses. Add it to hair conditioners for dandruff and hair loss and to keep it healthy.

Caution: Rosemary can be too stimulating and may increase blood pressure.

Sandalwood

Latin name: *Santalum album*

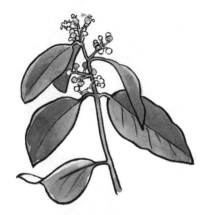

Description: One of the oldest perfume materials, sandalwood essential oil has been in use at least 2,000 years. Parasitic on surrounding trees for its first seven years, the oil is not distilled from the roots and heartwood until the tree is at least 30 years old. Mysore, India, produces the best quality oil, which is grown in plantations and regulated by the government, but a usually inferior oil from a different species of sandalwood tree (*Santalum spicatum*) is available from Indonesia and Australia.

Scent: Soft, warm, woody, and balsamic.

Uses: Sandalwood is a major remedy in Ayurvedic medicine, where its most important uses is to sedate the nervous system, subduing nervousness, anxiety, and insomnia and reducing nerve pain. Researchers found that it even relaxes brain waves. Suitable for all complexion types, the antifungal and bacteria-fighting oil is useful on rashes, inflammation, acne, and dry, dehydrated, or chapped skin. Sandalwood also repairs skin damage and encourages new cell growth. It increases the production of white blood cells to help the body rid itself of infection and aids with digestion. As a massage oil, it can be rubbed over reproductive organs, bladder infections, and on hemorrhoids. A sandalwood syrup or chest balm helps relieve persistent coughs and sore throat. The oil also is a fixative that retains the scent in potpourri, perfume, and other fragrant products. Cosmetically, it both moisturizes dry hair and regulates oily hair Sandalwood is known to be an effective aphrodisiac.

Tea Tree

Latin name: *Melaleuca alternifolia*

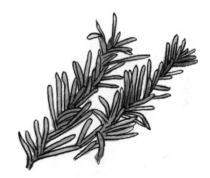

Description: The leaves of this medium-size Australian tree look similar to its relative, the eucalyptus. Its interesting bark peels off the trunk, giving tea tree the nickname "paper-bark" tree. With at least 300 species and subspecies, several different ones probably are sold as tea tree oil. Other oils that are produced are the harsher, less expensive cajeput (*Melaleuca cajuputi*) and the sweeter niaouli (*Melaleuca viridiflora*), which aromatherapists consider more effective on viral infections such as herpes blisters.

Scent: The sharp and camphorlike scent is very similar to eucalyptus. Many people say it smells "medicinal." You will know it if you run into poor quality oil; it smells like melted rubber.

Uses: The essential oil is an all-purpose antiseptic whose use is supported by medical studies. It's effective against bacteria, fungi, and viruses, including those that cause flu, colds, herpes blisters, shingles, candida, thrush, and chicken pox. As a bonus, it stimulates the immune system and increases the production of white blood cells. It is mostly used to treat mouth, urinary tract, and vaginal infections, but it hastens the healing of wounds, diaper rash, acne, and insect bites. It protects the skin from radiation burns, encourages the regeneration of scar tissue, and reduces swelling. The presence of blood and pus from infection increase its antiseptic properties. Use it in compresses, salves, massage oil, and aromatherapy washes. Cosmetically, it can be found in shampoos and skin care products as an oil-controlling agent.

Thuja

Latin name: *Thuja occidentalis*

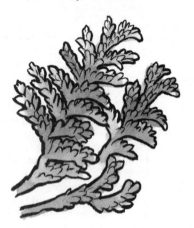

Description: Known as cedar leaf or arborvitae, the essential oil is distilled from the leaves, twigs, or bark of this small, evergreen tree.

Uses: Thuja essential oil is one of the best natural remedies to eliminate warts. In a massage oil, it also treats conditions involving congestion of blood in the pelvic region, enlarged prostate, and urinary infections.

Caution: Thuja contains compound thujene and thujone, which irritant skin and act on the nervous system, so it should not be used by anyone who is prone to seizures. Use it only in small amounts.

Thyme

Latin name: *Thymus vulgaris*

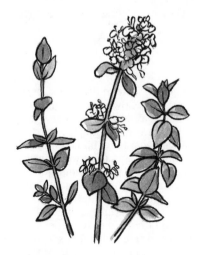

Description: This fragrant, culinary ground cover has at least a hundred varieties. Most thyme essential oil is produced from the common thyme that is used to season foods. The oil is red after it is distilled once, but a second distillation yields a clear oil that has removed the color. Both thyme oils are available.

Scent: The herbaceous, strong, hot, and sharp fragrance led Rudyard Kipling to write of the "wind-bit thyme that smells like the perfume of the dawn in paradise." Ancient Greeks complimented each other by saying that one smelled of thyme.

Uses: The essential oil is used in a compress, salve, or cream to fight or to prevent serious viral or fungal infection from a wound, gum, or mouth infection. The compound thymol, which is in the essential oil, is one of the strongest antiseptics known. It increases the production of white blood cells in the body, relieves indigestion, and, when used in a liniment, can warm and relax sore muscles. It is an ingredient in numerous drugstore gargles, mouthwashes, cough drops, and vapor chest rubs. These products include Listerine mouthwash and Vick's VapoRub.

Caution: Thyme essential oil can irritate the skin and mucus membranes as well as increase blood pressure, so use it in low doses. Red thyme oil is even stronger than the white, so it's rarely used, except to increase the heat of a liniment. Both thyme oils should not be used by pregnant women or children. Thyme does destroy intestinal worms, but the essential oil should never be taken internally. Instead, use the herb in the form of a tea or tincture.

Valerian

Latin name: *Valeriana officinalis*

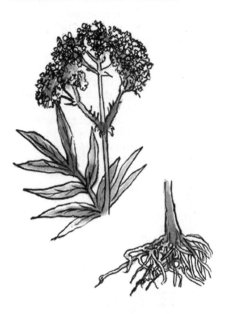

Description: The tall, thin stalks bear a round flower head of small, pink-white flowers. Well over 100 species of valerian are native to North America, Europe, India, and the Far East. Each has a little different chemistry makeup and so also a slightly different scent. An oil that smells more woodsy is available from the Japanese "kesso root" and also from the Indian valerian *(Valeriana wallichi).* Another commercial essential oil that's closely related to valerian is spikenard *(Nardosachus jatamansi).* (When you compare their scents, you can tell the resemblance.) The essential oil is either distilled or solvent-extracted.

Scent: Valerian's scent is nose-wrinkling potent — enough to have it compared to the smell of old socks. Surprisingly, valerian's used as an earthy, forest fragrance in soaps and colognes, as well as tobacco, soft drinks, and liqueurs, but only in very small amounts.

Uses: Similar to drinking a tea made from the roots, the scent alone of valerian has a sedative effect, so it's used to treat nervous conditions, headaches, insomnia, muscle pain, tension, and some forms of anxiety. You need to use a light hand in aromatherapy blends. Perhaps that's why it's not as popular as some other sedative essential oils, although it is one of the most effective. Valerian (which contains a chemistry similar to catnip) also attracts cats and rats (and, I discovered, gophers!). It's thought that valerian in the pockets of the historic Pied Piper of Hamelin, not music, is what caused the rats to follow him out of the city.

Vanilla

Latin Name: *Vanilla planifolia*

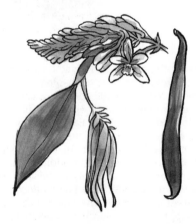

Description: This tropical orchid is a Mexican native that is now also grown in Tahiti, Java, and Madagascar. The essential oil is extracted from the vanilla bean with solvents into a thick, dark brown absolute. There is a variety of different-smelling essential oils, but it takes a good quality to obtain a true vanilla fragrance.

Scent: Vanilla's sweet, honeylike, and distinct scent is familiar to people worldwide from its popular use as a food flavoring. Researchers found that the scent is the closest to mother's milk.

Uses: The healing attributes of vanilla's fragrance are emotional, producing feelings of happiness and pleasant childhood memories. It also doubles as an aphrodisiac, depending upon what other essential oils are blended with it.

Vetivert

Latin name: *Vetiveria zizanoides*

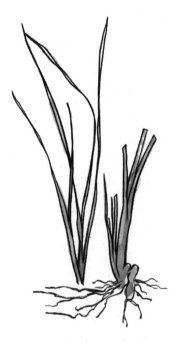

Description: Vetivert, also called vetiver, is a clump of thin, grasslike leaves. Its roots are spindly, but intensely aromatic. In India, they are woven into fans and screens called tatties for doors and windows. These are sprinkled with water on hot days to cool the air and so that the breeze blows the scent through the room. (An inferior oil is made from the used screens!) India inspired the famous British vetivert colognes and perfumes of the 19th century.

Scent: Heavy, bitter, and very earthy, some people bluntly say that the smell of vetivert resembles dirt. Many find the scent unappealing, but the oil is a crucial ingredient in fine perfumes where its heaviness brings out the sweet smell of other essential oils.

Uses: Vetivert's essential oil is used to heal acne, wounds, and cracked and excessively dry skin. It is also helpful for notably dry hair and to regulate oily hair. It helps fight bacteria and other infections by increasing the production of the body's white blood cells. The scent is relaxing and an antidepressant. The East Indians say that it cools the mind, as well as the body, of excessive heat. In a lotion or massage oil, it eases muscular pain, sprains, and stimulates circulation. In addition, it's used in conditions of liver congestion. A scent fixative, it retains its fragrance for a long time and is used in small amounts to keep the scent in perfumes and other aromatic products.

Ylang Ylang

Latin name: *Cananga odorata*

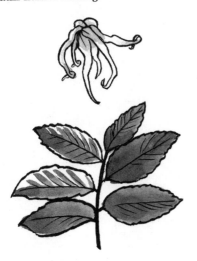

Description: The tall ylang ylang tree originated in the Philippines, but is now grown throughout tropical Asia for the perfume trade and even used as a flavoring in beverages and desserts. The name, meaning "flower of flowers," describes the sweet, yellow blooms, which produce the essential oil. The oil varies greatly due to climatic and botanical differences. As a result, you can find several commercial grades with distinctly different smells.

Scent: The scent is intensely sweet, heady, floral, slightly spicy, with overtone of narcissus or banana. Most people prefer it blended with other scents to mellow its intensity.

Uses: Aromatherapists find that ylang ylang is one of the most relaxing fragrances to both mind and body. It also slightly lowers blood pressure and serves as a natural antidepressant. However, studies show that the scent is both stimulating and relaxing to brain waves, and also is known for its aphrodisiac properties. Like many natural remedies, it seems to energize or relax one, depending upon the individual's needs. Use it in a bath or massage oil or simply sniff it when you need to completely chill out or when you experience insomnia. It balances oil production when used as a hair conditioner, and people in the Philippines and tropical Asia use it to protect their hair from the damages of swimming in salt water. It's good for all skin types, but especially those with combination skin.

Caution: High concentrations can produce headaches or nausea, so use lightly.

Part V
The Appendix

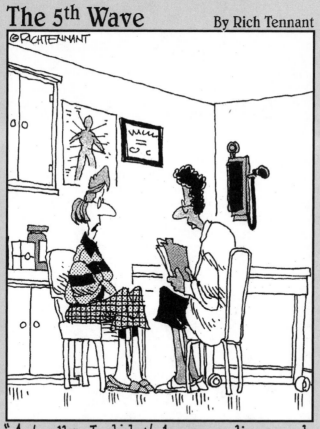

The 5th Wave   By Rich Tennant

"Actually, I didn't become dizzy and nauseous until I started inhaling the scent strips in the waiting room magazines."

In this part

In case aromatherapy is a new subject to you, the
Appendix comes in might handy. You can use the
extensive resource guide for buying aromatherapy products or the materials to make them, locating education
seminars, and getting whatever else is important in your
exploration of aromatherapy.

Appendix

Aromatherapy Resources

· ·

*N*ow that I've convinced you about the benefits and pleasures of using aromatherapy, you're certainly ready to try it out. To help you find just what you need, this resource section contains places to go where you can find out more (including aromatherapy tours) about aromatherapy and discover companies that sell their products through the mail. I also list organizations, aromatherapy publications, and a selection of the best Web sites. It's worth the price of the book just to have this great guide! If you want to know which seminars and conferences I'm involved with, check out my author bio at the front of this book.

Aromatherapy Educational Opportunities

Here are some places where you can find reliable aromatherapy education.

Organizations

National Association for Holistic Aromatherapy (NAHA)
836 Hanley Industrial Court
St. Louis, MO 63144
888-ASK-NAHA
www.naha.org

This national organization is composed of aromatherapy businesses and professionals and is open to everyone (annual dues are $45 or $100 professional). Membership includes a subscription to the quarterly *Scentsitivity* magazine and a copy of their Source/Practitioner Directory. They also sponsor a conference (see the section "Aromatherapy conferences").

American Herb Association (AHA)
PO Box 1673
Nevada City, CA 95959
530-265-9552
www.jps.net/ahaherb.com

This group covers herbalism and aromatherapy in its American Herb Association Quarterly Newsletter. Membership ($20 annual) is open to everyone. AHA also offers a Directory of Herbal and Aromatherapy Education in North America ($3.50) and a Directory of Mail-Order Herbal and Aromatherapy Products ($4).

United Plant Savers
PO Box 420
East Barre, VT 05649
802-479-9825

Not aromatherapy specifically, but a worthwhile cause started by herbalists to save healing plants, fragrant and otherwise. The group has a newsletter to keep you posted on the status of North American herbs.

Worldwide aromatherapy organizations

These organizations supply lists of qualified aromatherapists (some charge for this). Most provide information on training courses. Please send a large stamped envelope with all inquiries.

Aromatherapy Organizations Council
(Umbrella organization for the U.K.)
3 Latymer Close
Baraybrooke
Market Harborough
Leicester, LE16 8LN
United Kingdom
0185-843-4242

Aromatherapy Trades Council
P.O. Box 38
Romford
Essex RM1 2DN
United Kingdom
0170-239-0625

The International Federation of Aromatherapists
1/390 Burnwood Road
Hawthorne
Melbourne, Victoria 3122
Australia
612-819-2502

New Zealand Register of Holistic Aromatherapists
9-5242-198
e-mail: nzaromas@xtra.co.nz

Aromatherapy conferences

Wholistic Aromatherapy Conference
Pacific Institute of Aromatherapy
PO Box 6723
San Rafael, CA 94903
415-479-9121

Annual fall conference in San Francisco, California.

The World of Aromatherapy
National Association of Holistic Aromatherapy
836 Hanley Industrial Court
St. Louis, MO 63144
888-ASK NAHA

Bi-annual, fall conference in a different location every year.

Aromatherapy tours

The Aromatic Plant Project
219 Carl St.
San Francisco, CA 94117

On-site distillation workshops to make hydrosols with Jeanne Rose scheduled throughout the summer. The project promotes the growing and distillation of plants and public education about the usefulness of hydrosols and has a newsletter, *AROMAtherapy 2037.*

Fragrant Harvest
Harlalka 801 Park Way
El Cerrito, CA 94530
members.aol.com/somanath/fragrant.html

Christopher McMahon with Ramakant Harlalka of Bombay lead two small tours a year to India to explore its aromatic traditions. They're working throughout India and in Oman setting up essential oils distillers to help small farmers learn how to distill high quality essential oils and hydrosols. Profits from tours support the project.

Aromatherapy Institute & Research Aroma Camp
P.O. Box 2354
Fair Oaks, CA 95628
916-965-7546

Aroma Tours
105 Queens Parade, Clifton Hill
3068, Victoria, Australia
3-9481-1933
www.dbm.com.au/aroma

Tours of the lavender fields and processing plants in Provence, France.

Australasian College of Herbal Studies
Dorene Peterson
PO Box 57
Lake Oswego, OR 97034
503-635-6652

Tours of Provence, France, including instructional workshops.

The Turkey Rose Pilgrimage
The Ol-Factory
91 Front St.
Sowerby Thirsk
UK YO7 IJP
1845-523-452

Aromatherapy publications

The Aromatic Thymes
18-4 East Dundee Road, Suite 200
Barrington, IL 60010
847-526-0456

Sensitivity Newsletter
(National Association for Holistic Aromatherapy)
836 Hanley Industrial Court
St. Louis, MO 63144
314-963-2071

The Aromatherapy Quarterly (USA)
P.O. Box 421
Inverness, CA 94937-0421
415-663-9519

The Aromatherapy Quarterly (UK)
5 Ranelagh Ave.
London, SW13 0BY
United Kingdom
0181-392-1691

Aromatherapy Times
Stanford House
2-4 Chiswick High Road
London, W4 1TH
United Kingdom
0181-742-2605

International Journal of Aromatherapy
P.O. Box 746
Hove
East Sussex, BN3 3XA
United Kingdom
0127-377-2479

Aromatherapy World
ISPA House
82 Ashby Road
Hinckley
Leicester, LE 10 1SN
United Kingdom
0145-563-7987

Perfumer and Flavorist
The Journal of Essential Oil Research
Allured Publishing
362 South Schmlae Rd.
Carol Stream, IL 60188
708-653-2155

Worldwide education opportunities

The Institute of Traditional Herbal Medicine and Aromatherapy
12 Prentices Lane
Woodbridge
Suffolk IP12 4LF
United Kingdom
0139-438-8386

The Tisserand Institute (also sells aromatherapy products)
65 Church Road
Hove
East Sussex BN3 2BD
United Kingdom
0127-332-5666
www.tisserand.com

The International Society of Professional Aromatherapists
ISPA House
82 Ashby Road
Hinckley
Leicester, LE 10 1SN
United Kingdom
0145-563-7987

International Federation of Aromatherapists
Stanford House
2-4 Chiswick High Road
London, W4 1TH
United Kingdom
0181-742-2605

The Register of Qualified Aromatherapists
52 Barrack Lane
Aldwick, Bognor Regis
West Sussex PO21 4DD
United Kingdom
0124-326-2035

Aromatherapy schools and seminars

Amrita's Foundation for Aromatherapy Research & Education
Sheryl Ryan
1900 W. Stone Ave.
Fairfield, IA 52556
515-469-6190

Ann Berwick Aromatherapy
Box 4996
Boulder, CO 80306

Artemis Institute of Natural Therapies
Peter Holmes
PO Box 1824
Boulder, CO 80306
303-443-9289

Blue Sky Foundation
Kathi Keville, instructor
220 Oak St.
Grafton, WI 53024
414-376-1011

Aromatherapy Institute & Research
Victoria Edwards
Box 2354
Fair Oaks, CA 95628
916-965-7546
leydet.com

Aromatherapy Studies Course
Jeanne Rose
219 Carl St.
San Francisco, CA 94117
415-564-6785

The Atlantic Institute of Aromatherapy
Sylla Hanger
16018 Saddlestring Drive
Tampa, FL 33618
813-265-2222

Australasian College of Herbal Studies
Dorene Peterson
PO Box 57
Lake Oswego, OR 97034
800-487-8839
www.herbrf.com
(Correspondence course)

Center for Holistic Botanical Studies
Susanne Wissell
Box 4015
Westford, MA 01886
978-692-7880

College of Botanical Healing Arts
Elizabeth Jones
1821 17th Ave.
Santa Cruz, CA 95062
831-462-1807

The Institute of Dynamic Aromatherapy
Jade Shutes
Unit 98, 936 Peace Portal Drive
Blaine, WA 98231
800-260-7401

Institute of Integrative Aromatherapy
Valerie Cooksley
PO Box 18
Issaquah, WA 98027
887 FMEDICA

Michael Scholes
1830 S. Robertson Blvd. #203
Los Angeles, CA 90035
800-677-2368

Mindy Green
4133 Amber St.
Boulder, CO
303-447-9552

Morris Institute of Natural Therapies
Mercedes Hnizdo
3108 RT 10 West
Denville, NJ 07834
201-989-8939

Natural Healing Institute of Naturopathy
PO Box 230294
Encinitas, CA 92023
800-599-Heal (4325)

Pacific Institute of Aromatherapy
Kurt Schnaubelt
PO Box 6723
San Rafael, CA 94903
415-479-9121

Oak Valley Herb Farm
Kathi Keville
PO Box 2482
Nevada City, CA 95959
www.jps.net/ahaherb.com

West Wind School of Aromatherapy
17 Leslie St.
PO Box 133
Toronto, Ontario M4M 3H9
416-466-9670

Web Sites

Purdue University has an incredible site for researching the practical dimensions of growing aromatic and medicinal crops. It's a treasure house of information on this subject: newcrop.hort.edu/newcrop/default.html

JP Manheimer's essential oil calendar contains extensive information about the seasonal harvest of aromatic crops around the world: `www.manheimer.com/html/cropchar.htm`

This site explores perfume products of the ancient world, especially the Middle East and Southeast Asia: `sarasvati.simple.net.com/dictionary/000perfumeproducts.htm`

The following is a nice site with basic information about aromatherapy: `www.geocities.com/~aromaWeb`

This gem of a Web site from Dr. James Duke is for folks deeply interested in the ethnobotanical uses and phytochemical constituents of aromatic and medicinal plants: `www.ars-grin.gov/duk/index.html`

You can find exquisite botanical illustrations of many aromatic and medicinal plants at this site: `www.mobot.org/MOBOT/research/library/kohler/taxa.html`

This is one of the finest sites existing with in-depth information on spices and their uses: `www-ang.krunigraz.ac.at/~katzer/engl`

This database contains an extraordinary amount of useful research information about a great variety of aromatic and medicinal plants. It's an excellent research site: `www.scs.leeds.ac.uk/pfaf/D_intro.html`

This nice site from Frontier Herb Company contains a great deal of information on aromatherapy-related subjects: `www.frontierherb.com/aromatherapy`

Graham Sorenson's site from Frontier Herb Companycontains a good deal of information on aromatherapy and aromatherapy links: `www.fragrant.demon.co.uk`

Christopher McMahon's Web site is devoted almost entirely to India's aromatic traditions, ancient and modern. It contains a wealth of information on individual fragrant plants, descriptions of aromatic explorations of India, and fragrance-related Web links: `members.aol.com/somanath/fragrant.html`

Aromatherapy Items You Can Purchase

The following are mail-order companies that I've carefully selected because they offer products made with pure, natural essential oils — something that you don't always find even when you shop in a natural-food store.

Keep in mind the following when you're looking at these listings:

- ✔ I indicate which companies export products with an asterisk. You can order from these places even if you live in another country.

- ✔ www is the first letters indicating a company's Web site on the World Wide Web. Use the Web site to locate them if you're computer's hooked up to the Internet. Most companies with a Web site list their catalog, and many times you can order directly through your computer.

Essential oils

Elizabeth Van Buren, Inc.
303 Potrero St. #33
Santa Cruz, CA 95060
800-710-7759

Quality essential oils, individually (including a starter kit) and therapeutic (dieting, menopause, PMS, sports, and so on), and emotional blends are available. You can find scented body lotions and massage oils, plus unscented ones to add your own oils, and an aroma lamp and candle. Its partner is Spectrix, who is available to analyze essential oils for purity.

Flower Essence Society
PO Box 459
Nevada City, CA 95959
530-265-9170

These folks sell essential oils and their own line of flower essences, in some cases, combined together as in their four Seasons of the Soul body oils, which also contain herbs.

JPT Aromatherapy
1901 Brule St.
South Lake Tahoe, CA 95150
888-278-7364

Essential oils (many organically grown), massage and vegetable oils, 40 floral waters, four types of diffusers, and aroma lockets are available.

Original Swiss Aromatics
PO Box 6723
San Rafael, CA 94903
415-479-9121

These quality essential oils are produced exclusively for aromatherapy rather than the industrial market. This company also has products designed for individual skin types.

Oshadhi USA
1340 G Industrial Ave.
Petaluma, CA 94952
888-OSHADHI
www.oshadhiusa.com

This company offers an extensive selection of high quality essential oils (some organically grown) and nearly 100 very nice blends. They also sell colognes, body oils, aftershave, and three electric diffuser models.

Simpler's Botanical Co.
PO Box 2534
Sebastopol, CA 95473
800-6 JASMIN
www.botanical.com/mtrose

This line of essential oils includes a number of organically grown oils. The geranium and lavender hydrosols produced in Northern California's wine country are out of this world. They also sell organically grown lavender from Provence, France, and herbal tinctures and salves.

Snow Lotus*
PO Box 1824
Boulder, CO 80306
800-682-8827
www.snowlotus.org

The selection of essential oils (some organically grown) includes some unusual ones, such as rhododendron, tagette, and may chang. They also carry six hydrosols.

White Lotus Aromatics
801 Park Way
El Cerrito, CA 94530
fax: 510-527-2138
members.aol.com/somanath/fragrant.html

This exclusive line of quality essential oils are direct from distillers, mostly in India. A price list is $2, refundable with order.

Aromatherapy products

California Baby
217 S. Linden Drive
Beverly Hills, CA 90212
310-277-6430

The baby oil bubble bath (complete with a bubble blower), shampoo, and powder contain decyl polyglucose as an alternative to sodium lauryl sulfate. A set of bath drops are designed for increasing immunity, easing a cold, or relieving crankiness.

Essena Aromatherapy
Los Angeles, CA
323-655-5950
InBeauty.com and BeautyJungle.com

This is a full line of natural aromatherapy facial care products for salons and spas. (Facials are given at their full service salon in Los Angeles, California.)

Essensa*
230 West 41st St. #1600
New York, NY 10036
800-932-0168
www.essensa.com

This complete line of facial care products use herbal extracts and natural essential oils. They also give seminars for spa professionals.

Essential Oil Products
5633 Paradise Drive
Corte Madera, CA 94925
800-570-3775
www.eoproducts.com

The shampoo, conditioner, shower gel, and hand cream in elegant, blue plastic bottles are wonderfully scented with lemon verbena essential oil and offer milder alternative to sodium lauryl sulfate. The golden citrus lip balm contains healing carrot seed oil and goldenseal. An aromatherapy Foot Care Kit has foot salts, balm, and a scrub.

Herbal Health, Inc.
Box 330411
Fort Worth, TX 76163
www.aromahealthTexas.com

Essential oils and flower essences are sold separately and in combination. Many flowers that aren't available as natural essential oils, such as gardenia, lilac, and magnolia, along with five different antique roses, are extracted into alcohol. The hydrosols also include unusual ones such as lemongrass, thyme, and yarrow.

Jeanne Rose Aromatherapy*
219 Carl St.
San Francisco, CA 94117
415-564-6785

A highlight of this company is its assortment of exquisite hydrosols. It also offers essential oils, a dozen aromatherapy kits, such as ones for sports, kids, stress, women's, and travel, and Jeanne Rose's numerous aromatherapy and herb books.

Ultra Scent
PO Box 1123
North Bend, WA 98045
425-831-7977

These elegant plug-in, fan/heater diffusers allow you to switch scents. One model has a timer, so it does so automatically.

Herbal and aromatherapy products

Harvest Moon Herbs
432 Ridge St.
Reno, NV 89501
775-329-6999

These aromatic products include oils for sore muscles, massage, baby, energizing, and menstrual cramps. You can also purchase facial herbs, bath salts for different emotions, lip balm, liniment, bug repellents, and pillows for tired eyes, babies, and dreaming.

Herbalina Gardens
PO Box 2378
Grass Valley, CA 95945
800-934-GLOW
www.herbalinagardens.com

All these products (the body lotion, bubble bath, shampoo, mists, facial scrub, eye therapy, and baby and mother massage oils, and hydrosols) are very nice.

Lily of Colorado
PO Box 12471
Denver, CO 80212
800-333-LILY
www.lilyofcolorado.com

This line of skin care products is made with pure essential oils and with herbs organically grown on its farm. Its home spa contains what you need to give yourself a facial.

Linnie's Herbal Products
1212 Lake View Drive
Colfax, CA 95713
(catalog $1, no phone orders)

Besides soaps, bath powders, massage oils, and eight skin balms made from organically grown, fragrant herbs and essential oils, this company carries furniture polish, a catnip toy for your cat, insect and moth repellents, and books and supplies to make your own products.

Lunar Farms Herbals*
#3 Highland
Gilmer, TX 75644
800-687-1052
www.herbworld.com/lunarfarms

Salves made with aromatic, organically grown herbs include rose petal comfrey salve. There are also herbal scrub bags, dream pillows, and aromatherapy mineral bath salts.

Oak Valley Herb Farm
PO Box 2482
Nevada City, CA 95959
www.jps.net/ahaherb.com
(catalog $1 refundable with order, no phone orders)

This company sells aromatherapy combined with organically grown herbs products in muscle relaxants, massage oils, pregnant belly oil, salves, and tinctures and many other products. It also carries herbal oils like St. John's wort and calendula, essential oils at good prices, and signed copies of Kathi Keville's 11 books on herbs and aromatherapy (including the one you're reading and *Pocket Guide to Aromatherapy*).

Scentsuous Beauty
PO Box 2
Sebastopol, CA 95473
707-824-1365

The fragrances and textures of these natural "sensual face and body care products" are wonderful. They include edible body elixirs, spritzers, and honeys, with x-rated names like "lust dust." You can also get a signed copy of the beautifully illustrated *Botanical Erotica: Arousing the Body, Mind, and Spirit,* by Diana DeLuca (Healing Arts Press) with recipes for sensual foods and body-care products.

Wild Sage Botanicals
PO Bo 631
Lyons, CO 80540

This complete line of natural facial products includes eye cream, masks, and lip balm. It also has body, bath, and hair oils, insect repellent, bath salts, an oil with helichrysum essential oil to treat scars, and moist heat, scented pillows for back and shoulders.

Wise Woman Herbals
99 Harvey Rd.
Worthington, MA 01098
www.wiseways.com

This company offers essential oils combined with flower essences and herbs in products such as body oils, burn spray, and vinegar hair rinses.

Worldwide aromatherapy products

Amyris Essential Oils
Simpson's Yard
Harrogate
North Yorkshire HG2 0NL
United Kingdom
0142-353-8886
www.amyris.com

Online store with essential oils, vegetable oils, cosmetics, shampoo, and soap.

Aromatherapy International, Ltd.
Banks House
Lane Burton Overy
Leicester LE8 9DD
United Kingdom
0116-259-3103

Essential oils (some organically grown), vegetable oils, hydrosols, and supplies.

Quinessence Aromatherapy
Forest Court
Linden Way
Coalville, LE67 3JY
United Kingdom
0153-083-8358
www.quinessence.com

Essential oils, vegetable oils, electric and ceramic diffusers, bottles, and jars.

Echo Essential Oils
44 Chestnut Drive
Congleton CW12 2UB
United Kingdom
0126-027-7680

Essential oils, vegetable oils, unscented creams, shampoo, starter kits, and presentation boxes.

Fragrant Earth
Orchard Court
Magdalene Street
Glastonbury, Somerset BA6 9EW
United Kingdom
0145-883-1216
www.fragrant-earth.com

Organically grown essential oils, vegetable oils, and hydrosols.

Shirley Price Aromatherapy, Ltd.
Essential House
Upper Bond Street
Hinckley, LE10 1RS
United Kingdom
0145-561-5059

Essential oils and aromatherapy products.

Floral France
42 Chemin des Aubepines
06130 Grasse, France
4937-78819

Essential Oils Supply Catalogs

Cheryl's Herbs*
836 Hanley Ind. Ct.
St. Louis, MO 63144
800-231-5971
www.cherylsherbs.com

Lots of good stuff here with nine hydrosols, several diffusers, essential oils in a variety of sizes, dried herbs, vegetable oils, and herbal oils. The company has a line of various liquid cleaning products, soaps, and shampoo (made with decyl polyglucose), including a cedarwood hydrosol. It sells many of Jeanne Rose's aromatherapy products.

Lavender Lane
7337, #1 Roseville Road
Sacramento, CA 95842
916-334-4400

These folks carry a large selection of glass and plastic ware for herbal and aromatherapy products, including perfume, spray, dropper, and cobalt blue bottles. They also carry vegetable and some essential oils, and unscented incense sticks.

Leydet Aromatics*
Box 2354
Fair Oaks, CA 95628
916-965-7546
www.leydet.com

This large selection of high-quality products includes essential oils, hydrosols, massage and bath oils and natural perfumes, oils for different facial types, and two dozen special blends for emotional conditions to put in a diffuser. They also sell manufacturing supplies including alcohols, vegetable oils, aloe vera, clays, glycerin and glass (including cobalt blue) and plastic bottles.

Mountain Rose Herbs*
20618 High St.
North San Juan, Ca 95960
800-879-3337

This catalog is an exhaustive list of quality aromatherapy (as well as herbal) items: Essential oils, hydrosols, complexion waters, vegetable oils, salves, herbal oils (St. John's wort, calendula, arnica, black walnut hull, and more), books, incense, flea collars, mosquito repellent, dog shampoo, dream pillow, tea tree toothpaste, tooth powder, soap, glass (including cobalt blue) and plastic containers, and dried herbs.

SKS Bottle & Packaging, Inc.
3 Knabner Road
Mechanicville, NY 12118
518-899-7488
www.sks.bottle.com

This varied selection of glass and plastic bottles and jars includes a couple dozen elegant cobalt blue bottles.

Essential Oil Diffusers

Aroma Land
1326 Rufina Circle
Santa Fe, NM 87505
800-933-5267
www.aromaland.com

This fun selection of aromatherapy products includes over a dozen creative designs of candle diffusers and several electric diffusers, as well as scented candles, a ceramic candle ring and a variety of small clay diffusers (including a Buddha!) that sit on a shelf or attach to a wall. There are also necklaces of a tiny vial enclosed in rainforest wood (from a preserve), a wallet-sized case to carry your oils, essential and vegetable oils, incense, and a series of aromatherapy "decoder" wheels for quick information access.

Aroma Therapeutix*
PO Box 2908
Seal Beach, CA 90740
800-308-6284

This company sells electric and nebulizing diffusers (including one for your car), candles, and light bulb rings. They also have a variety of aromatherapy lines including sprays, bath salts, natural perfume, lavender eye pillow, inhalers and roll-ons for sinus or to affect emotions, jojoba, orange and rose waters, dropper, pipettes (for dispensing drops), and a few fancy bottles.

Amrita Aromatherapy
1900 West Stone Ave.
Fairfield, IA 52556
515-472-9136
www.amrita.noet

Essential, massage, and facial oils, cleansers, and creams, a set of essential oils for children, and herbal tinctures combined with essential oils and flower essences are specialties of this company. It also carries plug-in, clay, and its own nebulizing diffusers, as well as books.

Specialty Items

Aroma Naturals
1202 McGraw Ave.
Irvine, CA 92614
800-46 AROMA
www.aromanaturals.com

This complete line of very fragrant aromatherapy candles are in various scents and sizes — even a travel candle in a can and votives. Made with natural essential oils and vegetable waxes rather than paraffin, they smell great even when not burning! To go with the votives are ceramic candle diffusers.

The Boston Jojoba Company
PO Box 771
Middleton, MA 01949
800-265-5622
www.bostonjojoba.com

Here's the place to go for unrefined jojoba (vegetable oil substitute that doesn't spoil) with almost no scent. You can find facts on jojoba on their Web site.

J.R. Martinez*
3208 Garfield Ave.
Alameda, CA 94501
510-865-6361

A unique pen, Plume De Parfum, holds 1.8 ounce of essential oil or hydrosol in a small sprayer in the pen's top. Of course, it's my favorite pen to use at book signings!

Latifa Rainbow*
12 Lochness Lane
San Rafael, CA 94901
415-457-9794
www.comfort@wenet.net

The company sells extra heavy moist packs filled with grains and six aromatic, relaxing herbs (they smell divine!), and you can heat them in your microwave. There are three styles each of shoulder collars and eye packs (a great relief after a few hours sitting at a computer), as well as wrist, knee, and lumbar pack, and even slippers, all covered in attractive materials.

Incense

Auromere Ayurvedic Imports
2621 West Highway 12
Lodi, CA 95242
800-735-4691

This company has a selection of stick incense from India and Ayurvedic soaps, toothpaste, and massage oils that contain natural essential oils.

Shoyeido Corporation*
1700 38th St.
Boulder, CO 80301
303-786-8000

Shoyeido Incense Co.
Karasuma Nijo, Nakagyo-ku*
Kyoto 604, Japan
81-75-212-5590

Japanische Raucherstachen von Shoyeido*
Hohenzollermring 26
D-22763 Hamburg, Germany
49-(0)40 39 76 49

This company sells a very fine incense in stick, pressed, or coiled form — all beautifully packaged and made with natural and traditional materials for therapeutic use. It also offers sachets made with 300-year-old recipes to carry or put in a drawer. The simple incense burners include a burner to heat wood chips.

Aroma Jewelry

Nature's Geometry
PO Box 662
Graton, CA 95444
707-829-0799
www.naturesgeometry.com
(Germany: PrimaVera Life. 837-68080)

Elegant, sculpted gemstones on necklaces with a small depression large enough to hold a couple drops of your favorite essential oil, but that doesn't leak. (Also produce "Aromatherapy Journeys," a global travel log of peoples' relationships to and use of fragrant plants.)

Spiritwinds
11186 White Oak Way
Nevada City, CA 95959
530-265-0786
www.spiritwinds.com

You have to see these unique necklaces to appreciate them, but I try to describe them. They're rainforest nuts and seeds crafted and polished by indigenous peoples (who receive a share of profits) and hold a tiny vial of essential oil (one of six scents for your emotions). Beneath a lattice circle inset is a scented pad. Some have tiny chimes dangling from them. Also available are clay goddess necklaces to scent with a special oil (and outdoor wind chimes, too).

Soap

Sun Feather*
Natural Soap Company
1551 State Hwy. 72
Potsdam, NY 13676
315-265-3648
www.sunsoap.com

These attractive soaps are scented with natural essential oils and sold cloth-wrapped or as soap balls. There are far too many choices to list, but my favorites are Aphrodite, erotica, gardener's soaps, and three Native American blends. Even more unusual are chocolate and java soaps and shampoo bars made from real soap for people, horses, dogs, and cats. Washy Squashy is kid's molding soap in lemon, mint, and tangerine scents. There are also bug repellents and a soapmaking kit.

Vermont Soap Works
616 Exchange St.
Middlebury, VT 05753
802-388-4302
www.vtsoap.com

This company offers mild, low alkaline bar soaps scented with natural essential oils and herbs. They also make Fruit and Vegie Wash, Non-Toxic Cleaner with rosemary extract, and liquid soaps and body gel made from real soap instead of synthetics.

Essential Oil Distillers

Benzalco
1291 Cumberland Ave.
West Lafayette, IN 47906
765-497-1313
www.benzalco.com

The two-quart, table top, Clevenger water-distillation kits ($1,000) may be best for making hydrosols because they process only seven ounces of herb, which yields less than a teaspoon of oil. A two-gallon size is also available for larger production.

FloraGenics
8698 Elk Grove Blvd. #3-220
Elk Grove, CA 95624
916-685-5611
www.floragenics.com

You can choose from six sizes of portable, glass essential oil distillers — all the way to a two-quart still ($200) that produces approximately less than a teaspoon of oil up to the 20-gallon deluxe size ($1,400) work very well. A larger commercial model is being designed. They come with plenty of accessories, and you can also order replacement parts, along with glass pipettes, vials, and other items. I use their small unit for in-class demos, but you'll want something larger for any real production.

Index

• N •

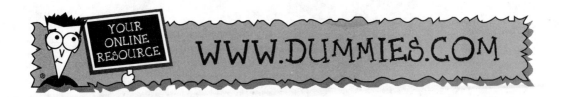

YOUR ONLINE RESOURCE

WWW.DUMMIES.COM

Discover Dummies Online!

The Dummies Web Site is your fun and friendly online resource for the latest information about ...For Dummies® books and your favorite topics. The Web site is the place to communicate with us, exchange ideas with other ...For Dummies readers, chat with authors, and have fun!

Ten Fun and Useful Things You Can Do at www.dummies.com

1. Win free ...For Dummies books and more!
2. Register your book and be entered in a prize drawing.
3. Meet your favorite authors through the IDG Books Author Chat Series.
4. Exchange helpful information with other ...For Dummies readers.
5. Discover other great ...For Dummies books you must have!
6. Purchase Dummieswear™ exclusively from our Web site.
7. Buy ...For Dummies books online.
8. Talk to us. Make comments, ask questions, get answers!
9. Download free software.
10. Find additional useful resources from authors.

Link directly to these ten fun and useful things at
http://www.dummies.com/10useful

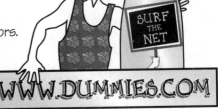

WWW.DUMMIES.COM

SURF THE NET

For other technology titles from IDG Books Worldwide, go to
www.idgbooks.com

Not on the Web yet? It's easy to get started with Dummies 101®: The Internet For Windows® 98 or The Internet For Dummies®, 6th Edition, at local retailers everywhere.

IDG BOOKS WORLDWIDE

Find other ...For Dummies books on these topics:
Business • Career • Databases • Food & Beverage • Games • Gardening • Graphics • Hardware
Health & Fitness • Internet and the World Wide Web • Networking • Office Suites
Operating Systems • Personal Finance • Pets • Programming • Recreation • Sports
Spreadsheets • Teacher Resources • Test Prep • Word Processing

IDG BOOKS WORLDWIDE
BOOK REGISTRATION

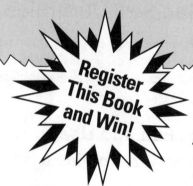

Register
This Book
and Win!

We want to hear from you!

Visit **http://my2cents.dummies.com** to register this book and tell us how you liked it!

✔ Get entered in our monthly prize giveaway.

✔ Give us feedback about this book — tell us what you like best, what you like least, or maybe what you'd like to ask the author and us to change!

✔ Let us know any other *...For Dummies*® topics that interest you.

Your feedback helps us determine what books to publish, tells us what coverage to add as we revise our books, and lets us know whether we're meeting your needs as a *...For Dummies* reader. You're our most valuable resource, and what you have to say is important to us!

Not on the Web yet? It's easy to get started with *Dummies 101*®: *The Internet For Windows*® *98* or *The Internet For Dummies*®, 6th Edition, at local retailers everywhere.

Or let us know what you think by sending us a letter at the following address:

...For Dummies Book Registration
Dummies Press
7260 Shadeland Station, Suite 100
Indianapolis, IN 46256-3945
Fax 317-596-5498

™

BESTSELLING
BOOK SERIES